T0252871

Home-Prepared
Dog and Cat Diets

Second Edition

Home-Prepared Dog and Cat Diets

Second Edition

by Patricia A. Schenck, DVM, PhD

WILEY-BLACKWELL

A John Wiley & Sons, Ltd., Publication

Edition first published 2010
© 2010 Patricia A. Schenck

Blackwell Publishing was acquired by John Wiley & Sons in February 2007. Blackwell's publishing program has been merged with Wiley's global Scientific, Technical, and Medical business to form Wiley-Blackwell.

Editorial Office
2121 State Avenue, Ames, Iowa 50014-8300, USA

For details of our global editorial offices, for customer services, and for information about how to apply for permission to reuse the copyright material in this book, please see our website at www.wiley.com/wiley-blackwell.

Authorization to photocopy items for internal or personal use, or the internal or personal use of specific clients, is granted by Blackwell Publishing, provided that the base fee is paid directly to the Copyright Clearance Center, 222 Rosewood Drive, Danvers, MA 01923. For those organizations that have been granted a photocopy license by CCC, a separate system of payments has been arranged. The fee codes for users of the Transactional Reporting Service are ISBN-13: 978-0-8138-0119-3/2010.

Designations used by companies to distinguish their products are often claimed as trademarks. All brand names and product names used in this book are trade names, service marks, trademarks or registered trademarks of their respective owners. The publisher is not associated with any product or vendor mentioned in this book. This publication is designed to provide accurate and authoritative information in regard to the subject matter covered. It is sold on the understanding that the publisher is not engaged in rendering professional services. If professional advice or other expert assistance is required, the services of a competent professional should be sought.

Library of Congress Cataloging-in-Publication Data

Schenck, Patricia A.
   Home-prepared dog and cat diets / by Patricia A. Schenck. – 2nd ed.
      p. cm.
   Rev. ed. of: Home-prepared dog & cat diets / Donald R. Strombeck. 1st ed. 1999.
   Includes bibliographical references and index.
   ISBN-13: 978-0-8138-0119-3 (alk. paper)
   ISBN-10: 0-8138-0119-2 (alk. paper)
1. Dogs–Food–Recipes. 2. Cats–Food–Recipes. 3. Dogs–Nutrition.
4. Cats–Nutrition. 5. Dogs–Diseases–Diet therapy. 6. Cats–Diseases–Diet
therapy. I. Strombeck, Donald R. Home-prepared dog & cat diets. II. Title.
   SF427.4.S77 2010
   636.7'085–dc22

                                                                2009051075

A catalog record for this book is available from the U.S. Library of Congress.

Set in 10 on 13pt Palatino by Toppan Best-set Premedia Limited

Disclaimer
The publisher and the author make no representations or warranties with respect to the accuracy or completeness of the contents of this work and specifically disclaim all warranties, including without limitation warranties of fitness for a particular purpose. No warranty may be created or extended by sales or promotional materials. The advice and strategies contained herein may not be suitable for every situation. This work is sold with the understanding that the publisher is not engaged in rendering legal, accounting, or other professional services. If professional assistance is required, the services of a competent professional person should be sought. Neither the publisher nor the author shall be liable for damages arising herefrom. The fact that an organization or Website is referred to in this work as a citation and/or a potential source of further information does not mean that the author or the publisher endorses the information the organization or Website may provide or recommendations it may make. Further, readers should be aware that Internet Websites listed in this work may have changed or disappeared between when this work was written and when it is read.

1   2010

TABLE OF CONTENTS

See the supporting companion Web site for this book: www.wiley.com/go/schenck

PREFACE

Diet is an important consideration in the care of a pet and is a major factor in health and life expectancy. *Home-Prepared Dog and Cat Diets* is a unique handbook in that it provides an introduction to nutrition of the healthy dog and cat as well as an extensive discussion of medical disorders that can be treated in part by dietary management. Recipes are provided for making home-prepared diets for both healthy pets and pets with special conditions. These diets have been formulated with a sophisticated computer program to ensure that they are balanced and complete, according to the Association of American Feed Control Officials (AAFCO) guidelines. Many diets have been carefully formulated for specific health problems according to current veterinary recommendations. Diets that have been designed for some special conditions may not be complete and balanced because of necessary diet restrictions. This is noted in the recipe, and these diets should be fed under the direct supervision of your veterinarian.

This edition of *Home-Prepared Dog and Cat Diets* has been thoroughly updated. Chapters have been expanded and completely rewritten to reflect nutritional recommendations based on current research. New chapters have been added on feeding the puppy and kitten, feeding the pregnant or lactating dog or cat, feeding the senior pet, feeding the performance dog, and the role of diet in pets with cancer. For ease of use, diets have been removed from individual chapters and are now found in Section II of the book. Nutrient content for protein, fat, carbohydrate, and fiber have been provided for every diet, along with the nutrient density. Diets can easily be adjusted for any size dog or cat, and exact ingested nutrient amounts can be calculated. Diets are cross-referenced for special conditions, by chapter, and also by protein source, making it simple to find a diet to suit the needs of most dogs or cats. Detailed directions are given regarding food safety and proper preparation of diets.

With the information presented in this book, pet owners will have an excellent background in nutrition of the dog and cat. If the diet directions are carefully followed, owners can safely prepare balanced diets for their healthy pets. Diets for pets with special conditions should be thoroughly discussed with the pet's veterinarian to ensure the proper management of the pet with special needs.

ACKNOWLEDGMENTS

This book is dedicated to all the four-legged critters in my life that have reminded me why I wanted to be a part of the veterinary profession. Thanks also to all my four-legged taste-testers that willingly evaluated many of the recipes. Special thanks to my friend Christopher Hamilton for his proofreading and typing skills and for helping me maintain my sanity throughout this project. Special thanks also to my mother for proofreading recipes and helping prepare diets. Lastly, I am grateful to my parents for a lifetime of love and support.

Home-Prepared Dog and Cat Diets

Second Edition

SECTION I
Nutrition and Dietary Management

CHAPTER 1
Homemade Diets

In the United States, there are more than 140 million dogs and cats. The vast majority of pets receive more than 90% of their calories from commercially prepared pet food. There is an increasing interest in feeding home-prepared foods to pets for a variety of reasons. In a recent telephone survey, owners of 635 dogs and 469 cats were questioned regarding diets fed to their pets. More dogs received noncommercial foods (table scraps, leftovers, or homemade foods) as compared to cats. Noncommercial foods were a part of the diet in 31% of dogs and 13% of cats and comprised at least one-fourth of the diet for 17% of dogs and 6% of cats. About 3% of pets were exclusively fed homemade diets, and 7% of dogs received homemade food for at least half of their diet. Treats of some kind were given daily to 57% of dogs and 26% of cats. Supplements were given to 13% of dogs and 6% of cats and were reported to include multivitamins, fatty acids, chondroprotective agents, vitamin C, yeast, taurine, zinc, calcium, and antioxidants, among others.

For humans, food consumption has social and cultural connotations. With the humanization of pets, owners may associate social and cultural behaviors with their pets. In the telephone survey, owners said that cuddling or petting their animals and talking to the pets were the most common activities shared with their dogs or cats. Dog owners were more likely to walk or run with their pets, play with toys together, play fetch, ride in the car together, participate in obedience or agility training, and go to work together as compared to cat owners. Other activities that both dog and cat owners shared with their pets included watching their pets play, grooming their pets, watching television with their pets, and eating with their pets. As pets are treated more as "humans," many owners may feel that their pets should share the food customs of humans.

There are many reasons suggested as to why a homemade pet diet is desired. Some owners wish to feed natural or organic foods or vegan or vegetarian foods. Many wish to cook for their pets and provide a varied diet. Others may find commercial pet food labels and ingredients confusing and want to avoid additives, preservatives, chemicals, or certain ingredients found in pet foods. In the previously mentioned telephone survey, owners feeding noncommercial pet foods had less trust in their veterinarian to provide sound nutritional advice and felt that dogs and cats needed a variety of different foods in their diet. Owners feeding noncommercial pet foods were more likely to feel that processed foods for pets were unhealthy, that cooking destroys nutrients in pet foods, and that organic foods were safer and healthier than other foods. Owners that fed noncommercial food were more likely to feel that dogs and cats need more meat than is provided in commercial products, that information on pet food labels is misleading, and that additives in pet foods have unhealthy side effects. They were less likely to trust pet food manufacturers to provide nutritionally sound products and less likely to feel that ingredients in commercial pet foods were wholesome and nutritious. They are less likely to believe that pets live longer today because of good nutrition from commercial products, that commercial products contain necessary nutrition, and that pet food companies place a high priority on pet health and wellbeing. Owners feeding noncommercial foods were more likely to believe that raw bones could be safely fed to pets, that raw meat provides better nutrition than cooked foods, and that foods sold for human consumption provide better nutrition than do commercial pet foods. Owners feeding noncommercial foods also enjoyed preparing foods for their pets more than did owners feeding commercial pet foods.

Problems Associated with Homemade Diets

Veterinarians are the most commonly cited source for pet nutritional information; however, about 17% of pet owners cite the Internet as their primary source for pet nutritional information. Unfortunately, there is a considerable amount of misinformation present on the Internet, and it can be difficult to determine which information is trustworthy. In the telephone survey discussed previously, less than one-third of owners used a homemade diet recipe specifically designed for pets. In another survey, 90% of the homemade elimination diets used by veterinarians were not balanced and were not nutritionally adequate to support adult maintenance. In another study comparing the nutritional adequacy of commercial diets to homemade diets, calcium, the calcium/phosphorus ratio, and vitamins A and E were below current recommendations for nutritional adequacy in homemade diets. Potassium, copper, and zinc concentrations were also inadequate in homemade diets.

Feeding unbalanced homemade diets can lead to complications, including osteodystrophy, osteopenia, nutritional secondary hyperparathyroidism, and pansteatitis. Meat sources are typically high in phosphorus and low in calcium; if no calcium source is added to the diet, the calcium concentration is typically inadequate and the calcium/phosphorus ratio is too low. Nutritional secondary hyperparathyroidism occurs when the parathyroid hormone concentration elevates in an attempt to raise the serum calcium concentration, and loss of bone density results. For further discussion of nutritional secondary hyperparathyroidism see Chapter 17, Diet and Endocrine Disease. Deficiency of dietary vitamin D can lead to type I rickets, characterized by osteodystrophy. Deficiencies in calcium and vitamin D are especially problematic in young, growing dogs, requiring a proper balance of calcium and phosphorus for bone growth. Certain ingredients can be very high in a particular vitamin and cause problems if not a part of a balanced diet. Liver is very high in vitamin A, and vitamin A toxicity can result in pets fed unbalanced diets based on liver. Pansteatitis (yellow fat disease) has been documented in cats fed diets with a high oily fish content and inadequate in vitamin E.

Some recipes call for the use of raw ingredients. Raw ingredients often contain bacteria that would normally be destroyed by cooking (see Chapter 2, Food Safety). The practice of feeding uncooked diets should be discouraged.

Formulating a Homemade Diet

Formulating a diet is a difficult task. The first step in doing so is to determine the nutritional requirements of the animal, and these requirements are based on species, life-stage, and the animal's special needs. The Nutrient Research Council (NRC) publishes a book about the nutritional requirements for various species, and these requirements serve as guidelines. The Association of American Feed Control

Officials (AAFCO) provides suggested nutrient profiles for dog and cat foods (see Chapter 3, Nutrients). Once the desired levels of nutrients are decided, then ingredients must be chosen that, in combination, will provide proper amounts of protein, fat, vitamins, and minerals. Nutrient databases must be maintained to provide the accurate nutritional analysis of each ingredient. Sophisticated computer programs containing human food ingredients are available (The Food Processor SQL, ESHA Research, Salem, Oregon), but these programs provide only a nutritional analysis of the combination of ingredients; they do not formulate a diet. The analysis of the combined ingredients must be compared to the suggested nutrient profile. If there are deficiencies or excesses, alterations to ingredients must be made and nutritional adequacy reevaluated. This can be a long and tedious process.

Some veterinary nutritionists offer a food formulation service or are available on the telephone for dietary consultations. Some of the veterinary nutritionists providing this service are listed in Table 1.1.

Assessing a Homemade Diet Recipe

When assessing a homemade diet recipe, there are some guidelines that can be quickly assessed. First, the five food groups (protein, carbohydrate, fat, vitamins, minerals) should appear in the recipe. Second, the carbohydrate source should be present in a higher or equal quantity to that of the protein source. Carbohydrate sources include rice, barley, lentils, potato, pasta, couscous, or quinoa. In cat foods, the carbohydrate-to-protein ratio should be 1:1 or 2:1, and in dog foods the ratio should be 2:1 to 3:1. Third, the protein source should be identified. Fourth, a fat source should be identified. Fat could take the form of an added vegetable oil or could be included in the meat source (chicken skin, fat in undrained ground beef, etc.). Fifth, a calcium or calcium/phosphorus supplement should be present. Calcium carbonate (baking soda) or bone meal (source of calcium and phosphorus) should also be present. Lastly, a source of vitamins and minerals should be present, typically in the form of a multivitamin tablet. For cat diets, a source of taurine should be present.

Choosing a Homemade Diet

There are many homemade recipe diets presented in the second section of this book. The first step in choosing a diet is to pick a species-

Table 1.1. Veterinary nutritionists offering nutritional consultation and/or homemade diet formulation.

Veterinary Nutritional Consultations, Inc.

http://www.petdiets.com

Diet formulation and nutrition consultation

DVM Consulting

1-888-3Homemade

http://balanceit.com

Diet formulation

Nutrition Support Service

Michigan State University College of Veterinary Medicine, East Lansing, MI

http://cvm.msu.edu/hospital/services/nutrition-support-service-1

Patients must be seen by the nutrition service at MSU

Nutrition Support Service

The Ohio State University College of Veterinary Medicine, Columbus, OH

http://www.vet.ohio-state.edu/2727.htm

Nutrition consultation and healthy weight clinic

Clinical Nutrition Service

North Carolina State University, College of Veterinary Medicine, Raleigh, NC

(919) 531-6871

Korinn_saker@ncsu.edu

MJ Ryan Veterinary Hospital of the University of Pennsylvania

On-Line Nutrition Consultation Service for Veterinarians

http://www.vet.upenn.edu/RyanHospital/SpecialtyCareServices/
    Nutrition/NutritionConsults/tabid/1380/Default.aspx

This service is for veterinarians only.

Georgia Veterinary Specialists

Susan G. Wynn, DVM

(404)-459-0903

http://www.susanwynn.com

Diet formulation for healthy pets; diet formulation for special health issues
    requires a veterinarian referral.

University of Florida, College of Veterinary Medicine

Richard Hill, MA, VetMB, PhD, DACVIM, DACVN, MRCVS

(352) 392-2226

Table 1.1. *(cont.)*

Homemade diet formulation for Florida veterinarians. Pet must visit the
University of Florida if there are special health issues.

Veterinary Nutrition Center

The University of Tennessee College of Veterinary Medicine

(865) 974-8387

http://www.vet.utk.edu/clinical/sacs/index.php

Nutrition Support Service

William R. Pritchard Veterinary Medical Teaching Hospital

University of California, Davis

(530) 752-7892

http://www.vetmed.ucdavis.edu/vmth/small_animal/nutrition/default.
cfm

Clinical Nutrition Specialty Service

University of Missouri Veterinary Medical Teaching Hospital

http://www.vmth.missouri.edu/clin_nu.htm

University of Minnesota College of Veterinary Medicine

St. Paul, MN

http://www.cvm.umn.edu/VMC/

Nutritional consultations. Pet must visit the Clinic or be referred by a
veterinarian if there are special health issues.

---

appropriate diet for the life stage of the dog or cat (adult, growth,
senior, reproduction, performance). Dog diets should not be fed to
cats, as these diets will not contain the specific and unique nutrients
that cats need. Cat diets should not be fed to dogs because these diets
will usually provide some nutrients in excess for dogs. The second
step is to determine if there are any special needs of the pet (weight
loss, allergy, renal disease, heart disease, etc.). If special needs are
present, then a diet specific for that condition should be chosen. A
variety of diets using different combinations of ingredients are presented for each life stage and special condition so that substitutions
are not necessary. It is best to provide the pet with a variety of dietary
ingredients over time to ensure a proper mix of nutrients. The majority
of diets in this book have been formulated to be balanced and nutritionally complete. However, some diets, such as those formulated for
renal disease and other conditions are not nutritionally complete
because of the severe dietary restrictions needed in some conditions.

If a diet is not nutritionally complete, this is stated in the diet recipe. These diets should *only* be fed to dogs or cats with that *specific* special condition and should *not* be fed to healthy pets.

Diet Preparation

Diets should be prepared according to the recipe given, with no substitutions, additions, or omissions. Each ingredient in the diet is important and provides specific necessary nutrients. Proper preparation of homemade diets requires time and effort. An accurate kitchen scale that measures in grams and ounces is required for diet preparation. Ingredients should be carefully measured to provide the proper combination of nutrients.

Individual ingredients in the diet (such as meat and the carbohydrate source) should be cooked separately. Meat should be cooked for a minimum of 10 minutes at 180°F. Chicken and ground beef, in particular, should be well cooked to prevent bacterial contamination. The use of raw ingredients is not recommended due to the increased risk for foodborne illness (see Chapter 2, Food Safety). Carbohydrate sources such as potatoes should be cooked to improve their digestibility. Vegetables should be washed and then cooked prior to use.

Once the food ingredients have been cooked, they should be measured and combined. Any salt in the recipe can be added at this time, but other vitamins and mineral supplements should not be added yet. Once the food ingredients are combined, the ingredients should be mixed in a blender to ensure their even distribution. This will prevent the pet from picking out certain dietary ingredients and not consuming others. An unbalanced diet will be consumed if ingredients are separate and the pet does not eat the entire mixture. Vitamin and mineral supplements should be crushed to a powder form and added after the food sources have been cooked and combined.

Homemade diets do not contain preservatives and are high in moisture, thus they are highly susceptible to bacterial and fungal contamination if left at room temperature for more than a few hours. The recipes in this book have been designed to be prepared in small batches to minimize the amount of food prepared but not required for feeding. Any prepared diet that is not being consumed immediately should be stored in an airtight container in the refrigerator for no more than a few days. If preparation of a larger batch of food is desired, then the recipe should be prepared up to the point of vitamin and mineral supplement addition and stored frozen. When ready to feed, the portion of diet can be thawed, weighed, and the appropriate amount of vitamins and minerals can be added prior to feeding. Before feeding any food that has been stored in the refrigerator or freezer, the color, odor, and consistency should be checked. If there are changes, or there is visible mold growth, the food should be discarded.

Vitamin and mineral supplements are present in small quantities, but they are a very important part of the diet. Supplements should be included as stated in each recipe and not substituted or omitted. For example, many diets include both iodized salt and a salt substitute (potassium chloride). Iodized salt is important as a source of iodine and sodium, and salt substitute is included as a source of potassium. Both are equally important for inclusion in the diet. Bone meal is included in diets because it is an excellent source of calcium and phosphorus, and calcium carbonate (baking soda) is included as a calcium source. Some recipes call for one-half of a vitamin or mineral tablet. In general, these are human products that are not meant to be cut in half, so each half may not be exactly half of the vitamins called for in the recipe. However, over the course of several days, the proper amounts of vitamins and minerals will be fed overall.

Prior to feeding, the diet should be warmed to just below body temperature (about 100°F). Especially if food is being warmed in the microwave, the food should be checked for hot spots, as the food may heat unevenly. A small amount of water can be added at this time, if necessary. When feeding, the food should not sit out at room temperature for more than a few hours. Any food not consumed should be removed and discarded. Bowls used for serving should be washed thoroughly after each use.

Monitoring

When feeding a homemade diet, monitoring is important, and the pet should be examined by a veterinarian at least twice yearly. Body weight, body condition score, and activity level should routinely be monitored so that adjustments to the amount of diet fed can be made. Hair and skin should be monitored, as these are good indicators of nutritional status. In addition, stool quality should be assessed. The prepared diets can also be evaluated by a laboratory for nutritional adequacy. Some laboratories providing this service are listed in Table 1.2.

Table 1.2. Selected commercial feed testing laboratories for pet food analysis.

Diagnostic Center for Population and Animal Health

Michigan State University, Lansing MI

Thomas H. Herdt, DVM, MS

herdt@cvm.msu.edu

http://www.animalhealth.msu.edu

Barrow-Agee Laboratories

Memphis, TN

(901) 332-1590

http://www.balabs.com

Eurofins Scientific, Inc.

Des Moines, IA

(515) 265-1461

http://eurofinsUS.com

Holmes Laboratory, Inc.

Millersburg, OH

(800) 344-1101

http://www.holmeslab.com

Midwest Laboratories, Inc.

Omaha, NE

(402) 334-7770

http://www.midwestlabs.com

Additional Reading

Diquelou A, Chaput C, Benoit E, and Priymenko N. 2005. Hypocalcaemia due to nutritional calcium deficiency and hypoparathyroidism in an adult dog. Vet Rec 156:45–48.

Freeman LM, Abood SK, Fascetti AJ, Fleeman LM, Michel KE, Laflamme DP, et al. 2006. Disease prevalence among dogs and cats in the United States and Australia and proportions of dogs and cats that receive therapeutic diets or dietary supplements. J Amer Vet Med Assoc 229:531–534.

Laflamme DP, Abood SK, Fascetti AJ, Fleeman LM, Freeman LM, Michel KE, et al. 2008. Pet feeding practices of dog and cat owners in the United States and Australia. Amer Vet Med Assoc 232:687–694.

Leon A, Bain SA, and Levick WR. 1992. Hypokalaemic episodic polymyopathy in cats fed a vegetarian diet. Aust Vet J 69(10):249–254.

Michel KE. 2006. Unconventional diets for dogs and cats. Vet Clin Small Anim 36:1269–1281.

Michel KE, Willoughby KN, Abood SK, Fascetti AJ, Fleeman LM, Freeman LM, et al. 2008. J Amer Vet Med Assoc 233:1699–1703.

Niza MMRE, Vilela CL, and Ferreira LMA. 2003. Feline pansteatitis revisited: hazards of unbalanced home-made diets. J Fel Med Surg 5:271–277.

Polizopoulou ZS, Kazakos G, Patsikas MN, and Roubies N. 2005. Hypervitaminosis A in the cat: a case report and review of the literature. J Fel Med Surg 7:363–368.

Streiff EL, Zwischenberger B, Butterwick RF, Wagner E, Iben C, and Bauer JE. 2002. A comparison of the nutritional adequacy of home-prepared and commercial diets for dogs. J Nutr 132:1698S–1700S.

Taylor MB, Geiger DA, Saker KE, and Larson MM. 2009. Diffuse osteopenia and myelopathy in a puppy fed a diet composed of an organic premix and raw ground beef. J Amer Vet Med Assoc 234:1041–1048.

CHAPTER 2
Food Safety

Foodborne illness affects more than 24 million people in the United States every year, and pets can also become ill from contaminated food. There are two different types of foodborne illness: food infections and food toxicosis. Food infection occurs when bacterial cells are ingested and then invade tissues. These cells then replicate, and after an incubation period, clinical disease results. The incubation period is typically 12 hours to 10 days, and examples include infection with *Salmonella*, *Escherichia coli*, *Neorickettsia*, *Vibrio*, *Yersinia*, and *Campylobacter*. Food intoxication or "food poisoning" results from the ingestion of food containing microbial toxins. Clinical signs usually appear within 6 hours of ingestion, and examples include infection with *Clostridium botulinum*, *Bacillus cereus*, *Staphylococcus aureus*, mycotoxins, metals, and biogenic amines.

Most cases of foodborne illness occur when spoiled foods, improperly cooked foods, or garbage is consumed. Foodborne illness is common in the racing greyhound industry as most of the diet is comprised of raw meat in many cases. Raw meats can contain large numbers of bacteria that are ingested, causing illness. Even foods purchased for human consumption can be contaminated with bacteria. In one study where 981 raw meat samples were obtained from grocery stores, *Enterococcus* was isolated as a bacterial contaminant in 97% of the pork samples and in 100% of the ground beef samples. In a study of 240 meat samples from grocery stores, *Salmonella* was found as a contaminant in 22% of the poultry samples and in 2% of the beef samples. *E. coli* was a contaminant in 37% of beef, 41% of chicken, 33% of pork, 48% of turkey, 3% of fish, and 4% of shellfish samples. Ground meat products were more likely to be contaminated with bacteria compared to nonground meats. Fastidious hygiene and preparation methods along with adequate storage and cooking of homemade diets are important in the prevention of foodborne illness.

When foodborne illness is suspected, history is very important. Potential for exposure to garbage or sources of pesticides or other toxic chemicals should be reviewed. Dogs are more prone to foodborne illness because they are more likely to eat garbage or consume dead animals. Young dogs may be more at risk because younger dogs tend to eat garbage more frequently than adult dogs. Older dogs or immunocompromised dogs are at higher risk for foodborne illness because their immune systems are less able to fight a bacterial infection. The risk of foodborne illness is higher during warm weather, hunting season, and during the Thanksgiving and Christmas holidays. Dogs allowed to freely roam outdoors have an increased exposure to dead animal tissues, pesticides, and garbage.

In addition, methods of food preparation and storage should be carefully reviewed, including types of containers used for storage. Samples of vomit, feces, and urine should be collected and frozen so that they may be tested for bacteria, pesticides, metals, and other toxic substances. The entire quantity of food in the original storage container should be retained or the ingredients used in the preparation of the diet should be stored for analysis.

Causes of Foodborne Illness

■ Mycotoxins

Mycotoxins are metabolites from mold and can cause a variety of symptoms. Grains such as corn or wheat are most commonly affected with mycotoxins, but cheeses, nuts, and fruits may also contain mycotoxins. Mycotoxins are produced while grains are growing or are in storage, and warm temperatures with high humidity generally favor mold growth. The major mycotoxin-producing fungi are *Aspergillus* and *Fusarium*.

Aflatoxin is a mycotoxin produced by *Aspergillus*. Corn, peanuts, and grains are the most common sources, and dogs and cats are very sensitive to low levels of aflatoxin. Clinical signs of aflatoxicosis include loss of appetite, lethargy, vomiting, jaundice, diarrhea, abdominal effusion, or sudden death. The liver is the primary organ affected, so an increase in serum liver enzyme activity, a decrease in serum protein, and an increase in serum bilirubin are commonly seen. Once affected, the survival rate is poor. In a recent outbreak of aflatoxicosis in dogs, 64% did not survive, even with extensive treatment. Aflatoxins are very stable and are not destroyed by cooking. Grains used for food manufacturing are routinely tested for aflatoxins.

Vomitoxin is a mycotoxin produced by *Fusarium*. The chemical name for vomitoxin is deoxynivalenol (DON), and vomitoxin most commonly affects wheat and barley. Like aflatoxin, vomitoxin is heat stable and is not destroyed by cooking. Dogs and pigs are the most sensitive to vomitoxin at very low concentrations. The most common signs of vomitoxin ingestion are vomiting and diarrhea. Many dogs can detect the odor from vomitoxin in the feed and will refuse to eat food contaminated with vomitoxin.

■ Bacteria

Salmonella

Salmonella are gram-negative bacteria that affect many species, including mammals, birds, reptiles, and amphibians. *Salmonella* infects humans, and transmission from animals to humans can occur; thus, it is a zoonotic disease. *Salmonella* is normally present in the intestinal tract, and healthy dogs and cats are fairly resistant to infection.

Exposure to *Salmonella* is most commonly through fecal contamination of food or water and is indicative of inadequate cooking or poor hygiene in food preparation. Racing greyhounds are commonly affected as they are routinely fed raw meats that are often contaminated with *Salmonella*. In a recent Canadian study, 166 raw diets for dogs were evaluated for the presence of *Salmonella*. Overall, *Salmonella* was isolated in 21% of the diets, and 67% of these diets contained chicken. Some of the *Salmonella* strains isolated were also resistant to many antimicrobials, which is of major concern.

Clinical signs of *Salmonella* infection include loss of appetite, lethargy, diarrhea, gastroenteritis, chronic fever, conjunctivitis, abortion, and pneumonia. Young animals or old animals that may have decreased immune function are at highest risk. In a recent case report, two cats from the same household were affected with *Salmonella*. One cat was 10 weeks old, and the other was almost 15 years old. Both cats were fed raw diets containing beef, and *Salmonella* was isolated from both the diet and the tissues from the cats. Neither cat survived.

Cases of human salmonellosis due to direct contact with infected animals are well documented. Humans at highest risk of infection and mortality are children younger than 9 years of age and the elderly.

Human exposure can occur by direct contact with pets consuming contaminated diets. In a recent study, 40 dogs consuming raw diets were evaluated for fecal shedding of *Salmonella* and were compared to 160 dogs not consuming a raw diet. Fecal shedding of *Salmonella* was found in up to 25% of dogs consuming raw diets. All dogs enrolled in this study routinely worked as therapy dogs visiting human patients in health-care facilities or retirement homes. As a result of this study, the recommendation was made that dogs consuming raw diets should be excluded from therapy programs due to the increased risk of *Salmonella* exposure for human patients.

Clostridium botulinum

Clostridium botulinum are gram-positive, anaerobic bacteria that are commonly found in the soil. These bacteria commonly contaminate raw meat, dead animal tissues, and vegetables. With anaerobic conditions (as in uncooked meat), *Clostridium botulinum* can produce an extremely potent toxin that, when ingested, can block the neurotransmitter acetylcholine. Clinical signs occur between 12 hours and 6 days after ingestion of the toxin. The most common clinical sign is paralysis starting in the rear limbs and progressing to all four limbs. The toxin is heat sensitive, and heating at 212°F for 10 minutes is sufficient to destroy the toxin.

Staphylococcus aureus

Staphylococcus species are commonly found on the skin of humans and other animals. Ingestion of *Staphylococcus aureus* (*S. aureus*) is the most common cause of foodborne illness in humans. Ingestion of toxin produced by *S. aureus* typically will cause nausea and vomiting within 2 to 4 hours, with spontaneous recovery in 24 to 48 hours. Dogs and cats are fairly resistant to the *S. aureus* enterotoxin. *S. aureus* bacteria are easily destroyed by heating, but the toxin produced can survive heating and the canning process.

Escherichia coli

E. coli is a common foodborne pathogen in people, but its role in foodborne illness in dogs and cats is unclear. *E. coli* has been implicated in a syndrome in racing greyhounds that is characterized by ulceration of the extremities and kidney damage.

Bacillus cereus

B. cereus is found in soil, grains, cereal products, and other foods, and it is commonly found in uncooked rice. *B. cereus* causes vomiting and diarrhea in people, but it is not a significant pathogen in dogs and cats. However, if pet food is exposed to moisture and warm temperatures, these bacteria can rapidly reproduce. Thus, pet diets containing a high amount of water (such as homemade diets) should not be exposed to high ambient temperatures for a prolonged period of time.

■ Rickettsia

Neorickettsia helminthoeca is a rickettsia that causes salmon poisoning. Raw salmon can contain a parasitic fluke, *Nanophyetus salmincola*. When this fluke is ingested in raw salmon, it matures in about a week and attaches to the intestinal lining. The rickettsia in the fluke can then invade the bloodstream and cause an acute infection. Clinical signs include vomiting, bloody diarrhea, fever, dehydration, and enlarged lymph nodes. Mortality can be high if treatment is not initiated early in the course of the infection.

■ Biogenic Amines

Biogenic amines are produced when bacteria decarboxylate amino acids in dead animal tissues. Biogenic amines include histamine, putrescine, and cadaverine. Histamine is commonly found in spoiled fish and is involved in scombroid fish poisoning. Scombroid fish include tuna, mackerel, and sardines. Histamine causes an allergic-type reaction, and clinical signs include flushing, nausea, diarrhea, rash, facial swelling, disorientation, and respiratory distress. Scombroid fish poisoning is rarely fatal.

■ Metals

Metals can accumulate in plants and animal tissues, and food can serve as a source of contamination. Metal contamination can also occur during food preparation. Most metal toxicities in dogs and cats involve lead, zinc, cadmium, and arsenic. With careful preparation of homemade diets, the potential for metal toxicity is low.

■ Other Sources

Chocolate
Feeding chocolate to pets should be avoided. Chocolate contains theobromine, which is a compound similar to caffeine. The dog is very

sensitive to even a small amount of theobromine because it is not metabolized very rapidly. The half-life of theobromine in humans is 6 hours, whereas it is 17.5 hours in the dog.

In the dog, a very small amount of theobromine can be potentially fatal, and a theobromine dose of 45 mg/lb body weight can be toxic. A 1-oz square of baking chocolate contains approximately 346 mg of theobromine. Cocoa powder contains an even higher level of theobromine. Semisweet and milk chocolate contain lower amounts of theobromine; however, consumption of just 8 oz of semisweet chocolate can be lethal for a midsized dog. One to 1.5 lb of milk chocolate can be fatal for a 25-lb dog. A dog could easily consume this much chocolate.

Clinical signs of theobromine toxicity include vomiting, diarrhea, restlessness, muscle tremors, and urinary incontinence. The treatment is to induce vomiting, as there is no specific antidote.

Onions and Garlic

Onions contain *n*-propyl disulfide, which, when ingested, can damage the lipid membranes of red blood cells. This membrane damage results in the irreversible denaturing of hemoglobin, and Heinz bodies are produced in the red blood cells. Heinz body anemia, in which red blood cells are destroyed, is the result. Dogs and cats are susceptible to Heinz body anemia, and ingestion of as little as 5–10 g onions/kg body weight can cause anemia. In one study, all dogs fed 30 g onions/kg body weight/day for 3 days exhibited severe anemia. Heinz body anemia has also occurred in cats. Garlic is also a member of the onion family, and chronic ingestion has caused anemia and dermatitis in dogs. The feeding of onions and garlic to pets should be restricted.

Grapes and Raisins

Recently, toxicity from ingesting grapes or raisins has been described. Following ingestion of what appears to be a trivial quantity of raisins or grapes, some dogs develop clinical signs of acute renal failure within 48 hours. In four dogs originally described with acute renal failure from eating grapes or raisins, ingestion was estimated to be from 0.41 to 1.1 oz of grapes or raisins per kilogram of body weight.

Not all dogs that consume grapes or raisins develop clinical signs of acute renal failure. Of 132 dogs that had ingested grapes or raisins, 33% developed acute renal failure and 25% had no clinical signs. The cause of renal failure associated with grapes or raisins is unknown, but it is speculated that ochratoxin may be a toxic component. An increase in serum calcium is common and was detected in 93% of dogs. Of 40 dogs with acute renal failure from ingestion of grapes or raisins, 42% failed to survive, even with extensive treatment. For those that do survive, therapy is intensive and requires several weeks of hospitalization. Aggressive treatment has been recommended for any dogs suspected of having ingested large, or even small, quantities of grapes or raisins, including induction of vomiting, gastric lavage, and administration of activated charcoal.

Bovine Spongiform Encephalopathy (BSE)

Bovine spongiform encephalopathy (BSE) is the technical name for mad cow disease, which can affect cattle. It is caused by a modified type of protein called a *prion protein*, which has some very unusual characteristics. The disease has a very long incubation period, from 3 to 9 years. Prion proteins affect the brain, giving the infected brain a spongelike appearance. Thus, BSE is a slowly progressive degenerative disease of the nervous system. Affected cattle show incoordination, aggression, nervousness, and loss of body weight. There is no treatment, and most die within 6 months.

Prion diseases are found in a number of species, including cows, humans, sheep, goats, mink, elk, mule deer, and cats. A prion-type disease has recently been described in cats in the United Kingdom, but no cases have been seen in the United States. In sheep, the disease is called scrapie, and in mink it is called transmissible mink encephalopathy (TME).

Prion proteins are located in nervous system tissues (brain and spinal cord), and the disease is transmitted by eating these tissues. In Britain, cows contracted BSE by eating scrapie-infected sheep meal. People may be infected with prion disease by eating brains and nervous tissue from infected animals. Striated muscle meats, fat, and milk are not infective since these tissues do not contain the BSE-causing agent. The potential for BSE to infect dogs and cats is very low.

Prevention of Foodborne Illness

The prevention of foodborne illness involves limiting exposure to garbage and dead animal tissue and proper preparation and storage of foods. Any food that is moldy, discolored, or has an off odor should not be used. All utensils and bowls used to prepare food should be clean and washed after every use. Bowls used for feeding should be washed daily. All homemade diets should be cooked for a minimum of 10 minutes at 180°F, and the internal temperature of any cooked meat should be verified with a meat thermometer. When feeding, any food that is not consumed within 2 to 4 hours should be thrown away if the ambient temperature is above 50°F. Prepared diets should be kept refrigerated prior to feeding and should not be kept more than 5 days. Food should be stored covered and should be inspected for mold growth prior to feeding.

Additional Reading

Miller EP, Cullor JS. 2000. Food safety. In *Small Animal Clinical Nutrition*, 4th edition. Hand MS, Thatcher CD, Remillard RL, Roudebush P (Eds). Mark Morris Institute, Topeka, pp. 183–200.

Remillard RL, Paragon B-M, Crane SW, Debraekeleer J, Cowell CS. 2000. Making pet foods at home. In *Small Animal Clinical Nutrition*, 4th edition. Hand MS, Thatcher CD, Remillard RL, Roudebush P (Eds). Mark Morris Institute, Topeka, pp. 163–182.

CHAPTER 3
Nutrients

Expression of Nutrient Content

The nutrients present in diets can be expressed in a number of different ways. The guaranteed analysis on a pet food label expresses nutrient levels on an "as-fed" basis. To arrive at these values, the nutrients have been measured in the finished product and represent what is being consumed by the pet. The amount of water is not taken into account in this determination, and dry pet foods will appear to have much higher percentages of nutrients than canned products that contain a considerable amount of water. Homemade diets typically have a high water content, and thus the percentages of nutrients will appear low on an as-fed basis.

A better way to compare diets is to look at nutrients on a dry matter (DM) basis. For this determination, the amount of water in each diet is taken into account. The values represent the percentage of a particular nutrient if no water were present in the diet; thus, it is a percentage of the dry matter of the diet. In this manner, percentages of nutrients can be compared independently of the amount of water present in the finished product. For example, a dry diet may contain 18% protein on an as-fed basis and contain 10% water (which means that there is 90% dry matter). Divide the 18% protein by 90% DM and multiply by 100% to get a protein content of 20% on a dry matter basis (sometimes expressed as 20% DM). A wet diet may contain 8% protein on an as-fed basis and contain 60% water (which means there is 40% dry matter). Divide the 8% protein by 40% DM and multiply by 100% to get a protein content of 20% on a dry matter basis. Thus, these two diets contain the same amount of protein on a dry matter basis, even though they appear be quite different when considered on an as fed basis.

A more accurate method of comparing foods is to calculate the amount of nutrient on a "metabolizable energy" (ME) basis. The ME basis gives an indication of the nutrient density of the diet. Using this method, nutrients are expressed as a percentage or as grams per 1000 kcal of ME. For example, a homemade diet may contain 11% protein on an as-fed basis, and this diet provides 1600 kcal/1000 g (or 160 kcal/100 g) of prepared diet. The 11% protein represents 11 g protein/100 g prepared diet, so if we divide the 11 g protein/100 g diet by 160 kcal/100 g diet, this diet provides 0.06875 g protein/kcal; or multiplying by 1000, we get 68.75 g protein/1000 kcal. Dogs and cats consume a diet based on their energy needs. Thus, in this manner the exact amounts of nutrient consumed can be determined.

Another way of expressing protein, carbohydrate, and fat is to look at the percentages of the total kilocalories in the diet provided by each of these nutrients. For example, a homemade diet may contain 11% protein, 6% fat, and 45% carbohydrate on an as-fed basis, with 63% water (37% DM). On a DM basis, the percentage of protein is essentially 30% (30% protein DM), the percentage of fat is 16% (16% fat DM), and the percentage of carbohydrate is 45% (45% carbohydrate DM). Protein and carbohydrate provide approximately 3.5 kcal/g, and fat provides approximately 8.5 kcal/g. Thus, the energy provided by protein is 30% times 3.5 kcal/g, or 105 kcal, and the energy provided by fat and carbohydrate are 136 kcal and 157.5 kcal, respectively, for a total of 398.5 kcal. The percentage of energy in the diet from protein is then 105 kcal/398.5 kcal * 100%, or approximately 26%. The percentage of energy in the diet from fat and carbohydrate is 34% and 40%, respectively.

Ingredient Selection

Ingredients used to formulate diets should be foods with high digestibility and biological value. Overall, the digestibility of ingredients for human consumption is high. As the quality of ingredients used in diets increases, so does the digestibility, and digestibility of 89% for protein, 95% for fat, and 88% for carbohydrates are possible. Diets with low digestibility tend to produce increased flatulence and larger stool volumes. In general, ingredients of animal origin are better digested by dogs and cats than are ingredients of plant origin.

Homemade diets can be formulated using basic information on the nutrient composition for all food ingredients. This information provides the content of calories, protein, fat, carbohydrate, fiber, amino acids, vitamins, and minerals for each ingredient included in the diet. Nutrient composition of foods can be obtained from the U.S. Department of Agriculture (USDA) or from sophisticated human diet formulation software (Food Processor SQL, ESHA Research, Salem, OR). Dietary requirements for the dog and cat are published yearly by the Association of American Feed Control Officials (AAFCO). Dietary requirements are determined by the Canine and Feline Nutrition Expert subcommittees of AAFCO, and these values differ from those of the National Research Council (NRC) Committee on Animal Nutrition. The NRC establishes minimum nutrients needed for growth based on highly purified diets. The AAFCO requirements take into account differences in ingredient digestibility and sources of vitamins and minerals. The AAFCO Dog and Cat Food Nutrient Profiles are used to substantiate the adequacy of foods that are "complete and balanced." Minimum levels and maximum levels for some nutrients have been determined. Nutrient levels are expressed on a DM basis and are also corrected for ME of the diet. Nutrient requirements for dogs can be found in Tables 3.1 and 3.2 and for cats in Tables 3.3 and 3.4.

Formulating a complete and balanced homemade diet is not a simple task due to the fact that many amino acids, vitamins, and minerals must be considered. Most human diet programs such as those found on the Internet are inadequate for use in formulating pet diets.

Review of Nutrients

■ Proteins

Proteins have many functions. They are important in muscle function, are the major structural components of collagen, are enzymes that catalyze metabolic reactions, and serve as hormones. Proteins also act as carrier substances in the blood and contribute to the regulation of acid-base balance. In addition, proteins are important in immune system function.

Proteins are composed of 22 different amino acids, most of which can be synthesized in the body (nonessential amino acids). However,

Table 3.1. AAFCO dog food nutrient profiles based on dry matter.[a]

Nutrients	Units DM Basis	Growth & Reproduction Minimum	Adult Maintenance Minimum	Maximum
Crude protein	%	22.0	18.0	
Arginine	%	0.62	0.51	
Histidine	%	0.22	0.18	
Isoleucine	%	0.45	0.37	
Leucine	%	0.72	0.59	
Lysine	%	0.77	0.63	
Methionine-cystine	%	0.53	0.43	
Phenylalanine-tyrosine	%	0.89	0.73	
Threonine	%	0.58	0.48	
Tryptophan	%	0.20	0.16	
Valine	%	1.48	0.39	
Crude fat	%	8.0	5.0	
Linoleic acid	%	1.0	1.0	
Minerals				
Calcium	%	1.0	0.6	2.5
Phosphorus	%	0.8	0.5	1.6
Ca/P Ratio	%	1:1	1:1	2:1
Potassium	%	0.6	0.6	
Sodium	%	0.3	0.06	
Chloride	%	0.45	0.09	
Magnesium	%	0.04	0.04	0.3
Iron	mg/kg	80	80	3,000
Copper	mg/kg	7.3	7.3	250
Manganese	mg/kg	5.0	5.0	
Zinc	mg/kg	120	120	1,000
Iodine	mg/kg	1.5	1.5	50
Selenium	mg/kg	0.11	0.11	2
Vitamins & Other				
Vitamin A	IU/kg	5,000	5,000	250,000
Vitamin D	IU/kg	500	500	5,000

Table 3.1. *(cont.)*

Nutrients	Units DM Basis	Growth & Reproduction Minimum	Adult Maintenance Minimum	Maximum
Vitamin E	IU/kg	50	50	1,000
Thiamine	mg/kg	1.0	1.0	
Riboflavin	mg/kg	2.2	2.2	
Pantothenic acid	mg/kg	10	10	
Niacin	mg/kg	11.4	11.4	
Pyridoxine	mg/kg	1.0	1.0	
Folic acid	mg/kg	0.18	0.18	
Vitamin B_{12}	mg/kg	0.022	0.022	
Choline	mg/kg	1,200	1,200	

DM, dry matter.
[a]Presumes an energy density of 3500 kcal ME/kg.
Adapted from the Official Publication of the Association of American Feed Control Officials, Inc.

Table 3.2. AAFCO Dog food nutrient profiles based on calorie content.[a]

Nutrients	Units per 1000 kcal ME	Growth & Reproduction Minimum	Adult Maintenance Minimum	Maximum
Crude protein	g	62.9	51.4	
Arginine	g	1.77	1.46	
Histidine	g	0.63	0.51	
Isoleucine	g	1.29	1.06	
Leucine	g	2.06	1.69	
Lysine	g	2.2	1.80	
Methionine-cystine	g	1.51	1.23	
Phenylalanine-tyrosine	g	2.54	2.09	
Threonine	g	1.66	1.37	
Tryptophan	g	0.57	0.46	
Valine	g	1.37	1.11	
Crude fat	g	22.9	14.3	
Linoleic acid	g	2.9	2.9	

Table 3.2. *(cont.)*

Nutrients	Units per 1000 kcal ME	Growth & Reproduction Minimum	Adult Maintenance Minimum	Maximum
Minerals				
Calcium	g	2.9	1.7	7.1
Phosphorus	g	2.3	1.4	4.6
Potassium	g	1.7	1.7	
Sodium	g	0.86	0.17	
Chloride	g	1.29	0.26	
Magnesium	g	0.11	0.11	0.86
Iron	mg	23	23	857
Copper	mg	2.1	2.1	71
Manganese	mg	1.4	1.4	
Zinc	mg	34	34	286
Iodine	mg	0.43	0.43	14
Selenium	mg	0.03	0.03	0.57
Vitamins & Others				
Vitamin A	IU	1429	1429	71429
Vitamin D	IU	143	143	1429
Vitamin E	IU	14	14	286
Thiamine	mg	0.29	0.29	
Riboflavin	mg	0.63	0.63	
Pantothenic acid	mg	2.9	2.9	
Niacin	mg	3.3	3.3	
Pyridoxine	mg	0.29	0.29	
Folic acid	mg	0.05	0.05	
Vitamin B_{12}	mg	0.006	0.006	
Choline	mg	343	343	

ME, metabolizable energy.

[a]Presumes an energy density greater than 4000 kcal ME/kg DM.

Adapted from the Official Publication of the Association of American Feed Control Officials, Inc.

Table 3.3. AAFCO cat food nutrient profiles based on dry matter.[a]

Nutrients	Units DM Basis	Growth & Reproduction Minimum	Adult Maintenance Minimum	Maximum
Crude protein	%	30.0	26.0	
Arginine	%	1.25	1.04	
Histidine	%	0.31	0.31	
Isoleucine	%	0.52	0.52	
Leucine	%	1.25	1.25	
Lysine	%	1.20	0.83	
Methionine-cystine	%	1.10	1.10	
Methionine	%	0.62	0.62	1.5
Phenylalanine-tyrosine	%	0.88	0.88	
Phenylalanine	%	0.42	0.42	
Threonine	%	0.73	0.73	
Tryptophan	%	0.25	0.16	
Valine	%	0.62	0.62	
Crude fat	%	9.0	9.0	
Linoleic acid	%	0.5	0.5	
Arachidonic acid	%	0.02	0.02	
Minerals				
Calcium	%	1.0	0.6	
Phosphorus	%	0.8	0.5	
Potassium	%	0.6	0.6	
Sodium	%	0.2	0.2	
Chloride	%	0.3	0.3	
Magnesium	%	0.08	0.04	
Iron	%	80	80	
Copper (extruded)	mg/kg	15	5	
Copper (canned)	mg/kg	5	5	
Manganese	mg/kg	7.5	7.5	
Zinc	mg/kg	75	75	
Iodine	mg/kg	0.35	0.35	2,000
Selenium	mg/kg	0.1	0.1	

Table 3.3. *(cont.)*

Nutrients	Units DM Basis	Growth & Reproduction Minimum	Adult Maintenance Minimum	Maximum
Vitamins & Others				
Vitamin A	IU/kg	9,000	5,000	750,000
Vitamin D	IU/kg	750	500	10,000
Vitamin E	IU/kg	30	30	
Vitamin K	mg/kg	0.1	0.1	
Thiamine	mg/kg	5.0	5.0	
Riboflavin	mg/kg	4.0	4.0	
Pantothenic acid	mg/kg	5.0	5.0	
Niacin	mg/kg	60	60	
Pyridoxine	mg/kg	4.0	4.0	
Folic acid	mg/kg	0.8	0.8	
Biotin	mg/kg	0.07	0.07	
Vitamin B_{12}	mg/kg	0.02	0.02	
Choline	mg/kg	2,400	2,400	
Taurine (extruded)	%	0.10	0.10	
Taurine (canned)	%	0.20	0.20	

DM, dry matter.
[a]Presumes an energy density of 4000 kcal ME/kg.
Adapted from the Official Publication of the Association of American Feed Control Officials, Inc.

Table 3.4. **AAFCO cat food nutrient profiles based on calorie content.**[a]

Nutrients	Units per 1000 kcal ME	Growth & Reproduction Minimum	Adult Maintenance Minimum	Maximum
Crude protein	g	75	65	
Arginine	g	3.10	2.60	
Histidine	g	0.78	0.78	
Isoleucine	g	1.30	1.30	
Leucine	g	3.10	3.10	
Lysine	g	3.00	2.08	

Table 3.4. *(cont.)*

Nutrients	Units per 1000 kcal ME	Growth & Reproduction Minimum	Adult Maintenance Minimum	Maximum
Methionine-cystine	g	2.75	2.75	
Methionine	g	1.55	0.55	3.75
Phenylalanine-tyrosine	g	2.20	2.20	
Phenylalanine	g	1.05	1.05	
Threonine	g	1.83	1.83	
Tryptophan	g	0.63	0.40	
Valine	g	1.55	1.55	
Crude fat	g	22.5	22.5	
Linoleic acid	g	1.25	1.25	
Arachidonic acid	g	0.05	0.05	
Minerals				
Calcium	g	2.5	1.5	
Phosphorus	g	2.0	1.25	
Potassium	g	1.5	1.5	
Sodium	g	0.5	0.5	
Chloride	g	0.75	0.75	
Magnesium	g	0.2	0.10	
Iron	mg	20.0	20.0	
Copper (extruded)	mg	3.75	1.25	
Copper (canned)	mg	1.25	1.25	
Manganese	mg	1.90	1.90	
Zinc	mg	18.8	18.8	
Iodine	mg	0.09	0.09	500
Selenium	mg	0.03	0.03	
Vitamins & Others				
Vitamin A	IU	2,250	1,250	187,500
Vitamin D	IU	188	125	2,500

Table 3.4. *(cont.)*

Nutrients	Units per 1000 kcal ME	Growth & Reproduction Minimum	Adult Maintenance Minimum	Maximum
Vitamin E	IU	7.5	7.5	
Vitamin K	mg	0.03	0.03	
Thiamine	mg	1.25	1.25	
Riboflavin	mg	1.00	1.00	
Pantothenic acid	mg	1.25	1.25	
Niacin	mg	15	15	
Pyridoxine	mg	1.0	1.0	
Folic acid	mg	0.20	0.20	
Biotin	mg	0.018	0.018	
Vitamin B_{12}	mg	0.005	0.005	
Choline	mg	600	600	
Taurine (extruded)	g	0.25	0.25	
Taurine (canned)	g	0.50	0.50	

DM, dry matter.
[a]Presumes an energy density greater than 4500 kcal ME/kg DM.
Adapted from the Official Publication of the Association of American Feed Control Officials, Inc.

10 amino acids cannot be made in the body, and these are termed *essential amino acids* (Table 3.5). These amino acids must be provided by the diet. An essential amino acid is one that the body cannot synthesize at a rate fast enough (from constituents normally in the diet) for normal growth or maintenance.

Dietary protein is the principal source of nitrogen and provides the amino acids that are used for protein synthesis. Nitrogen is necessary for the synthesis of the nonessential amino acids and other molecules such as purines, nucleic acids, pyrimidines, and neurotransmitters.

The nutritional value of protein depends on its amino acid composition as well as on the efficiency of its digestion, absorption, and utilization. The use of amino acids for protein synthesis depends on the availability to cells of all amino acids in the right proportion and at the right time. The diet must provide these amino acids; otherwise,

Table 3.5. Amino acids in dogs and cats.

Essential Amino Acids	Nonessential Amino Acids
Arginine	Alanine
Histidine	Asparagine
Isoleucine	Aspartate
Leucine	Cysteine
Lysine	Glutamate
Methionine	Glutamine
Phenylalanine	Glycine
Taurine (only required by cats)	Hydroxylysine
Tryptophan	Hydroxyproline
Threonine	Proline
Valine	Serine
	Tryptophan

the body mobilizes them from protein in its tissues. Plants can make all the amino acids they require by synthesizing them from simple nitrogenous compounds such as ammonia and nitrates. Animals require most of their dietary nitrogen to be in the form of specific amino acids.

Different protein sources have different levels of essential amino acids. Organ and muscle meats, whole egg, and soybeans are examples of protein sources with high levels of essential amino acids in the proper proportions. When evaluating a diet, one must also be aware of how digestible the protein is. Organ and muscle meat protein is more digestible than soybean meal. Proteins provide approximately 3.5 kcal/g ME.

Taurine is an amino acid required only by the cat. Most animals can synthesize adequate taurine from methionine and cysteine. Taurine plays important roles in myocardial and retinal function. Cats can synthesize a small amount of taurine, but they have a high demand for it. Cats can use only taurine for bile salt formation and cannot switch to using glycine when taurine is limited. Taurine is continually lost in the cat, and thus there is a dietary requirement for taurine. Taurine is present only in animal tissues, with high concentrations found in shellfish. Poultry, meat, and fish also contain taurine. Because of the cat's requirement for taurine, diets formulated for dogs should not be fed to cats, as those diets may not contain adequate amounts of this amino acid.

Biological Value of Proteins

Biological value describes how efficiently a protein is used. This value is high for proteins from meat, eggs, and dairy products. Dogs and cats digest these proteins efficiently, and they provide amino acids in proportions suitable for tissue protein synthesis. In contrast, the biological value of most plant proteins is low due to insufficiencies of specific amino acids and lower digestibility. Careful balancing of proteins from plant sources can improve the protein quality of the diet and make them suitable for meeting nutritional needs. Diets must contain more proteins when their biological value is lower or when they have less than an ideal amino acid profile.

Protein Requirement

The protein requirement is difficult to determine due to the multiple factors that affect it. Protein quality, amino acid composition, diet energy density, activity level, and nutritional status can all affect the protein requirement. If very high-quality synthetic proteins are fed, the requirement for protein in adult dogs is between 4% and 7% of ME. If lower quality protein sources are used, the protein requirement may be as high as 20% of ME. Growing animals have a higher protein requirement. AAFCO requires that canine diets contain 18% protein for maintenance and 22% protein for growth and reproduction.

Cats have a substantially higher protein requirement; approximately 24% DM protein or 17% of ME is required. AAFCO requires that feline diets contain 26% DM protein for maintenance and 30% DM protein for growth and reproduction.

Dynamic State of Body Proteins

Adult animals have ongoing requirements for dietary protein because body proteins are in a dynamic state; the body continually degrades and rebuilds them. Some proteins, such as in the gastrointestinal mucosa, turn over rapidly, while others, such as in tendons and ligaments, turn over slowly. During protein degradation and rebuilding, the body does not completely reuse the amino acids released. Dietary amino acids replace those lost during degradation.

When caloric intake is inadequate to meet energy requirements, body proteins are catabolized and used for energy. When the diet provides all nutrients needed for energy requirements, amino acids requirements are less, and minimal protein is degraded. During disease with fevers, infection, and trauma, extensive body protein can be lost in much greater amounts than with starvation. Release is augmented by hormones such as cortisol to promote body protein breakdown.

Except during growth, the amount of protein or nitrogen in the body should remain stable; the animal is in nitrogen balance. When the intake of nitrogen exceeds excretion, there is positive balance and the animal stores nitrogen. With a negative balance, body protein is degraded.

Nitrogen balance is not only the result of having the proper amount of protein in the diet. The balance also depends on the quality of protein. To maintain balance, more protein is required when its biological value is low and less when that value is high.

Formulation of Diets to Meet Amino Acid Needs

Requirements for dietary protein are based on (1) an animal's nitrogen requirements, (2) an animal's amino acid requirements, and (3) the dietary protein's amino acid composition. Nitrogen requirements are expressed as crude protein requirements. When a diet satisfies these requirements, it is necessary to find the first limiting amino acid. Dietary levels of that amino acid indicate the least amount of protein necessary to satisfy all essential amino acids. When a diet satisfies requirements for the first limiting amino acid, it satisfies all other amino acid requirements.

For example, wheat grain protein is low in lysine, and the sulfur-containing amino acids (such as methionine) are deficient for puppies. An additional source of protein containing lysine and the sulfur amino acids must be added to provide the proper amounts of all amino acids. If wheat was fed without any other added protein or amino acids, the amount fed would have to more than double.

Besides calculating the protein and amino acid requirements, it is necessary to determine their availability. The minimal protein requirement is known only after calculating the digestibility of the dietary protein. Feeding trials give information on protein digestibility; it is not possible to determine the biological value of a protein from amino acid or protein analysis of a food. Digestibility and utilization vary greatly for different proteins. Nonprotein nutrients (such as fiber) in the diet can influence the digestibility and utilization. Cooking improves the digestibility of proteins, although sometimes heat can decrease digestibility, especially if protein is cooked with sugars.

■ Carbohydrates

Carbohydrates include starches, sugars, and fiber and provide a primary source of energy for most pet foods. Dietary carbohydrate contributes approximately 3.5 kcal ME per gram of carbohydrate. Carbohydrate sources in pet foods typically include rice, corn, potato, wheat, soybean, oats, barley, quinoa, and sorghum. Vegetables are also considered a source of carbohydrate but are much less digestible than the common starches due to their fiber content. The most soluble and digestible carbohydrates are starches and sugars in plants. The source and type of processing determines the carbohydrate's digestibility. Rice is highly digestible by dogs and cats, but raw wheat, oats, and potato are poorly digested. Corn has a poorer digestibility as compared to rice. Cooking increases the digestibility of all starches, especially potato starch.

Sugars are sometimes included in pet foods and can be highly digestible in small quantities. Sucrose is found in molasses, honey, maple syrup, sugar, fruits, and vegetables. Sucrase present in the small intestine hydrolyzes sucrose to glucose and fructose. Lactose is usually found only in milk products and is digested by lactase. The activity of lactase decreases when there is little lactose in the diet. Excess sugars are not completely digested and can cause diarrhea.

Carbohydrate is stored in limited quantity in the body as glycogen. If excess carbohydrate is consumed, most is stored in the body as fat. Even though dogs and cats have no established dietary requirement for carbohydrates, carbohydrate is protein sparing. As long as there is adequate dietary carbohydrate, carbohydrate will be used as the energy source, which allows protein to be used for growth and tissue repair rather than energy.

Dogs usually tolerate high levels of carbohydrate with no problem; however, cats tolerate less dietary starch. If excessive carbohydrate is fed, diarrhea can result because the small intestine cannot digest and absorb all the carbohydrate present. Some dogs can also have insufficient enzyme activity in the small intestine for proper digestion of carbohydrate. The cat is a true carnivore, and the natural diet is mostly protein and fat and is very low in carbohydrate. Carnivores can convert amino acids and glycerol for glucose, and cats can maintain normal blood glucose levels on starvation diets better than other animals. Cats are also able to store more glycogen in their liver when fed a high-protein diet.

Dogs may not readily digest galactosides, which are carbohydrates found in dairy products and soybeans. Galactosides are digested by unique intestinal enzymes specific for galactosides, and this enzyme activity may be low if little galactoside has been fed. New foods containing this carbohydrate should be introduced gradually into the diet to prevent diarrhea.

Longer-chain carbohydrates (oligosaccharides) containing galactose, such as rhamnose, stachyose, and verbacose, form about half the carbohydrate in soybeans. These carbohydrates are not digested in the small intestine and are fermented in the colon by bacteria. Fermentation produces gas, so flatulence is not uncommon. This fermentation also produces short-chain fatty acids (SCFA) that help support nutrition for the colon and promote water and salt absorption.

■ Dietary Fiber

Dietary fiber affects carbohydrate digestion and absorption. Dietary fiber consists of plant materials such as cellulose, hemicellulose, lignin, and pectins. Nonplant cell wall sources of fiber include gums, mucilages, algal polysaccharides, and modified cellulose.

Dietary fibers are insoluble or soluble. Insoluble fibers consist primarily of cellulose and some hemicelluloses. They also include lignin, which represents a small part of dietary total fiber. Insoluble fibers are the structural building material of cell walls. Insoluble fiber is found in whole wheat flour, bran, grains, and vegetables. The bonds present in insoluble fibers cannot be broken down by the enzymes in the intestinal tract and thus cannot be absorbed. Water-soluble fibers are all other nonstructural and indigestible plant carbohydrates. Soluble fibers such as pectin, guar gum, and carboxymethylcellulose absorb water and form gels; they slow gastric emptying, reduce nutrient absorption, and increase intestinal transit rate. Increased dietary fiber reduces digestibility of carbohydrates, proteins, and fats and affects absorption for some vitamins and minerals. Water-insoluble fibers such as wheat cereal bran and cellulose reduce digestion and absorption the least.

Fiber increases fecal volume and promotes more frequent defecation. Fiber from cereal grains also increases fecal volume by absorbing water.

Bacteria present in the large intestine have the ability to partially break down some fiber sources. This fermentation creates short-chain fatty acids (SCFA) such as acetate, propionate, and butyrate. Soluble fibers are highly fermentable, whereas insoluble fibers are not fermented. Beet pulp, rice bran, and some gums are moderately fermented. Pectin, guar gum, oat bran, and some vegetable fibers are readily fermented.

The SCFAs produced during fiber fermentation do not contribute significantly to the energy provided by the diet. However, they do serve as an energy source for the intestinal epithelial cells. Fatty acids also promote colonic salt and water absorption. Excess fermentable fiber results in diarrhea caused by large amounts of SCFAs.

Fiber is rarely added to homemade diets, yet these diets provide enough fiber to supply colonic nutritional needs. In the wild, dogs and cats consume diets containing very little fiber. Thus, dogs and cats probably have a low requirement for fiber. Homemade diets typically contain less than 1.4% fiber unless they contain large amounts of vegetables, beans, peas, or bran-rich cereals.

The amount of dietary fiber can be altered for different conditions; for example, an increased amount is often recommended for diets designed for weight reduction. Fiber reduces the digestibility of other nutrients and may reduce appetite or hunger by filling the stomach. If fiber is increased, then there must be added attention to the rest of the diet to ensure that it is balanced and that enough will be consumed to meet nutritional needs. Increased fiber can also cause an increase in stool volume.

■ Fats

Dietary fat contributes approximately 8.5 kcal ME per gram of fat. Digestibility of fat is typically high and can be greater than 90%. In dogs, the minimum nutrient requirement for fat is 5% of the diet in adults, and 8% for growth and reproduction. In cats, the minimum nutrient requirement for fat is 9% for all life stages. As fat increases in the diet, the energy content rapidly increases. Since most pets will eat to satisfy their caloric needs, providing an energy-dense diet with higher fat content will typically decrease the volume of food ingested. High-fat diets are important to supply the energy needs of very active dogs, hard-working dogs (e.g., sled dogs), and lactating animals.

Dietary fat contributes to the palatability of the diet, and the texture and "mouth-feel" of the diet. Fat can provide a significant portion the diet's energy and is also important for the absorption of fat-soluble vitamins. Most relatively sedentary house pets do not require high levels of fat in their diet to maintain good body condition. Feeding highly palatable diets that are high in fat can contribute to overeating and obesity. Excessive dietary fat can overwhelm digestion and cause steatorrhea (the passage of undigested fat). Excess dietary fat reduces food consumption, which can cause deficiency of other nutrients unless those dietary levels increase. Protein, iodine, and thiamin levels should especially be augmented when dietary fat increases.

Essential Fatty Acids

Dietary fat is necessary as a source of essential fatty acids. In the dog, linoleic acid and linolenic acid are required in the diet. In cats,

Table 3.6. Omega-3 Fatty Acid Content in Selected Ingredients.

Ingredient	Grams Omega-3 Fatty Acids in 100 g of Ingredient[a]
Salmon	0–1.5
Mackerel	2.2
Herring	1.4
Albacore tuna	0.5
Trout	0.6
Whitefish	1.5
Menhaden oil	23.2
Flaxseed oil	53.3
Cod liver oil	18.8
Canola oil	11.1
Soybean oil	6.8
Sardines	3.5
Wheat germ oil	6.9
Butter	0.3
Lard	1.0

[a]Adapted from Food Processor SQL (ESHA Research).

linoleic acid, linolenic acid, and arachidonic acid are required because cats cannot convert linoleic acid to arachidonic acid. Linoleic and arachidonic acid are omega-6 fatty acids, and linolenic acid is an omega-3 fatty acid. Fat sources differ greatly in their concentrations of omega-6 and omega-3 fatty acids. Omega-6 fatty acids can be found in meat products, egg yolks, and vegetable oils. Arachidonic acid, however, is found almost entirely in meat sources (small amounts are found in borage oil and evening primrose oil). Omega-3 fatty acids are present in high levels in fish oils (Table 3.6); they can also be found in flaxseed oil, wheat germ oil, canola oil, and soybean oil. Fish sources of omega-3 fatty acids provide long-chain omega-3 fatty acids (eicosapentaenoic acid [EPA] and docosahexaenoic acid [DHA]), which are used in metabolism. Plant sources (flaxseed, canola, soybean, wheat germ) contain high levels of linolenic acid, which needs to be converted to EPA and DHA for metabolism. Cats are unable to convert linolenic acid to EPA and DHA and thus should be supplemented with a fish source of omega-3 fatty acids. The omega-3 fatty acids from fish oils are more effective than those from plant sources.

Considerable research is ongoing to investigate the ideal ratio of dietary omega-6 to omega-3 fatty acids and the use of omega-3 fatty acids in the treatment of disease. Some have suggested that an optimal dietary omega-6/omega-3 fatty acid ratio is between 4:1 and 10:1. Research has also suggested that not only is the ratio of omega-6 to omega-3 fatty acids important, but the actual amounts are equally as important at the cellular level. The use of omega-3 fatty acids to modulate inflammation is a major focus of research. Omega-6 fatty acids are utilized in the synthesis of compounds that strongly promote inflammation. Omega-3 fatty acids are utilized in the synthesis of similar compounds, but these compounds are much weaker regarding promoting inflammation. Thus, there is the potential to decrease the inflammatory response with dietary omega-3 fatty acids.

In dogs, linoleic acid should be provided at 1% of the dry weight of the diet for maintenance, growth, and reproduction (about 2% of calories). Cats require 0.50% DM linoleic acid and 0.02% DM arachidonic acid in a diet containing 4000 kcal ME/kg. If cat diets do not contain adequate arachidonic acid, decreases in platelets and platelet function is observed, and queens fail to deliver living kittens. Decreased growth rate, poor coat condition, and impaired wound healing have also been seen with arachidonic acid deficiency in cats.

Fatty Acid Deficiency and Excess

Low-fat diets are not very palatable, thus essential fatty acid deficiency is not common in dogs and cats and usually only occurs with a long period of deficiency. Diets that have adequate levels of fat when formulated but that have been stored improperly can result in fatty acid deficiency. Oxidation of fats in foods occurs when the food is exposed to high temperatures or high-humidity conditions. This oxidation is termed *rancidity*. In commercial pet foods, antioxidants are typically added to help prevent the oxidation of fats; homemade diets usually do not have antioxidants (preservatives) added, so they should be made in very small batches and stored properly to prevent rancidity.

High-fat diets are relatively safe for dogs and cats. In humans, atherosclerosis can be a result of high-fat diets; however, due to major differences in lipoprotein metabolism, dogs and cats rarely develop atherosclerosis unless there is an underlying condition altering lipid metabolism (hypothyroidism, diabetes mellitus, or primary lipid defects). If polyunsaturated fats are present in excess, there is an increase in the vitamin E requirement. In cats, pansteatitis (yellow fat disease) can occur if the diet is high in polyunsaturated fats and low in vitamin E. Feeding a high-fat diet can potentially cause pancreatitis, but this association is not clear. Many dogs with pancreatitis have a history of eating a fat-rich diet or consuming fatty meat scraps. However, normal dogs fed a 70% fat diet do not usually develop acute pancreatitis.

High-fat diets can result in maldigestion or malabsorption, where unabsorbed fat enters the colon; normally, very little fat reaches this point. Bacteria that normally live in the colon transform dietary fats to fatty compounds that are essentially the same as the active ingredient in castor oil (ricinoleic acid). By making one small change in normal fat, bacteria convert it to a potent laxative. Ricinoleic-like compounds damage the colonic mucosa, stimulate colonic water secretion, and stimulate intestinal motility, all of which contribute to diarrhea. Therefore, most diets recommended for the management of chronic diarrhea are low in fat, even for dogs and cats with no loss in their ability to digest and absorb fats.

■ Water

The most essential nutrient for dogs and cats is water. A dog can lose all its body fat and one-half its protein and still survive. Signs of deficiencies of other nutrients can take long periods of time to develop; however, this is not the case with a deficiency of water. In dogs, clinical signs of water deficiency can occur with as little as a 5% loss of body water. Death can occur if 15% of body water is lost. A supply of fresh, good-quality water should be available at all times. The average dog requires between 50 and 90 mL water per kilogram of body weight per day (approximately 1 to 2 cups per 10 lb body weight per day).

Cats are better able to tolerate a lack of water than are dogs. This is in part due to the cat's greater ability to concentrate urine and prevent water loss. Cats require between 10 and 45 mL water per kilogram of body weight per day (approximately ¼ to 1 cup per 10 lb body weight per day).

■ Vitamins and Minerals

Vitamins and minerals are important components of an animal's diet and are required for the normal functioning of every body system. Vitamins are separated into two groups: fat-soluble and water-soluble vitamins. Fat-soluble vitamins include vitamins A, D, E, and K and are stored within the fat of the body. Water-soluble vitamins are the B vitamins (B_{12}, thiamin, riboflavin, and pyridoxine), vitamin C, pantothenic acid, biotin, niacin, folic acid, and choline. Excesses of the water-soluble vitamins are excreted in the urine. Minerals are classified as macrominerals and microminerals. Microminerals are present in very small quantities in the body and include iron, zinc, copper, manganese, iodine, and selenium. Macrominerals are present in slightly higher concentrations and include calcium, phosphorus, magnesium, potassium, sodium, and chlorine.

Interactions between minerals occur, so oversupplementation of one particular mineral may result in a deficiency of another mineral. Well-formulated pet foods are developed to keep vitamins and minerals in proper balance. Many vitamins are destroyed very easily with cooking; therefore, vitamin supplements should be added to the diet after the other ingredients have been cooked.

Vitamins

Vitamin A

Vitamin A is a fat-soluble vitamin that is important in vision and maintenance of the skin. Signs of deficiency include decreased vision, skin lesions, and abnormal bone growth. Signs of toxicity include abnormal bone remodeling, lameness, and death. Fish liver oils contain high levels of vitamin A; milk, liver, and egg yolks also contain vitamin A. Dogs can convert carotenoid into vitamin A; however, cats are unable to produce vitamin A and must receive a source of vitamin A in their diet.

Vitamin D

Vitamin D is a fat-soluble vitamin that is required for normal bone growth. Signs of deficiency include bone malformations (rickets) characterized by bowing of the legs, thickening of the joints, and an increased incidence of fractures. Signs of toxicity include teeth abnormalities and bone deposition in soft tissues such as cartilage and muscle. There are few food sources rich in vitamin D; most foods contain very little. Cod liver oil is the most concentrated source; egg yolks, liver, and some fish contain a moderate amount. Dog and cats do not synthesize appreciable vitamin D in their skin with sunlight exposure, thus diets should be supplemented with vitamin D to ensure adequate intake. Vitamin D deficiency resulting in nutritional secondary hyperparathyroidism is one of the most common problems resulting from improperly formulated homemade diets.

Vitamin E

Vitamin E is a fat-soluble vitamin that acts as a biological antioxidant and is required for normal reproduction. A deficiency of vitamin

E can lead to decreased reproductive performance, retinal degeneration, and impairment of the immune system. There is no known toxicity. Food sources rich in vitamin E include wheat germ, corn oil, soybean oil, and sunflower oil. Egg yolk can provide some vitamin E as well.

Vitamin K

Vitamin K is a fat-soluble vitamin that is required for blood clotting. Vitamin K is not added to pet foods because the bacteria present in the intestine can synthesize all the vitamin K that is necessary. Hemorrhage is the major sign of vitamin K deficiency. There is no known toxicity. Foods with a high vitamin K concentration include green, leafy plants such as spinach, kale, cabbage, and cauliflower; liver and eggs are an adequate source. The large intestine bacteria can synthesize vitamin K, but antibiotics can interfere with vitamin K production.

Thiamin (Vitamin B_1)

Thiamin is very important in the functioning of the nervous system. Deficiencies are typically caused by a diet of raw fish, which contains thiaminase. Signs of deficiency include incoordination, weakness, and seizures. There is no known toxicity. Foods rich in thiamin include pork, beef, liver, wheat germ, whole grains, and legumes.

Riboflavin (Vitamin B_2)

Riboflavin is important in many enzyme reactions in metabolism. Signs of deficiency include decreased reproductive performance, dry skin, weakness, and anemia. There is no known toxicity. Foods rich in riboflavin include milk, kidney, liver, whole grains, and vegetables.

Pyridoxine (Vitamin B_6)

Pyridoxine is important in the formation of blood and in protein metabolism. Signs of deficiency include anemia and seizures. There is no known toxicity. Foods rich in pyridoxine include liver, kidney, fish, wheat germ, and whole grains.

Vitamin B_{12} (Cobalamin)

Vitamin B_{12} is important in the formation of blood and for synthesis of myelin. Deficiency probably does not occur except as an inherited disorder seen in some giant schnauzers and border collies. Concentrations may be low in some intestinal disorders. There is no known toxicity. Vitamin B$_{12}$ is found only in animal products, including meat, poultry, fish, and dairy products.

Vitamin C
Vitamin C is not required in the diet of dogs and cats because it is synthesized in the liver. Vitamin C is required in the diet of guinea pigs, primates (including humans), and a few other species. Vitamin C is important in collagen synthesis and in many other metabolic reactions, including proper functioning of the immune system. Signs of deficiency include impaired wound healing, greater susceptibility to infection (decreased immune function), and muscle and joint pain. There is no known toxicity.

Biotin
Biotin is necessary for protein and fatty acid metabolism. Signs of deficiency are rare, but may occur if a high quantity of raw egg whites (which contain avidin) are fed. Deficiency is not a problem if whole raw or cooked eggs are fed. Signs of deficiency include scaly skin, hair loss, and diarrhea. There is no known toxicity. Foods rich in biotin include eggs, liver, milk, legumes, and nuts. Antibiotic use can cause an increase in the biotin requirement because this decreases the bacterial population of the large intestine.

Folic Acid (Folate)
Folate is required for many metabolic reactions and the formation of blood. Signs of deficiency include anemia and bone marrow disorders. There is no known toxicity. Foods rich in folate include green, leafy vegetables, liver, and kidney. Folic acid can be synthesized by dogs and cats in the large intestine.

Choline
Choline is important for normal liver function and as a part of cell membranes. Choline can be synthesized by the body. Signs of deficiency include liver disease and prolonged blood-clotting time. An excess choline intake can result in diarrhea. Foods rich in choline include egg yolk, organ meat, legumes, dairy product, and grains.

Pantothenic Acid
Pantothenic acid is important in many enzyme reactions in metabolism. Signs of deficiency include scaly skin, hair loss, poor growth, and diarrhea. There is no known toxicity. Foods rich in pantothenic acid include liver, kidney, egg yolk, dairy products, and legumes.

Niacin

Niacin is important in many enzyme reactions in metabolism. Signs of deficiency include loss of appetite, bad breath, increased salivation, diarrhea, and emaciation. Excess intake results in itching and burning skin. Foods rich in niacin include meat, legumes, and grains. Dogs can synthesize adequate niacin from the amino acid tryptophan; cats, however, cannot synthesize niacin, and it must be supplied in the diet.

Minerals

Calcium

Calcium is important in the formation and maintenance of bones and teeth. Signs of deficiency include lameness, bone demineralization, and an increased incidence of fractures. During lactation, signs include seizures and tetany (eclampsia). Excess intake of calcium results in growth retardation and severe bone and joint abnormalities. The dietary calcium/phosphorus ratio is very important for proper skeletal development. Foods rich in calcium include dairy products and legumes; grains, meat, and organ tissue are very low in calcium.

Phosphorus

Phosphorus is important in the formation and maintenance of bones and teeth. A deficiency of phosphorus is very rare. A sign of deficiency is depraved appetite. Excess phosphorus ingestion usually results from feeding an all-meat diet, which results in a calcium deficiency. As well as signs of calcium deficiency, excess phosphorus promotes kidney damage. Foods rich in phosphorus include fish, meats, poultry, and organ meats.

Potassium

Potassium is important in maintenance of body water, many enzyme reactions, nerve impulses, and proper cardiac functioning. A lack of potassium results in the loss of appetite, weakness, head drooping, incoordination, and paralysis. Toxicity usually does not occur except in renal failure when potassium is not excreted. Excess potassium is toxic to the heart and can lead to death. Dietary sources rich in potassium include meats, poultry, fish, and most vegetables.

Sodium

Sodium is important in maintenance of body water and maintains nerve cells and muscle fibers. Signs of deficiency include a depraved appetite, weight loss, and slow growth. High levels of dietary sodium result in increased urinary excretion of sodium and increased water intake. Toxicity may result when dogs ingest a salt block or eat water-softener salt. Signs include seizures and death. Dietary sources rich in sodium include dairy products, meat, poultry, fish, and egg whites.

Chloride
Chloride is important in maintenance of body water and acid-base balance. Increases or decreases in body chlorine typically only occur in disease states such as prolonged vomiting, renal disease, etc. Foods rich in sodium are also rich in chloride.

Magnesium
Magnesium is important for normal muscle and nerve function. Signs of deficiency include weakness and seizures. Excess magnesium results in diarrhea and has been implicated as a cause of feline lower urinary tract disease. Foods rich in magnesium include whole grains, legumes, and dairy products.

Sulfur
Sulfur is required for the synthesis of chondroitin sulfate found in cartilage, insulin, heparin, and glutathione. It is a constituent of biotin and thiamin and the amino acids cystine and methionine. Sulfate present in the diet is poorly absorbed, but sulfur deficiency has not been demonstrated, most likely because of adequate dietary intake of cystine and methionine.

Iron
Iron is important in the formation of blood cells. Iron deficiency results in anemia and is typically caused by chronic blood loss rather than dietary deficiency. Signs of toxicity include weight loss, loss of appetite, and death. Foods rich in iron include liver, kidney, egg yolk, fish, legumes, and whole grains.

Copper
Copper is needed for iron transport and for the formation of blood cells. Copper deficiency results in anemia. An excess copper intake may result in liver disease. Liver is the richest dietary source of copper.

Manganese
Manganese is important for reproductive function and joint formation. Signs of deficiency include decreased reproductive performance, abortion, stiffness, and bone abnormalities. Excess manganese also

results in decreased reproductive performance. Foods rich in manganese include legumes and whole grains.

Zinc

Zinc is important for normal skin, sense of taste, and immune function. Signs of deficiency include crusty skin lesions, dry hair coat, fading hair color, growth retardation, poor reproductive performance, decreased testicular size, and diarrhea. Excess zinc intake results in vomiting and may cause calcium and copper deficiencies. Meat and eggs provide a highly absorbable source of zinc.

Iodine

Iodine is important for normal thyroid gland function. Signs of deficiency include thyroid disorders, hair loss, and drowsiness. Excess iodine intake also results in thyroid disorders.

Selenium

Selenium is important for normal muscle function. Signs of deficiency include skeletal disorders, weakness, and heart disease. Excess selenium may result in vomiting, weakness, and death. Foods rich in selenium include grains, meat, and fish.

Chromium

Chromium functions to enhance the activity of insulin. Low chromium intake may be associated with the development of diabetes.

Unique Nutritional Needs of Cats

Cats have a number of unique nutritional needs, and their diets must be formulated differently from canine diets. Feline diets must provide proteins containing essential amino acids for which cats have an absolute requirement. Dietary proteins must also provide more nitrogen than for most other animals because they do not conserve nitrogen as well as do other animals. Their enzyme activities for metabolizing amino acids are greater than in other animals, and that activity does not decrease when they eat a low-protein diet. Excess amino acid destruction continues, leaving insufficient amounts for making protein.

Cats need 18%–20% of total calories as protein for growth and 12%–13% for adult maintenance. Thus, cats need two to three times more protein than do most other animals under comparable circumstances. The 18%–20% of total calories for a growing kitten represents about 25% of the dry weight of the diet. Diets formulated for dogs contain inadequate protein for feeding cats.

Cats cannot synthesize the essential amino acid citrulline, which is low in any food; however, cats can convert arginine to citrulline. Therefore, feline diets must contain arginine to meet the need for citrulline. Cats fed a diet lacking arginine develop hyperammonemia and show clinical signs of illness within several hours. Ammonia accumulates because it is not converted to urea; arginine and citrulline are needed for that conversion. Cats have only a limited ability to synthesize the essential amino acid taurine from sulfur-containing amino acids. Therefore, a cat's diet must provide taurine; diets should also be rich in sulfur-containing amino acids. Diets low in protein, and therefore sulfur amino acids, are more likely to induce taurine deficiency.

Taurine is the most abundant free amino acid in the body. It is not incorporated into body proteins. Its many important functions include being a precursor for bile salts (both cats and dogs have an obligatory and continuous requirement for taurine to make bile salts to replace what is lost continuously in the feces). Taurine is also involved in growth and maturation of nervous tissue, maintenance of normal vision, normal heart function, and female reproduction. Taurine is found in all animal tissues, but not in plant materials.

Since taurine is free in animal tissues (not incorporated in proteins), it readily leaches out in water. Cooking meat in water and discarding the water can greatly reduce its taurine content. Proteins from plants such as soybeans and from animal products such as cottage cheese provide no taurine.

Within the last decade, two diseases, dilated cardiomyopathy and central retinal degeneration, appeared in cats fed diets containing insufficient taurine. In only some animals can these problems be reversed with taurine supplementation, so it is important that taurine is adequate in any feline diet.

Cats show low tolerance for the amino acid glutamic acid. Excess amounts cause sporadic vomiting and thiamin deficiency. Glutamic acid is abundant in vegetable proteins and is comparatively low in animal proteins.

Cats also have some unique vitamin needs. Cats do not have the ability to convert carotene to vitamin A. Lacking the enzyme for that conversion makes it necessary for cats to have vitamin A in their diet. Cats also do not have the capacity for converting tryptophan to niacin. Cats metabolize tryptophan too rapidly to other compounds; thus, the diet must provide niacin.

Additional Reading

Case LP, Carey DP, Hirakawa DA, Daristotle L. 2000. *Canine and Feline Nutrition: A Resource for Companion Animal Professionals,* 2nd edition. Mosby, St. Louis.

Gross KL, Wedekind KJ, Cowell CS, Schoenherr WD, Jewell DE, Zicker SC, et al. 2000. Nutrients. In *Small Animal Clinical Nutrition,* 4th edition. Hand MS, Thatcher CD, Remillard RL, Roudebush P (Eds). Mark Morris Institute, Topeka, KS, pp. 21–110.

Huber TL, Wilson RC, McGarity SA. 1986. Variations in digestibility of dry dog foods with identical label guaranteed analysis. J Am Anim Hosp Assoc 22:571–575.

Kallfelz FA. 1989. Evaluation and use of pet foods: General considerations in using pet foods for adult maintenance. Vet Clin North Am Small Anim Pract 19:387–403.

Kerl ME, Johnson PA. 2004. Nutritional plan: Matching diet to disease. Clin Tech in Sm Anim Pract 19(1):9–21.

National Research Council of the National Academies. 2006. *Nutrient Requirements of Dogs and Cats.* The National Academic Press, Washington DC.

CHAPTER 4
Canine and Feline Energy Requirements

All animals require a source of energy. Balance occurs when energy intake matches energy expenditure: a positive balance occurs when intake exceeds expenditure, and a negative balance occurs when expenditure exceeds intake. The resting energy requirement (RER) accounts for most energy expenditure and represents the energy required to sit quietly and maintain homeostasis of the body. Both the body surface area and body weight play a role in determining RER. In addition, muscle activity, stress, heat production to maintain body temperature, and meal digestion require energy and contribute to the energy requirement. The RER accounts for about 60% of daily energy expenditure, with about 30% energy expenditure from muscle activity. Total energy expenditure is impacted by gender, reproductive status, hormonal status, body composition, nutritional status, and age.

Calculating the exact energy requirement for dogs is very difficult because there is such a variety of size among different dog breeds. Energy expenditure is related to body surface area and weight; body surface area as related to body weight decreases as dogs get larger. Thus, there is not a linear relationship between body weight and energy expenditure. Calculating the energy requirements of cats is not as difficult as in dogs because there is not the size variation seen in different breeds of cats. In general, the energy requirement per pound of body weight is greatest for the very small breeds and the lowest for the largest breeds.

Determining Daily Energy Requirements

Energy is commonly expressed in units of calories or kilocalories (kcal). A calorie is the amount of heat energy required to raise the temperature of 1 gram (g) of water from 14.5°Celsius (C) to 15.5°C. This amount of energy is very small, so energy requirements are reported as kilocalories; 1 kcal equals 1000 calories. There is some confusion, as many people refer to kcal as Calories (with a capital C).

There are a number of formulas that have been used to calculate energy requirements for both dogs and cats. No formula is perfect, but linear formulas are the least accurate; with linear formulas, the energy needs of very small animals are underestimated, and they are overestimated for larger animals. One formula that works well for calculating RER is the formula

$$RER = 70 \times (\text{body weight in kilograms})^{0.75}$$

For weight, 1 kilogram (kg) is equivalent to 2.2 lb. To determine body weight in kilograms, take the body weight in pounds and divide by 2.2. With this basic formula, different multiplication factors can be used to estimate the energy needs of dogs and cats with different reproductive states, life stages, and activity levels.

Remember that these energy requirements are estimates and may need to be increased or decreased depending on the individual. Pets should be fed based on the estimated energy requirement and then monitored closely for weight gain or loss. Body condition should also be monitored. Body condition score (BCS) is based on a defined set of criteria so that a somewhat objective measurement of condition can be recorded over time. Body condition scoring can be done on a 5-point or a 9-point scale. With the 5-point BCS scale, BCS 1 represents a very thin animal: the ribs are easily palpable, with no fat cover, and are visible, and there is an exaggerated abdominal tuck. BCS 2 represents an underweight animal: the ribs are easily palpable, with minimal fat cover, and an abdominal tuck is present. BCS 3 represents the ideal body condition: ribs are palpable, with a slight fat cover, but not readily visible, and there is a slight abdominal tuck. BCS 4 represents an overweight animal: ribs are difficult to palpate and are covered by a moderate layer of fat, there is little abdominal tuck present, and the back may appear slightly broadened. BCS 5 represents an obese animal: ribs are very difficult to palpate under a thick fat layer, there is a pendulous ventral bulge, no waist is visible, and the back is markedly broadened.

Daily Energy Requirements for Dogs

■ Adult

The daily energy requirement for adult dogs is based on the resting energy requirement multiplied by a factor that takes into account whether the dog is intact or neutered. Neutering decreases the activity level and thus decreases the daily energy requirement. The daily energy requirements for intact adult dogs can be found in Table 4.1. For intact adult dogs, the daily energy requirement is calculated by the formula DER = 1.8 × RER. The daily energy requirements for neutered adult dogs can be found in Table 4.2. For neutered adult dogs, the daily energy requirement is calculated by the formula DER = 1.6 × RER.

Table 4.1. Daily energy requirements (DER) for intact adult dogs.[a]

BW (lb)	Daily kcal	BW (lb)	Daily kcal	BW (lb)	Daily kcal	BW (lb)	Daily kcal
1	70	53	1370	105	2288	157	3094
2	117	54	1389	106	2304	158	3108
3	159	55	1409	107	2321	159	3123
4	197	56	1428	108	2337	160	3138
5	233	57	1447	109	2353	161	3153
6	267	58	1466	110	2369	162	3167
7	300	59	1485	111	2385	163	3182
8	332	60	1504	112	2401	164	3197
9	362	61	1522	113	2417	165	3211
10	392	62	1541	114	2434	166	3226
11	421	63	1560	115	2449	167	3240
12	450	64	1578	116	2465	168	3255
13	478	65	1597	117	2481	169	3269
14	505	66	1615	118	2497	170	3284
15	532	67	1633	119	2513	171	3298
16	558	68	1652	120	2529	172	3313
17	584	69	16700	121	2545	173	3327
18	610	70	1688	122	2560	174	3342
19	635	71	1706	123	2576	175	3356
20	660	72	1724	124	2592	176	3370

Table 4.1. *(cont.)*

BW (lb)	Daily kcal	BW (lb)	Daily kcal	BW (lb)	Daily kcal	BW (lb)	Daily kcal
21	684	73	1742	125	2608	177	3385
22	709	74	1760	126	2623	178	3399
23	733	75	1778	127	2639	179	3413
24	756	76	1795	128	2654	180	3428
25	780	77	1813	129	2670	181	3442
26	803	78	1831	130	2685	182	3456
27	826	79	1848	131	2701	183	3470
28	849	80	1866	132	2716	184	3485
29	872	81	1883	133	2732	185	3499
30	894	82	1901	134	2747	186	3513
31	916	83	1918	135	2763	187	3527
32	938	84	1935	136	2778	188	3541
33	960	85	1953	137	2793	189	3555
34	982	86	19700	138	2808	190	3570
35	1004	87	1987	139	2824	191	3584
36	1025	88	2004	140	2839	192	3598
37	1046	89	2021	141	2854	193	3612
38	1068	90	2038	142	2869	194	3626
39	1089	91	2055	143	2884	195	3640
40	1109	92	2072	144	2900	196	3654
41	1130	93	2089	145	2915	197	3668
42	1151	94	2106	146	2930	198	3682
43	1171	95	2122	147	2945	199	3696
44	1192	96	2139	148	2960	200	3710
45	1212	97	2156	149	2975	205	3779
46	1232	98	2173	150	2990	210	3848
47	1252	99	2189	151	3005	215	3916
48	1272	100	2206	152	3020	220	3984
49	1292	101	2222	153	3034	225	4052
50	1312	102	2239	154	3049	230	41200
51	1331	103	2255	155	3064	240	4253
52	1351	104	2272	156	3079	250	4385

BW, body weight.
[a]DER = 1.8 × RER (resting energy requirement).

Table 4.2. Daily energy requirements (DER) for neutered adult dogs.[a]

BW (lb)	Daily kcal	BW (lb)	Daily kcal	BW (lb)	Daily kcal	BW (lb)	Daily kcal
1	62	53	1218	105	2034	157	2750
2	104	54	1235	106	2048	158	2763
3	141	55	1252	107	2063	159	2776
4	175	56	1269	108	2077	160	2789
5	207	57	1286	109	2092	161	2802
6	238	58	1303	110	2106	162	2815
7	267	59	1320	111	2120	163	2828
8	295	60	1337	112	2135	164	2841
9	322	61	1353	113	2149	165	2854
10	349	62	1370	114	2163	166	2867
11	374	63	1386	115	2177	167	2880
12	400	64	1403	116	2192	168	2893
13	424	65	1419	117	2206	169	2906
14	449	66	1436	118	2220	170	2919
15	473	67	1452	119	2234	171	2932
16	496	68	1468	120	2248	172	2945
17	519	69	1484	121	2262	173	2958
18	542	70	1500	122	2276	174	2970
19	564	71	1517	123	2290	175	2983
20	586	72	1532	124	2304	176	2996
21	608	73	1548	125	2318	177	3009
22	630	74	1564	126	2332	178	3021
23	651	75	1580	127	2346	179	3034
24	672	76	1596	128	2359	180	3047
25	693	77	1612	129	2373	181	3060
26	714	78	1627	130	2387	182	3072
27	734	79	1643	131	2401	183	3085
28	755	80	1659	132	2415	184	3098
29	775	81	1674	133	2428	185	3110
30	795	82	1690	134	2442	186	3123
31	815	83	1705	135	2456	187	3135
32	834	84	1720	136	2469	188	3148
33	854	85	1736	137	2483	189	3160
34	873	86	1751	138	2496	190	3173

Table 4.2. *(cont.)*

BW (lb)	Daily kcal	BW (lb)	Daily kcal	BW (lb)	Daily kcal	BW (lb)	Daily kcal
35	892	87	1766	139	2510	191	3185
36	911	88	1781	140	2523	192	3198
37	930	89	1797	141	2537	193	3210
38	949	90	1812	142	2550	194	3223
39	968	91	1827	143	2564	195	3235
40	986	92	1842	144	2577	196	3248
41	1005	93	1857	145	2591	197	3260
42	1023	94	1872	146	2604	198	3273
43	1041	95	1887	147	2618	199	3285
44	1059	96	1902	148	2631	200	3297
45	1077	97	1916	149	2644	205	3359
46	1095	98	1931	150	2657	210	3420
47	1113	99	1946	151	2671	215	3481
48	1131	100	1961	152	2684	220	3542
49	1148	101	1975	153	2697	225	3602
50	1166	102	1990	154	2710	230	3662
51	1183	103	2005	155	2724	240	3781
52	1201	104	2019	156	2737	250	3898

BW, body weight.
[a]DER = 1.6 × RER (resting energy requirement).

Weight Loss

For weight loss to occur, energy expenditure must be greater than the energy intake. The daily requirements for adult dogs that need to lose weight can be found in Table 4.3. The daily energy requirement for adult dogs that need to lose weight is calculated by the formula DER = 1.0 × RER.

Moderate and Heavy Work

Activity level has a significant impact on the daily energy requirement. Short bouts of exercise have a minimal impact on daily energy requirement, but dogs that regularly participate in strenuous exercise

Table 4.3. Daily energy requirements (DER) for weight loss in dogs.[a]

BW (lb)	Daily kcal	BW (lb)	Daily kcal	BW (lb)	Daily kcal	BW (lb)	Daily kcal
1	39	53	761	105	1271	157	1719
2	65	54	772	106	1280	158	1727
3	88	55	783	107	1289	159	1735
4	110	56	793	108	1298	160	1743
5	130	57	804	109	1307	161	1751
6	149	58	814	110	1316	162	1760
7	1677	59	825	111	1325	163	1768
8	184	60	835	112	1334	164	1776
9	201	61	846	113	1343	165	1784
10	218	62	856	114	1352	166	1792
11	234	63	867	115	1361	167	1800
12	2500	64	877	116	1370	168	1808
13	265	65	887	117	1379	169	1816
14	280	66	897	118	1387	170	1824
15	295	67	907	119	1396	171	1832
16	310	68	918	120	1405	172	1840
17	324	69	928	121	1414	173	1848
18	339	70	938	122	1422	174	1856
19	353	71	948	123	1431	175	1864
20	366	72	958	124	1440	176	1872
21	380	73	968	125	1449	177	1880
22	394	74	978	126	1457	178	1888
23	407	75	988	127	1466	179	1896
24	420	76	997	128	1475	180	1904
25	433	77	1007	129	1483	181	1912
26	466	78	1017	130	1492	182	1920
27	459	79	1027	131	1500	183	1928
28	472	80	1037	132	1509	184	1936
29	484	81	1046	133	1518	185	1944
30	497	82	1056	134	1526	186	1952
31	509	83	1066	135	1535	187	1960
32	521	84	1075	136	1543	188	1967
33	534	85	1085	137	1552	189	1975
34	546	86	1094	138	1560	190	1983

Table 4.3. *(cont.)*

BW (lb)	Daily kcal	BW (lb)	Daily kcal	BW (lb)	Daily kcal	BW (lb)	Daily kcal
35	558	87	1104	139	1569	191	1991
36	570	88	1113	140	1577	192	1999
37	581	89	1123	141	1586	193	2007
38	593	90	1132	142	1594	194	2014
39	605	91	1142	143	1602	195	2022
40	616	92	1151	144	1611	196	2030
41	628	93	1160	145	1619	197	2038
42	639	94	1170	146	1628	198	2045
43	651	95	1179	147	1636	199	2053
44	662	96	1188	148	1644	200	2061
45	673	97	1198	149	1653	205	2099
46	684	98	1207	150	1661	210	2138
47	696	99	1216	151	1669	215	2176
48	707	100	1225	152	1678	220	2214
49	718	101	1235	153	1686	225	2251
50	729	102	1244	154	1694	230	2289
51	740	103	1253	155	1702	240	2363
52	750	104	1262	156	1711	250	2436

BW, body weight.
[a]DER = 1 × RER (resting energy requirement).

require significantly higher levels of daily energy to meet their energy needs. Dogs that may have increased energy requirements include those that regularly participate in performance events such as agility or flyball or dogs that are routinely used for hunting. The daily energy requirements for adult dogs undergoing moderate work or heavy work can be found in Tables 4.4 and 4.5, respectively. The daily energy requirement for adult dogs undergoing moderate work is calculated by the formula DER = 3 × RER. The daily energy requirement for adult dogs undergoing heavy work is calculated by the formula DER = 4 × RER. Some dogs undergoing very strenuous activity, such as sled dogs in training and racing in long races, may have a daily energy requirement up to eight times the resting energy requirement (DER = 8 × RER).

Table 4.4. Daily energy requirements (DER) for adult dogs undergoing moderate work.[a]

BW (lb)	Daily kcal	BW (lb)	Daily kcal	BW (lb)	Daily kcal	BW (lb)	Daily kcal
1	116	53	2284	105	3813	157	5156
2	196	54	2316	106	3840	158	5181
3	265	55	2348	107	3868	159	5205
4	329	56	2380	108	3895	160	5230
5	389	57	2412	109	3922	161	5254
6	446	58	2443	110	3949	162	5279
7	500	59	2475	111	3976	163	5303
8	553	60	2506	112	4002	164	5328
9	604	61	2537	113	4029	165	5352
10	654	62	2569	114	4056	166	5376
11	702	63	2600	115	4082	167	5401
12	750	64	2630	116	4109	168	5425
13	796	65	2661	117	4136	169	5449
14	841	66	2692	118	4162	170	5473
15	886	67	2722	119	4189	171	5497
16	930	68	2753	120	4215	172	5521
17	973	69	2783	121	4241	173	5545
18	1016	70	2813	122	4267	174	5569
19	1058	71	2843	123	4294	175	5593
20	1099	72	2873	124	4320	176	5617
21	1140	73	2903	125	4346	177	5641
22	1181	74	2933	126	4372	178	5665
23	1221	75	2963	127	4398	179	5689
24	1261	76	2992	128	4424	180	5713
25	1300	77	3022	129	4450	181	5737
26	1339	78	3051	130	4476	182	5760
27	1377	79	3081	131	4501	183	5784
28	1415	80	3110	132	4527	184	5808
29	1453	81	3139	133	4553	185	5832
30	1490	82	3168	134	4579	186	5855
31	1527	83	3197	135	4604	187	5879
32	1564	84	3226	136	4630	188	5902
33	1601	85	3254	137	4655	189	5926

Table 4.4. *(cont.)*

BW (lb)	Daily kcal	BW (lb)	Daily kcal	BW (lb)	Daily kcal	BW (lb)	Daily kcal
34	1637	86	3283	138	4681	190	5949
35	1673	87	3312	139	4706	191	5973
36	1709	88	3340	140	4731	192	5996
37	1744	89	3369	141	4757	193	6020
38	1779	90	3397	142	4782	194	6043
39	1814	91	3425	143	4807	195	6066
40	1849	92	3453	144	4833	196	6090
41	1884	93	3481	145	4858	197	6113
42	1918	94	3510	146	4883	198	6136
43	1952	95	3537	147	4908	199	6159
44	1986	96	3565	148	4933	200	6183
45	2020	97	3593	149	4958	205	6298
46	2053	98	3621	150	4983	210	6413
47	2087	99	3649	151	5008	215	6527
48	2120	100	3676	152	5003	220	6641
49	2153	101	3704	153	5057	225	6754
50	2186	102	3731	154	5082	230	6866
51	2219	103	3759	155	5107	240	7089
52	2251	104	3786	156	5132	250	7309

BW, body weight.
[a]DER = 3 × RER (resting energy requirement).

Table 4.5. Daily energy requirements (DER) for adult dogs undergoing heavy work.[a]

BW (lb)	Daily kcal	BW (lb)	Daily kcal	BW (lb)	Daily kcal	BW (lb)	Daily kcal
1	155	53	3045	105	5084	157	6875
2	261	54	3088	106	5121	158	6908
3	353	55	3130	107	5157	159	6940
4	438	56	3173	108	5193	160	6973
5	518	57	3215	109	5229	161	7006
6	594	58	3258	110	5265	162	7038
7	667	59	3300	111	5301	163	7071
8	737	60	3342	112	5336	164	7104
9	805	61	3383	113	5372	165	7136

Table 4.5. *(cont.)*

BW (lb)	Daily kcal	BW (lb)	Daily kcal	BW (lb)	Daily kcal	BW (lb)	Daily kcal
10	872	62	3425	114	5408	166	7168
11	936	63	3466	115	5443	167	7201
12	999	64	3507	116	5479	168	7233
13	1061	65	3548	117	5514	169	7265
14	1122	66	3589	118	5549	170	7298
15	1181	67	3630	119	5585	171	7330
16	1240	68	3670	120	5620	172	7362
17	1298	69	3711	121	5655	173	7394
18	1355	70	3751	122	5690	174	7426
19	1411	71	3791	123	5725	175	7458
20	1466	72	3831	124	5760	176	7490
21	1521	73	3871	125	5795	177	7522
22	1575	74	3911	126	5829	178	7554
23	1628	75	3950	127	5864	179	7585
24	1681	76	3990	128	5899	180	7617
25	1733	77	4029	129	5933	181	7649
26	1785	78	4068	130	5968	182	7681
27	1836	79	4107	131	6002	183	7712
28	1887	80	4146	132	6036	184	7744
29	1937	81	4185	133	6071	185	7775
30	1987	82	4224	134	6105	186	7807
31	2036	83	4262	135	6139	187	7838
32	2085	84	4301	136	6173	188	7870
33	2134	85	4339	137	6207	189	7901
34	2182	86	4377	138	6241	190	7932
35	2230	87	4416	139	6275	191	7964
36	2278	88	4454	140	6309	192	7995
37	2325	89	4491	141	6342	193	8026
38	2372	90	4529	142	6376	194	8057
39	2419	91	4567	143	6410	195	8088
40	2465	92	4604	144	6443	196	8120
41	2511	93	4642	145	6477	197	8151
42	2557	94	4679	146	6510	198	8182
43	2603	95	4717	147	6544	199	8213

Table 4.5. (cont.)

BW (lb)	Daily kcal	BW (lb)	Daily kcal	BW (lb)	Daily kcal	BW (lb)	Daily kcal
44	2648	96	4754	148	6577	200	8244
45	2693	97	4791	149	6610	205	8398
46	2738	98	4828	150	6644	210	8551
47	2782	99	4865	151	6677	215	8703
48	2827	100	4902	152	6710	220	8854
49	2871	101	4938	153	6743	225	9005
50	2915	102	4975	154	6776	230	9155
51	2958	103	5012	155	6809	240	9451
52	3002	104	5048	156	6842	250	9745

BW, body weight.
[a]DER = 4 × RER (resting energy requirement).

■ Growth

Growing puppies require more daily energy than do adult dogs to support bone, muscle, and tissue growth. Puppies who weigh up to about 50% of their adult body weight have the highest energy requirement, as a considerable amount of growth is occurring during this period. The daily energy requirement for puppies up to 50% of their adult body weight is calculated by the formula DER = 3 × RER. As puppies get older, the rate of growth slows, and the daily energy requirement starts to decrease. The daily energy requirement for puppies that are 50%–80% of their adult body weight is calculated by the formula DER = 2.5 × RER. Older puppies are still growing, but at a much slower rate. The daily energy requirement for puppies that are 80%–100% of their adult body weight is calculated by the formula DER = 2 × RER. The daily energy requirements for puppies up to 50% of their adult body weight, for puppies 50%–80% of their adult body weight, and for puppies 80%–100% of their adult body weight can be found in Tables 4.6, 4.7, and 4.8, respectively.

For growing puppies, it is important to evaluate body condition on a weekly basis and to adjust dietary energy intake accordingly. Energy intake should be moderated, especially in puppies of large breeds. Maximal growth is not necessarily optimal growth. Rapid growth leads to abnormal skeletal development. A slower growth rate reduces

Table 4.6. Daily energy requirements (DER) for puppies up to 50% of their adult weight (about 5 months of age).[a]

BW (lb)	Daily kcal	BW (lb)	Daily kcal	BW (lb)	Daily kcal	BW (lb)	Daily kcal
1	116	53	2284	105	3813	157	5156
2	196	54	2316	106	3840	158	5181
3	265	55	2348	107	3868	159	5205
4	329	56	2380	108	3895	160	5230
5	389	57	2412	109	3922	161	5254
6	446	58	2443	110	3949	162	5279
7	500	59	2475	111	3976	163	5303
8	553	60	2506	112	4002	164	5328
9	604	61	2537	113	4029	165	5352
10	654	62	2569	114	4056	166	5376
11	702	63	2600	115	4082	167	5401
12	750	64	2630	116	4109	168	5425
13	796	65	2661	117	4136	169	5449
14	841	66	2692	118	4162	170	5473
15	886	67	2722	119	4189	171	5497
16	930	68	2753	120	4215	172	5521
17	973	69	2783	121	4241	173	5545
18	1016	70	2813	122	4267	174	5569
19	1058	71	2843	123	4294	175	5593
20	1099	72	2873	124	4320	176	5617
21	1140	73	2903	125	4346	177	5641
22	1181	74	2933	126	4372	178	5665
23	1221	75	2963	127	4398	179	5689
24	1261	76	2992	128	4424	180	5713
25	1300	77	3022	129	4450	181	5737
26	1339	78	3051	130	4476	182	5760
27	1377	79	3081	131	4501	183	5784
28	1415	80	3110	132	4527	184	5808
29	1453	81	3139	133	4553	185	5832
30	1490	82	3168	134	4579	186	5855
31	1527	83	3197	135	4604	187	5879
32	1564	84	3226	136	4630	188	5902
33	1601	85	3254	137	4655	189	5926

Table 4.6. *(cont.)*

BW (lb)	Daily kcal	BW (lb)	Daily kcal	BW (lb)	Daily kcal	BW (lb)	Daily kcal
34	1637	86	3283	138	4681	190	5949
35	1673	87	3312	139	4706	191	5973
36	1709	88	3340	140	4731	192	5996
37	1744	89	3369	141	4757	193	6020
38	1779	90	3397	142	4782	194	6043
39	1814	91	3425	143	4807	195	6066
40	1849	92	3453	144	4833	196	6090
41	1884	93	3481	145	4858	197	6114
42	1918	94	3510	146	4883	198	6136
43	1952	95	3537	147	4908	199	6159
44	1986	96	3565	148	4933	200	6183
45	2020	97	3593	149	4958	205	6298
46	2053	98	3621	150	4983	210	6413
47	2087	99	3649	151	5008	215	6527
48	2120	100	3676	152	5033	220	6641
49	2153	101	3704	153	5057	225	6754
50	2186	102	3731	154	5082	230	6866
51	2219	103	3759	155	5107	240	7089
52	2251	104	3786	156	5132	250	7309

BW, body weight.
[a]DER = 3 × RER (resting energy requirement).

Table 4.7. Daily energy requirement (DER) for puppies at 50%–80% of their adult weight.[a]

BW (lb)	Daily kcal	BW (lb)	Daily kcal	BW (lb)	Daily kcal	BW (lb)	Daily kcal
1	97	53	1903	105	3178	157	4297
2	163	54	1930	106	3200	158	4317
3	221	55	1957	107	3223	159	4338
4	274	56	1983	108	3246	160	4358
5	324	57	2010	109	3268	161	4379
6	371	58	2036	110	3291	162	4399
7	417	59	2062	111	3313	163	4419
8	461	60	2088	112	3335	164	4440

Table 4.7. *(cont.)*

BW (lb)	Daily kcal	BW (lb)	Daily kcal	BW (lb)	Daily kcal	BW (lb)	Daily kcal
9	503	61	2115	113	3358	165	4460
10	545	62	2140	114	3380	166	4480
11	585	63	2166	115	3402	167	4500
12	625	64	2192	116	3424	168	4521
13	663	65	2218	117	3446	169	4541
14	701	66	2243	118	3468	170	4561
15	738	67	2269	119	3490	171	4581
16	775	68	2294	120	3512	172	4601
17	811	69	2319	121	3534	173	4621
18	847	70	2344	122	3556	174	4641
19	882	71	2370	123	3578	175	4661
20	916	72	2395	124	3600	176	4681
21	950	73	2419	125	3622	177	4701
22	984	74	2444	126	3643	178	4721
23	1017	75	2469	127	3665	179	4741
24	1050	76	2494	128	3687	180	4761
25	1083	77	2518	129	3708	181	4781
26	1115	78	2543	130	3730	182	4800
27	1147	79	2567	131	3751	183	4820
28	1179	80	2591	132	3773	184	4840
29	1211	81	2616	133	3794	185	4860
30	1242	82	2640	134	3815	186	4879
31	1273	83	2664	135	3837	187	4899
32	1303	84	2688	136	3858	188	4919
33	1334	85	2712	137	3879	189	4938
34	1364	86	2736	138	3901	190	4958
35	1394	87	2760	139	3922	191	4977
36	1424	88	2783	140	3943	192	4997
37	1453	89	2807	141	3964	193	5016
38	1483	90	2831	142	3985	194	5036
39	1512	91	2854	143	4006	195	5055
40	1541	92	2878	144	4027	196	5075
41	1570	93	2901	145	4048	197	5094
42	1598	94	2925	146	4069	198	5114

Table 4.7. *(cont.)*

BW (lb)	Daily kcal	BW (lb)	Daily kcal	BW (lb)	Daily kcal	BW (lb)	Daily kcal
43	1627	95	2948	147	4090	199	5133
44	1655	96	2971	148	4111	200	5152
45	1683	97	2994	149	4132	205	5249
46	1711	98	3017	150	4152	210	5344
47	1739	99	3041	151	4173	215	5439
48	1767	100	3064	152	4194	220	5534
49	1794	101	3086	153	4214	225	5628
50	1822	102	3109	154	4235	230	5722
51	1849	103	3132	155	4256	240	5907
52	1876	104	3155	156	4276	250	6091

BW, body weight.
[a]DER = 2.5 × RER (resting energy requirement).

Table 4.8. Daily energy requirements (DER) for puppies 80%–100% of their adult weight.[a]

BW (lb)	Daily kcal	BW (lb)	Daily kcal	BW (lb)	Daily kcal	BW (lb)	Daily kcal
1	78	53	1522	105	2542	157	3437
2	130	54	1544	106	2560	158	3454
3	177	55	1565	107	2578	159	3470
4	219	56	1587	108	2596	160	3487
5	259	57	1608	109	2614	161	3503
6	297	58	1629	110	2632	162	3519
7	334	59	1650	111	2650	163	3536
8	369	60	1671	112	2668	164	3552
9	403	61	1692	113	2686	165	3568
10	436	62	1712	114	2704	166	3584
11	468	63	1733	115	2722	167	3600
12	500	64	1754	116	2739	168	3617
13	531	65	1774	117	2757	169	3633
14	561	66	1795	118	2775	170	3649
15	591	67	1815	119	2792	171	3665
16	620	68	1835	120	2810	172	3681
17	649	69	1855	121	2827	173	3697
18	677	70	1876	122	2845	174	3713
19	705	71	1896	123	2862	175	3729

Table 4.8. *(cont.)*

BW (lb)	Daily kcal	BW (lb)	Daily kcal	BW (lb)	Daily kcal	BW (lb)	Daily kcal
20	733	72	1916	124	2880	176	3745
21	760	73	1936	125	2897	177	3761
22	787	74	1955	126	2915	178	3777
23	814	75	1975	127	2932	179	3793
24	840	76	1995	128	2949	180	3809
25	866	77	2015	129	2967	181	3824
26	892	78	2034	130	2984	182	3840
27	918	79	2054	131	3001	183	3856
28	943	80	2073	132	3018	184	3872
29	969	81	2093	133	3035	185	3888
30	993	82	2112	134	3052	186	3903
31	1018	83	2131	135	3069	187	3919
32	1043	84	2150	136	3086	188	3935
33	1067	85	2170	137	3103	189	3951
34	1091	86	2189	138	3120	190	3966
35	1115	87	2208	139	3137	191	3982
36	1139	88	2227	140	3154	192	3997
37	1163	89	2246	141	3171	193	4013
38	1186	90	2265	142	3188	194	4029
39	1210	91	2283	143	3205	195	4044
40	1233	92	2302	144	3222	196	4060
41	1256	93	2321	145	3238	197	4075
42	1279	94	2340	146	3255	198	4091
43	1301	95	2358	147	3272	199	4106
44	1324	96	2377	148	3289	200	4122
45	1347	97	2395	149	3305	205	4199
46	1369	98	2414	150	3322	210	4275
47	1391	99	2432	151	3338	215	4352
48	1413	100	2451	152	3355	220	4427
49	1435	101	2469	153	3372	225	4502
50	1457	102	2487	154	3388	230	4577
51	1479	103	2506	155	3405	240	4726
52	1501	104	2524	156	3421	250	4873

BW, body weight.
[a]DER = 2 × RER (resting energy requirement).

the incidence of abnormalities and does not affect the ability of the puppy to attain its normal adult size. The goal of feeding is to provide all the essential nutrients while keeping the growing puppy "lean." Puppies should look trim, with only a slight layer of fat over the ribs. The puppy is too fat if the ribs cannot be felt with gentle pressure on the rib cage. The puppy is too thin if the ribs can be seen easily when the puppy moves.

■ Senior Dogs

It can be difficult to determine the energy needs of the senior pet. Dogs are considered to be senior when they have reached half their life expectancy; thus, most are considered to be senior at about 7 years of age. The daily energy requirement of a senior dog is very dependent on body condition, activity level, reproductive status, and the presence of underlying medical conditions. Many senior dogs are still very active in performance events, and some females may still be reproducing; thus, these seniors will have increased energy requirements. However, senior dogs are more prone to obesity and thus would require a lower daily energy requirement. As dogs get very old, the daily energy requirement may be higher because of decreased digestion of nutrients and underlying medical conditions.

For the healthy adult senior dog over 7 years of age with reduced activity level, the daily energy requirement should be decreased to avoid the occurrence of obesity. The daily energy requirement in this case is calculated by the formula DER = 1.1 × RER and can be found in Table 4.9. For older dogs that do not digest nutrients well or that have underlying medical conditions, the daily energy requirement could be similar to that for an intact adult dog (Table 4.1). Senior dogs must be monitored closely for body weight and body condition, with adjustment of daily energy intake as needed.

■ Gestation

Daily energy needs increase during gestation, and those needs are dependent on the prior nutritional status of the bitch, size of the bitch, and the number of fetuses carried by the bitch. During the first 5 to 6 weeks, most dogs do not require additional energy, although in about the sixth week of gestation the amount of energy fed could be increased. The daily energy requirement increases during the last few weeks of gestation, while the fetuses are rapidly growing. The daily energy requirement for the early weeks of gestation is calculated by the

Table 4.9. Daily energy requirement (DER) for healthy, inactive senior dogs.[a]

BW (lb)	Daily kcal	BW (lb)	Daily kcal	BW (lb)	Daily kcal	BW (lb)	Daily kcal
1	43	53	837	105	1398	157	1891
2	72	54	849	106	1408	158	1900
3	97	55	861	107	1418	159	1909
4	121	56	873	108	1428	160	1918
5	143	57	884	109	1438	161	1927
6	163	58	896	110	1448	162	1936
7	183	59	907	111	1458	163	1945
8	203	60	919	112	1468	164	1953
9	221	61	930	113	1477	165	1962
10	240	62	942	114	1487	166	1971
11	257	63	953	115	1497	167	1980
12	275	64	965	116	1507	168	1989
13	292	65	976	117	1516	169	1998
14	309	66	987	118	1526	170	2007
15	325	67	998	119	1536	171	2016
16	341	68	1009	120	1545	172	2025
17	357	69	1020	121	1555	173	2033
18	373	70	1032	122	1565	174	2042
19	388	71	1043	123	1574	175	2051
20	403	72	1054	124	1584	176	2060
21	418	73	1065	125	1594	177	2068
22	433	74	1075	126	1603	178	2077
23	448	75	1086	127	1613	179	2086
24	462	76	1097	128	1622	180	2095
25	477	77	1108	129	1632	181	2103
26	491	78	1119	130	1641	182	2112
27	505	79	1130	131	1651	183	2121
28	519	80	1140	132	1660	184	2130
29	533	81	1151	133	1669	185	2138
30	546	82	1162	134	1679	186	2147
31	560	83	1172	135	1688	187	2156
32	574	84	1183	136	1698	188	2164
33	587	85	1193	137	1707	189	2173

Table 4.9. *(cont.)*

BW (lb)	Daily kcal	BW (lb)	Daily kcal	BW (lb)	Daily kcal	BW (lb)	Daily kcal
34	600	86	1204	138	1716	190	2181
35	613	87	1214	139	1726	191	2190
36	626	88	1225	140	1735	192	2199
37	639	89	1235	141	1744	193	2207
38	652	90	1246	142	1753	194	2216
39	665	91	1256	143	1763	195	2224
40	678	92	1266	144	1772	196	2233
41	691	93	1277	145	1781	197	2241
42	703	94	1287	146	1790	198	2250
43	716	95	1297	147	1800	199	2258
44	728	96	1307	148	1809	200	2267
45	741	97	1318	149	1818	205	2309
46	753	98	1328	150	1827	210	2351
47	765	99	1338	151	1836	215	2393
48	777	100	1348	152	1845	220	2435
49	789	101	1358	153	1854	225	2476
50	801	102	1368	154	1863	230	2518
51	813	103	1378	155	1873	240	2599
52	825	104	1388	156	1882	250	2680

BW, body weight.
[a]DER = 1.1 × RER (resting energy requirement).

formula DER = 1.8 × RER. The daily energy requirement for the last weeks of gestation is calculated by the formula DER = 3 × RER. Daily energy requirements for early and late gestation in dogs are found in Tables 4.10 and 4.11, respectively.

■ Lactation

Milk production places the largest nutritional demands on the dam. She must metabolize very large amounts of nutrients in order to produce sufficient milk to support the growth of her puppies. Dams with a large litter may require four times more calories during lactation than they needed for maintenance. Peak milk production occurs when the puppies are 4–5 weeks of age, right before they are weaned. The daily energy requirement for lactation for dams nursing up to four

Table 4.10. Daily energy requirement (DER) for dogs in the first 6 weeks of gestation.[a]

BW (lb)	Daily kcal	BW (lb)	Daily kcal	BW (lb)	Daily kcal	BW (lb)	Daily kcal
1	70	53	1370	105	2288	157	3094
2	117	54	1389	106	2304	158	3108
3	159	55	1409	107	2321	159	3123
4	197	56	1428	108	2337	160	3138
5	233	57	1447	109	2353	161	3153
6	267	58	1466	110	2369	162	3167
7	300	59	1485	111	2385	163	3182
8	332	60	1504	112	2401	164	3197
9	362	61	1522	113	2417	165	3211
10	392	62	1541	114	2434	166	3226
11	421	63	1560	115	2449	167	3240
12	450	64	1578	116	2465	168	3255
13	478	65	1597	117	2481	169	3269
14	505	66	1615	118	2497	170	3284
15	532	67	1633	119	2513	171	3298
16	558	68	1652	120	2529	172	3313
17	584	69	1670	121	2545	173	3327
18	610	70	1688	122	2560	174	3342
19	635	71	1706	123	2576	175	3356
20	660	72	1724	124	2592	176	3370
21	684	73	1742	125	2608	177	3385
22	709	74	1760	126	2623	178	3399
23	733	75	1778	127	2639	179	3413
24	756	76	1795	128	2654	180	3428
25	780	77	1813	129	2670	181	3442
26	803	78	1831	130	2685	182	3456
27	826	79	1848	131	2701	183	3470
28	849	80	1866	132	2716	184	3485
29	872	81	1883	133	2732	185	3499
30	894	82	1901	134	2747	186	3513
31	916	83	1918	135	2763	187	3527
32	938	84	1935	136	2778	188	3541
33	960	85	1953	137	2793	189	3555

Table 4.10. *(cont.)*

BW (lb)	Daily kcal	BW (lb)	Daily kcal	BW (lb)	Daily kcal	BW (lb)	Daily kcal
34	982	86	1970	138	2808	190	3570
35	1004	87	1987	139	2824	191	3584
36	1025	88	2004	140	2839	192	3598
37	1046	89	2021	141	2854	193	3612
38	1068	90	2038	142	2869	194	3626
39	1089	91	2055	143	2884	195	3640
40	1109	92	2072	144	2900	196	3654
41	1130	93	2089	145	2915	197	3668
42	1151	94	2106	146	2930	198	3682
43	1171	95	2122	147	2945	199	3696
44	1192	96	2139	148	2960	200	3710
45	1212	97	2156	149	2975	205	3779
46	1232	98	2173	150	2990	210	3848
47	1252	99	2189	151	3005	215	3916
48	1272	100	2206	152	3020	220	3984
49	1292	101	2222	153	3034	225	4052
50	1312	102	2239	154	3049	230	4120
51	1331	103	2255	155	3064	240	4253
52	1351	104	2272	156	3079	250	4385

BW, body weight.
[a]DER = 1.8 × RER (resting energy requirement).

Table 4.11. Daily energy requirement (DER) for dogs in the last 3 weeks of gestation.[a]

BW (lb)	Daily kcal	BW (lb)	Daily kcal	BW (lb)	Daily kcal	BW (lb)	Daily kcal
1	116	53	2284	105	3813	157	5156
2	196	54	2316	106	38400	158	5181
3	265	55	2348	107	3868	159	5205
4	329	56	2380	108	3895	160	5230
5	389	57	2412	109	3922	161	5254
6	446	58	2443	110	3949	162	5279
7	500	59	2475	111	3976	163	5303
8	553	60	2506	112	4002	164	5328
9	604	61	2537	113	4029	165	5352

Table 4.11. *(cont.)*

BW (lb)	Daily kcal	BW (lb)	Daily kcal	BW (lb)	Daily kcal	BW (lb)	Daily kcal
10	654	62	2569	114	4056	166	5376
11	702	63	2600	115	4082	167	5401
12	750	64	2630	116	4109	168	5425
13	796	65	2661	117	4136	169	5449
14	841	66	2692	118	4162	170	5473
15	886	67	2722	119	4189	171	5497
16	930	68	2753	120	4215	172	5521
17	973	69	2783	121	4241	173	5545
18	1016	70	2813	122	4267	174	5569
19	1058	71	2843	123	4294	175	5593
20	1099	72	2873	124	4320	176	5617
21	11400	73	2903	125	4346	177	5641
22	1181	74	2933	126	4372	178	5665
23	1221	75	2963	127	4398	179	5689
24	1261	76	2992	128	4424	180	5713
25	1300	77	3022	129	4450	181	5737
26	1339	78	3051	130	4476	182	5760
27	1377	79	3081	131	4501	183	5784
28	1415	80	3110	132	4527	184	5808
29	1453	81	3139	133	4553	185	5832
30	1490	82	3168	134	4579	186	5855
31	1527	83	3197	135	4604	187	5879
32	1564	84	3226	136	4630	188	5902
33	1601	85	3254	137	4655	189	5926
34	1637	86	3283	138	4681	190	5949
35	1673	87	3312	139	4706	191	5973
36	1709	88	3340	140	4731	192	5996
37	1744	89	3369	141	4757	193	6020
38	1779	90	3397	142	4782	194	6043
39	1814	91	3425	143	4807	195	6066
40	1849	92	3453	144	4833	196	6090
41	1884	93	3481	145	4858	197	6113
42	1918	94	3510	146	4883	198	6136
43	1952	95	3537	147	4908	199	6159

Table 4.11. *(cont.)*

BW (lb)	Daily kcal	BW (lb)	Daily kcal	BW (lb)	Daily kcal	BW (lb)	Daily kcal
44	1986	96	3565	148	4933	200	6183
45	2020	97	3593	149	4958	205	6298
46	2053	98	3621	150	4983	210	6413
47	2087	99	3649	151	5008	215	6527
48	2120	100	3676	152	5033	220	6641
49	2153	101	3704	153	5057	225	6754
50	2186	102	3731	154	5082	230	6866
51	2219	103	3759	155	5107	240	7089
52	2251	104	3786	156	5132	250	7309

BW, body weight.
[a]DER = 3 × RER (resting energy requirement).

puppies is calculated by the formula DER = 4 × RER. The daily energy requirement for lactation for dams nursing more than four puppies is calculated by the formula DER = 6 × RER. If dams have very large litters, the daily energy requirement may be as high as eight times RER. Daily energy requirements for dogs during lactation are found in Tables 4.12 and 4.13.

Daily Energy Requirements for Cats

■ Adult

The daily energy requirement for adult cats is based on the resting energy requirement multiplied by a factor that takes into account whether the cat is intact, neutered, or breeding. Neutering decreases the activity level and thus decreases the daily energy requirement. The daily energy requirements for intact adult cats can be found in Table 4.14. For intact adult cats, the daily energy requirement is calculated by the formula DER = 1.4 × RER. The daily energy requirements for neutered adult cats can be found in Table 4.15. For neutered adult cats, the daily energy requirement is calculated by the formula DER = 1.2 × RER. Actively breeding male and female cats have a slightly higher daily energy requirement, and the daily energy requirement is calculated by the formula DER = 1.6 × RER. The daily energy requirement for breeding females and males can be found in Table 4.16.

Table 4.12. Daily energy requirement (DER) for lactating dogs with up to four puppies.[a]

BW (lb)	Daily kcal	BW (lb)	Daily kcal	BW (lb)	Daily kcal	BW (lb)	Daily kcal
1	155	53	3045	105	5084	157	6875
2	261	54	3088	106	5121	158	6908
3	353	55	3130	107	5157	159	6940
4	438	56	3173	108	5193	160	6973
5	518	57	3215	109	5229	161	7006
6	594	58	3258	110	5265	162	7038
7	667	59	3300	111	5301	163	7071
8	737	60	3342	112	5336	164	7104
9	805	61	3383	113	5372	165	7136
10	872	62	3425	114	5408	166	7168
11	936	63	3466	115	5443	167	7201
12	999	64	3507	116	5479	168	7233
13	1061	65	3548	117	5514	169	7265
14	1122	66	3589	118	5549	170	7298
15	1181	67	3630	119	5585	171	7330
16	1240	68	3670	120	5620	172	7362
17	1298	69	3711	121	5655	173	7394
18	1355	70	3751	122	5690	174	7426
19	1411	71	3791	123	5725	175	7458
20	1466	72	3831	124	5760	176	7490
21	1521	73	3871	125	5795	177	7522
22	1575	74	3911	126	5829	178	7554
23	1628	75	3950	127	5864	179	7585
24	1681	76	3990	128	5899	180	7617
25	1733	77	4029	129	5933	181	7649
26	1785	78	4068	130	5968	182	7681
27	1836	79	4107	131	6002	183	7712
28	1887	80	4146	132	6036	184	7744
29	1937	81	4185	133	6071	185	7775
30	1987	82	4224	134	6105	186	7807
31	2036	83	4262	135	6139	187	7838
32	2085	84	4301	136	6173	188	7870
33	2134	85	4339	137	6207	189	7901

Table 4.12. *(cont.)*

BW (lb)	Daily kcal	BW (lb)	Daily kcal	BW (lb)	Daily kcal	BW (lb)	Daily kcal
34	2182	86	4377	138	6241	190	7932
35	2230	87	4416	139	6275	191	7964
36	2278	88	4454	140	6309	192	7995
37	2325	89	4491	141	6342	193	8026
38	2372	90	4529	142	6376	194	8057
39	2419	91	4567	143	6410	195	8088
40	2465	92	4604	144	6443	196	8120
41	2511	93	4642	145	6477	197	8151
42	2557	94	4679	146	65100	198	8182
43	2603	95	4717	147	6544	199	8213
44	2648	96	4754	148	6577	200	8244
45	2693	97	4791	149	6610	205	8398
46	2738	98	4828	150	6644	210	8551
47	2782	99	4865	151	6677	215	8703
48	2827	100	4902	152	6710	220	8854
49	2871	101	4938	153	6743	225	9005
50	2915	102	4975	154	6776	230	9155
51	2958	103	5012	155	6809	240	9451
52	3002	104	5048	156	6842	250	9745

BW, body weight.
[a]DER = 4 × RER (resting energy requirement).

Table 4.13. Daily energy requirement (DER) for lactating dogs with more than four puppies.[a]

BW (lb)	Daily kcal	BW (lb)	Daily kcal	BW (lb)	Daily kcal	BW (lb)	Daily kcal
1	233	53	4567	105	7626	157	10312
2	391	54	4632	106	7681	158	10362
3	530	55	4696	107	7735	159	10411
4	656	56	4760	108	7789	160	10460
5	777	57	4823	109	7843	161	10509
6	891	58	4887	110	7897	162	10558
7	1001	59	4950	111	7951	163	10607
8	1106	60	5012	112	8005	164	10655

Table 4.13. *(cont.)*

BW (lb)	Daily kcal	BW (lb)	Daily kcal	BW (lb)	Daily kcal	BW (lb)	Daily kcal
9	1208	61	5075	113	8058	165	10704
10	1307	62	5137	114	8112	166	10753
11	1404	63	5199	115	8165	167	10801
12	1499	64	5261	116	8218	168	10850
13	1592	65	5323	117	8271	169	10898
14	1683	66	5384	118	8324	170	10946
15	1772	67	5445	119	8377	171	10995
16	1860	68	5506	120	8430	172	11043
17	1947	69	5566	121	8482	173	11091
18	2032	70	5627	122	8535	174	11139
19	2116	71	5687	123	8587	175	11187
20	2199	72	5747	124	8640	176	11235
21	2281	73	5807	125	8692	177	11283
22	2362	74	5866	126	8744	178	11330
23	2442	75	5926	127	8796	179	11378
24	2521	76	5985	128	8848	180	11426
25	2600	77	6044	129	8900	181	11473
26	2677	78	6102	130	8951	182	11521
27	2754	79	6161	131	9003	183	11568
28	2830	80	6219	132	9054	184	11616
29	2906	81	6278	133	9106	185	11663
30	2980	82	6336	134	9157	186	11710
31	3055	83	6394	135	9208	187	11757
32	3128	84	6451	136	9259	188	11805
33	3201	85	6509	137	9310	189	11852
34	3274	86	6566	138	9361	190	11899
35	3346	87	6623	139	9412	191	11946
36	3417	88	6680	140	9463	192	11992
37	3488	89	6737	141	9514	193	12039
38	3559	90	6794	142	9564	194	12086
39	3629	91	6850	143	9615	195	12133
40	3698	92	6907	144	9665	196	12179
41	3767	93	6963	145	9715	197	12226
42	3836	94	7019	146	9766	198	12272

Table 4.13. *(cont.)*

BW (lb)	Daily kcal	BW (lb)	Daily kcal	BW (lb)	Daily kcal	BW (lb)	Daily kcal
43	3904	95	7075	147	9816	199	12319
44	3972	96	7131	148	9866	200	12365
45	4040	97	7186	149	9916	205	12596
46	4107	98	7242	150	9966	210	12826
47	4174	99	7297	151	10015	215	13055
48	4240	100	7352	152	10065	220	13282
49	4306	101	7408	153	10115	225	13507
50	4372	102	7462	154	10164	230	13732
51	4437	103	7517	155	10214	240	14177
52	4502	104	7572	156	10263	250	14618

BW, body weight.
[a]DER = 6 × RER (resting energy requirement).

Table 4.14. Daily energy requirement (DER) for intact adult cats.[a]

BW (lb)	Daily kcal	BW (lb)	Daily kcal	BW (lb)	Daily kcal	BW (lb)	Daily kcal
1	54	7	233	13	371	19	494
2	91	8	258	14	393	20	513
3	124	9	282	15	414	21	532
4	153	10	305	16	434	22	551
5	181	11	328	17	454	23	570
6	208	12	350	18	474	24	588

BW, body weight.
[a]DER = 1.4 × RER (resting energy requirement).

Table 4.15. Daily energy requirement (DER) for neutered adult cats.[a]

BW (lb)	Daily kcal	BW (lb)	Daily kcal	BW (lb)	Daily kcal	BW (lb)	Daily kcal
1	47	7	200	13	318	19	423
2	78	8	221	14	337	20	440
3	106	9	242	15	354	21	456
4	132	10	262	16	372	22	472
5	155	11	281	17	389	23	488
6	178	12	300	18	406	24	504

BW, body weight.
[a]DER = 1.2 × RER (resting energy requirement).

Table 4.16. Daily energy requirement (DER) for breeding male and female cats.[a]

BW (lb)	Daily kcal	BW (lb)	Daily kcal	BW (lb)	Daily kcal	BW (lb)	Daily kcal
1	62	7	267	13	425	19	564
2	104	8	295	14	449	20	586
3	141	9	322	15	473	21	608
4	175	10	349	16	496	22	630
5	207	11	374	17	519	23	651
6	238	12	400	18	542	24	672

BW, body weight.
[a]DER = 1.6 × RER (resting energy requirement).

Table 4.17. Daily energy requirement (DER) for weight loss in cats.[a]

BW (lb)	Daily kcal	BW (lb)	Daily kcal	BW (lb)	Daily kcal	BW (lb)	Daily kcal
1	39	7	167	13	265	19	353
2	65	8	184	14	280	20	366
3	88	9	201	15	295	21	380
4	110	10	218	16	310	22	394
5	130	11	234	17	324	23	407
6	149	12	250	18	339	24	420

BW, body weight.
[a]DER = 1.0 × RER (resting energy requirement).

■ Weight Loss

For weight loss to occur, energy expenditure must be greater than the energy intake. The daily requirements for adult cats that need to lose weight can be found in Table 4.17. The daily energy requirement for adult cats that need to lose weight is calculated by the formula DER = 1.0 × RER.

■ Growth

Growing kittens require more daily energy than do adult cats to support bone, muscle, and tissue growth. Kittens up to 4 months of age have the highest energy requirement, as a considerable amount of growth is occurring during this period. The daily energy requirement for kittens up to 4 months of age is calculated by the formula DER = 4 × RER. As kittens get older, the rate of growth slows, and the daily energy requirement starts to decrease. The daily energy requirement for kittens 4–5 months of age is calculated by the formula DER = 3 × RER. Growth continues until about 12 months of age, but at a slower rate. The daily energy requirement for kittens 6–8 months of age is calculated by the formula DER = 2.5 × RER, and the requirement for kittens 9–12 months of age is calculated by the formula DER = 2 × RER. The daily energy requirements for kittens up to 4 months of age, 4–5 months of age, 6–8 months of age, and 9–12 months of age can be found in Tables 4.18, 4.19, 4.20, and 4.21, respectively.

Table 4.18. Daily energy requirement (DER) for kittens up to 4 months of age.[a]

BW (lb)	Daily kcal	BW (lb)	Daily kcal	BW (lb)	Daily kcal	BW (lb)	Daily kcal
1	155	7	667	13	1061	19	1411
2	261	8	737	14	1122	20	1466
3	353	9	805	15	1181	21	1521
4	438	10	872	16	1240	22	1575
5	518	11	936	17	1298	23	1628
6	594	12	999	18	1355	24	1681

BW, body weight.
[a]DER = 4 × RER (resting energy requirement).

Table 4.19. Daily energy requirement (DER) for kittens 4–5 months of age.[a]

BW (lb)	Daily kcal	BW (lb)	Daily kcal	BW (lb)	Daily kcal	BW (lb)	Daily kcal
1	116	7	500	13	796	19	1058
2	196	8	553	14	841	20	1099
3	265	9	604	15	886	21	1140
4	329	10	654	16	930	22	1181
5	389	11	702	17	973	23	1221
6	446	12	750	18	1016	24	1261

BW, body weight.
[a]DER = 3 × RER (resting energy requirement).

Table 4.20. Daily energy requirement (DER) for kittens 6–8 months of age.[a]

BW (lb)	Daily kcal	BW (lb)	Daily kcal	BW (lb)	Daily kcal	BW (lb)	Daily kcal
1	97	7	417	13	663	19	882
2	163	8	461	14	701	20	916
3	221	9	503	15	738	21	950
4	274	10	545	16	775	22	984
5	324	11	585	17	811	23	1017
6	371	12	625	18	847	24	1050

BW, body weight.
[a]DER = 2.5 × RER (resting energy requirement).

Table 4.21. Daily energy requirement (DER) for kittens 9–12 months of age.[a]

BW (lb)	Daily kcal	BW (lb)	Daily kcal	BW (lb)	Daily kcal	BW (lb)	Daily kcal
1	78	7	334	13	531	19	705
2	130	8	367	14	561	20	733
3	177	9	403	15	591	21	760
4	219	10	436	16	620	22	787
5	259	11	468	17	649	23	814
6	297	12	500	18	677	24	840

BW, body weight.
[a]DER = 2 × RER (resting energy requirement).

■ **Senior Cats**

It can be difficult to determine the energy needs of the senior cat. Cats are considered to be senior when they have reached half their life expectancy; thus, most are considered to be senior at about 7 years of age. The daily energy requirement of a senior cat is dependent on body condition, activity level, reproductive status, and the presence of underlying medical conditions. Senior cats are prone to obesity and thus require a lower daily energy requirement. As cats get very old, the daily energy requirement is actually higher because of a decrease in the ability to digest nutrients and underlying medical conditions.

For the adult senior cat over 7–11 years of age, the daily energy requirement should be decreased to avoid the occurrence of obesity.

Table 4.22. Daily energy requirement (DER) for senior cats 7–11 years of age.[a]

BW (lb)	Daily kcal	BW (lb)	Daily kcal	BW (lb)	Daily kcal	BW (lb)	Daily kcal
1	43	7	183	13	292	19	388
2	72	8	203	14	309	20	403
3	97	9	221	15	325	21	418
4	121	10	240	16	341	22	433
5	143	11	257	17	357	23	448
6	163	12	275	18	373	24	462

BW, body weight.
[a]DER = 1.1 × RER (resting energy requirement).

Table 4.23. Daily energy requirement (DER) for senior cats over 11 years of age.[a]

BW (lb)	Daily kcal	BW (lb)	Daily kcal	BW (lb)	Daily kcal	BW (lb)	Daily kcal
1	54	7	233	13	371	19	494
2	91	8	258	14	393	20	513
3	124	9	282	15	414	21	532
4	153	10	305	16	434	22	551
5	181	11	328	17	454	23	570
6	208	12	350	18	474	24	588

BW, body weight.
[a]DER = 1.4 × RER (resting energy requirement).

The daily energy requirement in this case is calculated by the formula DER = 1.1 × RER and can be found in Table 4.22. For senior cats over 12 years of age, the daily energy requirement is calculated by the formula DER = 1.4 × RER and is found in Table 4.23. Senior cats must be monitored closely for body weight and body condition, with adjustment of daily energy intake as needed.

■ Gestation

Daily energy needs increase during gestation, and those needs are dependent on the prior nutritional status of the female and the number of fetuses she is carrying. During gestation, the daily energy requirement increases gradually; thus, there should be a gradual increase in

Table 4.24. Daily energy requirement (DER) for cats in the final weeks of gestation.[a]

BW (lb)	Daily kcal	BW (lb)	Daily kcal	BW (lb)	Daily kcal	BW (lb)	Daily kcal
1	78	7	334	13	531	19	705
2	130	8	367	14	561	20	733
3	177	9	403	15	591	21	760
4	219	10	436	16	620	22	787
5	259	11	468	17	649	23	814
6	297	12	500	18	677	24	840

BW, body weight.
[a]DER = 2 × RER (resting energy requirement).

Table 4.25. Daily energy requirement (DER) for cats during the first 4 weeks of lactation.[a]

BW (lb)	Daily kcal	BW (lb)	Daily kcal	BW (lb)	Daily kcal	BW (lb)	Daily kcal
1	155	7	667	13	1061	19	1411
2	261	8	737	14	1122	20	1466
3	353	9	805	15	1181	21	1521
4	438	10	872	16	1240	22	1575
5	518	11	936	17	1298	23	1628
6	594	12	999	18	1355	24	1681

BW, body weight.
[a]DER = 4 × RER (resting energy requirement).

the amount of energy fed daily throughout gestation. By the final weeks of gestation, the daily energy requirement is calculated by the formula DER = 2 × RER. Daily energy requirements for late gestation in cats are found in Table 4.24.

■ Lactation

Milk production places the largest nutritional demands on the queen. She must metabolize very large amounts of nutrients in order to produce sufficient milk to support the growth of her kittens. Peak milk production occurs when the kittens are 4–5 weeks of age, right before they are weaned. The daily energy requirement for lactation for queens in the first 4 weeks of lactation is calculated by the formula DER = 4 × RER. The daily energy requirement for queens lactating for

Table 4.26. Daily energy requirement (DER) for cats lactating for longer than 4 weeks.[a]

BW (lb)	Daily kcal	BW (lb)	Daily kcal	BW (lb)	Daily kcal	BW (lb)	Daily kcal
1	233	7	1001	13	1592	19	2116
2	391	8	1106	14	1683	20	2199
3	530	9	1208	15	1772	21	2281
4	656	10	1307	16	1860	22	2362
5	777	11	1404	17	1947	23	2442
6	891	12	1499	18	2032	24	2521

BW, body weight.

[a]DER = 6 × RER (resting energy requirement).

more than 4 weeks is calculated by the formula DER = 6 × RER. Daily energy requirements for cats during lactation are found in Tables 4.25 and 4.26.

Additional Reading

Case LP, Carey DP, Hirakawa DA, Daristotle L. 2000. Energy balance. In *Canine and Feline Nutrition: A Resource for Companion Animal Professionals*, 2nd edition. Case LP, Carey DP, Hirakawa DA, Daristotle L (Eds.). Mosby, St. Louis, pp. 75–88.

Debraekeleer J, Gross KL, Zicker SC. 2000. Normal dogs. In *Small Animal Clinical Nutrition*, 4th edition. Hand MS, Thatcher CD, Remillard RL, Roudebush P (Eds.) Mark Morris Institute, Topeka, KS, pp. 211–260.

Kirk CA, Debraekeleer J, Armstrong PJ. 2000. Normal cats. In *Small Animal Clinical Nutrition*, 4th edition. Hand MS, Thatcher CD, Remillard RL, Roudebush P (Eds.). Mark Morris Institute, Topeka, KS, pp. 291–350.

National Research Council of the National Academies. 2006. *Nutrient Requirements of Dogs and Cats*. The National Academic Press, Washington DC.

Association of American Feed Control Officials. 2008 Official Publication. http://www.aafco.org

Remillard RL, Paragon B-M, Crane SW, Debraekeleer J, Cowell CS. 2000. Making pet foods at home. In *Small Animal Clinical Nutrition*, 4th edition. Hand MS, Thatcher CD, Remillard RL, Roudebush P (Eds.). Mark Morris Institute, Topeka, KS, pp. 163–182.

CHAPTER 5
Feeding the Healthy Adult Dog or Cat

Dogs and cats belong to the order Carnivora. Dogs are omnivores, as their nutritional needs can be met either by meat or plant sources. Cats are true carnivores because their nutritional requirements can only be met using meat sources in combination with plants.

Nutrition of the Dog

A number of factors must be taken into consideration when determining a diet for dogs. Reproductive status, breed activity level, age, stress, and environment all have an impact on nutritional requirements. Neutered dogs require less energy than do intact dogs, and energy needs are increased in pregnant or lactating females. Sedentary or overweight dogs need less energy than a normally active dog, and dogs participating in racing, hunting, or endurance work require more energy. Some breeds, such as Great Danes or Dalmatians, appear to have higher energy requirements, and some very large breeds, such as Newfoundlands, require less energy. Nutritional needs of young, growing dogs are different from those of adults, and older pets may require less energy. Stresses of boarding, event performance, or the presence of other pets in the house may impact the energy requirement. Dogs housed outside in cold temperatures require a higher energy intake. The energy requirements for different life stages and conditions can be found in Chapter 4.

▪ Water

Approximately 56% of an adult dog's body weight (BW) is water. Water deprivation can quickly lead to dehydration, and death can occur. The lack of water leads to death more quickly than a deficiency in any other nutrient, thus water is the most important of all nutrients.

▪ Protein

Proteins are composed of amino acids, and there are many amino acids that are required by the dog (see Chapter 3). Enough protein must be provided in the diet to meet these amino acid requirements. Protein provided in excess of that required is not stored as protein but is deaminated by the liver. The by-products of protein breakdown are excreted by the kidneys. The minimum requirement for protein is approximately 2.5 g protein/kg $BW^{0.75}$. For adult maintenance, the daily protein intake should be about 5.0 g protein/kg $BW^{0.75}$ or approximately 6.5 g protein/100 kcal. Diets should contain between 15% and 30% protein dry matter (DM; Table 5.1).

▪ Fat

Fat is an important source of energy and also provides essential fatty acids. Fat consumption is also necessary for absorption of the fat-soluble vitamins (A, D, E, K). In the dog, both linoleic acid and linolenic acid are required because these cannot be synthesized in the body. Linoleic acid is used for production of all the other omega-6 fatty acids, and linolenic acid is used for the production of all the other omega-3 fatty acids. Adequate intake of these essential fatty acids is necessary for normal skin and coat condition. Fat should comprise at least 5% DM of the diet, with 1% DM as linoleic acid.

Table 5.1. Dietary recommendations for healthy adult dogs.

Nutrient	Dietary Recommendation
Protein	15%–%30% DM
Fiber	≤5% DM
Fat	>5% DM; linoleic acid 1% DM
Calcium	0.5–0.8% DM
Ca/P ratio	1:1–2:1

DM, dry matter.

■ Fiber

Whether fiber is truly required in the diet is debated. Fiber does not provide any energy to the diet, thus as the fiber content of the diet increases, the energy density of the food decreases. Some fiber in the diet may be beneficial for gut health, and dietary fiber contributes to "feeling full." Less than 5% DM dietary fiber appears to be adequate.

■ Minerals

Calcium and phosphorus are important for bone health and must be maintained in a proper dietary ratio. Meat sources are high in phosphorus and low in calcium. Home-prepared diets typically will need to be supplemented with a source of calcium and/or phosphorus. Bone meal is often used to provide calcium and phosphorus and cannot be omitted from homemade diet recipes. Calcium should be provided in the diet at 0.5%–0.8% DM and phosphorus should be 0.4%–0.6% DM in the diet. It is probably wise to avoid feeding excessive phosphorus as this may accelerate the progression of renal disease.

In young, healthy dogs, a high intake of sodium does not appear to be harmful. However, in certain diseases (kidney disease, heart disease, obesity), sodium should be restricted because of the presence of hypertension. Sodium should be provided at 25–50 mg/kg BW/day or at 0.15%–0.4% DM in the diet.

Nutrition of the Cat

As in dogs, a number of factors need to be considered when determining a diet for a cat. Neutering decreases the energy requirement, and energy needs are increased in pregnant or lactating cats, as in dogs. Sedentary or obese cats require less energy. Cats do not participate in sporting activities as dogs do, but active or stressed cats may require more energy. There is not a great difference in body size of different breeds, but some breeds are more docile and therefore less active. Nutritional needs of cats differ with age, and young, growing kittens require more energy than the adult or senior cat. The energy requirement for different life stages and conditions in the cat can be found in Chapter 4.

■ Water

Water is the most important nutrient for the cat, although cats are able to better cope with water deprivation as compared to the dog. Cats have the ability to conserve total body water by producing highly concentrated urine. Even so, if there is not an adequate supply of water, cats can become dehydrated and die. In general, cats should drink about 1 mL of water per kilocalorie requirement. In other words, if a cat requires 200 kcal/day, then it should consume approximately 200 mL of water a day. Most homemade diets contain quite a high percentage of water, so if a homemade diet is fed, the cat may not need to consume much additional water.

■ Protein

Cats require a number of different amino acids in their diet (see Chapter 3). The amino acids found in meat sources are a better match for the cat's requirements than are the amino acids present in plant sources. Thus, most of the protein in the cat's diet should be from a meat source. In particular, taurine is required by the cat and is not found in plant sources. The recommended protein concentration in a diet for adult cats is 30%–45% DM (Table 5.2).

■ Fat

As in dogs, fat provides a good source of energy and is necessary for the absorption of fat-soluble vitamins. In the cat, linoleic acid, lino-

Table 5.2. Dietary recommendations for healthy adult cats.

Nutrient	Dietary Recommendation
Protein	30%–50% DM
Fiber	≤5% DM
Fat	>9% DM; linoleic acid 0.5% DM, arachidonic acid 0.02% DM
Calcium	0.5%–1.0% DM
Ca/P ratio	0.9:1–1.5:1
Potassium	0.6%–1.0% DM
Average urinary pH	6.2–6.5

DM, dry matter.

lenic acid, and arachidonic acid are essential fatty acids and must be provided in the diet. Arachidonic acid is only found in meat sources. Linoleic and linolenic acids are important for maintenance of the skin and coat. Arachidonic acid is important for normal platelet function and reproduction. Linolenic acid is an omega-3 fatty acid, and omega-3 fatty acids are required for proper neurological developments in neonates. Omega-3 fatty acids are prone to oxidation, and cats can develop pansteatitis from oxidized omega-3 fatty acids if there is not sufficient vitamin E in the diet. Dietary fat should be present at greater than 9% DM. There should be 0.5% DM linoleic acid and 0.02% DM arachidonic acid in the diet. Palatability of the diet appears to be best when dietary fat is about 25% DM.

■ Fiber

Cats do not require dietary fiber, but a small amount promotes normal GI function and helps maintain good stool quality. Dietary fiber should be present at less than 5% DM for normal cats, but the fiber content can be increased up to 15% DM for obese cats. Increased fiber content may also be beneficial for cats with hairballs.

■ Minerals

As in dogs, proper levels of calcium and phosphorus are necessary for bone health. Cats fed exclusively meats are at high risk for the development of nutritional secondary hyperparathyroidism, which results in a loss of bone density, lameness, and fractures. Meats are very low in calcium and high in phosphorus; this leads to a calcium deficiency. Even though the cat is a carnivore, ingredients other than meat must be provided in their diet to ensure that there is an adequate intake of calcium. Recommended calcium in the diet is 0.6% DM, and recommended dietary phosphorus is 0.5% DM. The calcium/phosphorus ratio should be maintained between 0.9:1 and 1.5:1 for optimal phosphorus availability. Restriction of dietary phosphorus is important in both renal disease and when struvite stones are present.

Excess sodium in the diet should be avoided due to the presence of hypertension. A dietary sodium level of 0.2%–0.5% DM is adequate, and chloride should be present at a minimum of 0.19% DM.

Potassium is a critical mineral in cats. High-protein foods promote the production of acidic urine, which increases the loss of potassium. Potassium should be fed at a level between 0.6% and 1.0% DM to prevent a potassium deficiency. Cats lose even more potassium when renal disease or diabetes mellitus is present, and higher levels of dietary potassium may be necessary in these conditions.

Magnesium is important in the development of struvite crystals in cats. To decrease the risk of struvite crystal formation, dietary magnesium should be less than 0.10% DM, or less than 20 mg/100 kcal. However, excessive restriction of magnesium is not recommended either, since this will predispose cats to the formation of oxalate stones.

Urine pH

The ingredients present in the diet and feeding practices determine the urinary pH. When the urinary pH is less than 6.5, the risk of developing struvite crystals is decreased. However, if the urine pH drops below 6.0, metabolic acidosis can occur, which leads to a decrease in bone density and an increased loss of calcium and potassium in the urine. Calcium oxalate stone formation is also promoted in very acidic urine. Free-choice feeding is best for a more constant urinary pH and avoids the large increase in urine pH seen 3 to 6 hours after a large meal is fed. Urine pH should be maintained between 6.2 and 6.5 in most cats.

■ Nutritional Issues Unique to the Cat

Cats have unique nutritional requirements that must be kept in mind when developing diets for them. Dog foods are not appropriate for cats and will not supply the particular nutrients that cats require. Vegetarian diets for cats are especially problematic. Protein content is typically low in plant sources so it may be difficult to acquire sufficient protein and amino acids. Taurine, which is required for cats, is not found in plants and thus must be supplemented when a vegetarian diet is fed. Carnitine is not a required amino acid, but it may be essential for growth. Carnitine is also not found in plant sources. Plant sources are typically low in methionine, lysine, and tryptophan, and diets must be formulated to include sufficient quantities of these amino acids. Glutamate is also found in high concentrations in plants, and some cats cannot tolerate diets high in glutamate. Arachidonic acid is an essential fatty acid for the cat, and it is found only in meat sources. If increased levels of omega-3 fatty acids are fed to cats, the vitamin E content should also be increased to prevent steatitis. Cats cannot utilize β-carotene, so vitamin A must be supplied in the diet. Vitamin B_{12} is not found in plant sources and must be added to vegetarian diets. Niacin should also be added to a vegetarian diet because the niacin present in plants is largely unavailable for absorption.

Many owners will give cats milk to drink. With age, lactose activity in the intestine decreases. Small amounts of milk may be tolerated by many cats, but milk ingestion can lead to diarrhea or GI discomfort.

Cats should not be fed onions, onion-based broth, or onion powder. Chemicals present in onions can oxidize hemoglobin in the cat, leading to red blood cell destruction and anemia. Spoiled fish should not be fed to cats. Histidine present in fish can convert to histamine with spoilage, and histamine ingestion causes salivation, vomiting, and diarrhea within 30 minutes. When fish is being fed to cats, it must be handled and stored properly to prevent spoilage.

Aberrant Behaviors in the Dog and Cat

Both dogs and cats will eat grass or other plants. Why they do so is not clear. Grass or plants are not readily digested and may be an irritant to the GI tract, resulting in vomiting. Many pets consume grass without vomiting, and it may be ingested just because they like the taste or texture.

Cats may commonly chew wool, and they may be attracted to the smell of lanolin present. Certain cat breeds such as Siamese and Burmese cats are more prone to wool chewing, thus there may be a genetic basis. Free-choice feeding or feeding a higher-fiber diet may help to eliminate wool chewing.

Dogs have a tendency to "get into the garbage." This behavior is probably normal, as dogs prefer the taste of certain chemicals that are produced in decomposing food. Unfortunately, decomposing foods can also contain a high number of bacteria, which is unhealthy if ingested. Garbage ingestion can result in vomiting, diarrhea, abdominal pain, shock, or death. Access to garbage should be prevented.

Coprophagia is the ingestion of feces by pets. Sometimes pets will ingest their own feces, but more commonly they will ingest the feces of other animals or species. This condition is common in dogs, but quite uncommon in cats. Coprophagia is a normal behavior in dams, who eat the feces of their young from birth to about 3 weeks of age. It is their way of keeping the nest area clean, and in the wild, helped to avoid attracting the attention of predators. Dogs in the wild may have also consumed the feces of herbivores because it is rich in many nutrients. Potential medical causes of coprophagia include intestinal parasites, intestinal malabsorption, hyperthyroidism, Cushing's disease, diabetes mellitus, or steroid administration. Complications associated with coprophagia include gastroenteritis and diarrhea, especially if cow feces are being consumed. Reinfection with intestinal parasites can also be a problem. The best treatment for coprophagia is to avoid exposure to feces. There are commercial products that can be added to the diet that are readily ingested but have an unpleasant taste when excreted in the stool. Meat tenderizer or pancreatic enzymes added to the diet may also be effective because these also cause feces to have an unpleasant taste. However, these products must be added to the diet of all dogs in the house. If the dog routinely eats feces, litter boxes should be kept clean at all times to minimize exposure to feces. If the dog eats its own stool or that of another animal, then it is best to walk the dog on a leash to prevent access. If the dog has the habit of eating its own feces, a food reward could be offered instead, before it has had the opportunity to eat stool. This way the dog learns to associate defecation with a treat.

Adult Dog Recipes

Adult Cat Recipes

Additional Reading

AAFCO. 2009 Official Publication. Association of American Feed Control Officials Inc. Available from: http://www.aafco.org.

Buffington CA, Holloway C, Abood SK (Eds). 2004. Normal dogs. In *Manual of Veterinary Dietetics*. Elsevier, St. Louis, pp. 9–26.

Buffington CA, Holloway C, Abood SK (Eds). 2004. Normal Cats. In *Manual of Veterinary Dietetics*. Elsevier, St. Louis, pp. 27–38.

Case LP, Carey DP, Hirakawa DA, Daristotle L (Eds). 2000. Feeding requirements for dogs. In *Canine and Feline Nutrition: A Resource for Companion Animal Professionals*, 2nd edition. Mosby, St. Louis, pp. 217–224.

Case LP, Carey DP, Hirakawa DA, Daristotle L (Eds). 2000. Adult maintenance. In *Canine and Feline Nutrition: A Resource for Companion Animal Professionals*, 2nd edition. Mosby, St. Louis, pp. 255–258.

Gray CM, Sellon RK, Freeman LM. 2004. Nutritional adequacy of two vegan diets for cats. J Am Vet Med Assoc 225(11):1670–1675.

Kirk CA, Debraekeleer J, Armstrong PJ. 2000. Normal cats. In *Small Animal Clinical Nutrition*, 4th edition. Hand MS, Thatcher CD, Remillard RL, Roudebush P (Eds). Mark Morris Institute, Topeka, KS, pp. 291–350.

Debraekeleer J, Gross KL, Zicker SC. 2000. Normal dogs. In *Small Animal Clinical Nutrition*, 4th edition. Hand MS, Thatcher CD, Remillard RL, Roudebush P (Eds). Mark Morris Institute, Topeka, KS, pp. 211–260.

Wakefield LA, Shofer FS, Michel KE. 2006. Evaluation of cats fed vegetarian diets and attitudes of their caregivers. J Am Vet Med Assoc 229(1):70–73.

CHAPTER 6
Feeding the Puppy or Kitten

Nutrition of the Growing Puppy

■ **Nursing Period**

Newborn puppies should be closely monitored for warmth and weight gain. During the first few weeks of life, puppies do not have a good ability to maintain their body temperature, and they have very little body fat. Thus, the environmental temperature should be maintained between 75° and 81°F to prevent hypothermia. If puppies become cold, the dam may reject the puppy and not allow it to nurse. Puppies should be weighed every day using an accurate gram scale. During the first week of life, puppies should gain about 8% of their current body weight daily. In the second week, puppies should gain about 6% of their current body weight per day, about 4% in the third week, and about 3.5% in the fourth week. Small breeds reach about 50% of their adult weight by 4 months of age, and larger breeds reach 50% of their adult weight by about 5 months of age. Adequate weight gain during the nursing period is a reflection of quality of milk, adequate intake of milk, and health status. If milk intake is inadequate, the puppy can easily develop a low glucose concentration. Puppies have very little reserve of fat or glycogen, and if there is inadequate milk intake, they are unable to maintain normal blood glucose concentrations. Puppies also can become dehydrated very rapidly.

Dam's milk is very digestible and high in calories. It is also high in protein, containing about twice as much protein as cow's milk. Puppies increase their fat stores rapidly after birth, and the dam's milk must contain adequate fat to support this. The fat content of milk is dependent on the dietary fat content of the food consumed by the dam, and it should be about 9% fat. Lactose is the primary carbohydrate in milk, but it is about 30% lower in dog's milk as compared to cow's milk. Lactose is easily absorbed after digestion. Colostrum is very high in calcium, but the calcium content decreases in subsequent milk. Milk is very low in iron, and puppies have a high iron requirement. Puppies can become iron deficient, especially if they are infected with fleas or have intestinal hookworms. Puppies should start to consume food at about 3 weeks of age to provide supplemental iron. For weaning, a diet designed for growth can be mixed with warm water and ground into gruel. The diet for weaning puppies should be highly digestible, and as intake increases, the amount of water can be decreased.

■ Postweaning Period

Energy

Young puppies have a high energy requirement and use about 50% of calories for growth. When puppies reach about 80% of their adult weight, only about 8%–10% of calories are used for growth. Thus, the energy requirement is highest in the youngest puppies and decreases as puppies reach maturity. Energy requirements for growing puppies can be found in Chapter 4.

Body condition should be closely monitored in growing puppies. If energy intake is excessive, puppies can become overweight or obese, and this increased weight can contribute to skeletal problems. Maintenance of lean body condition does not decrease adult size and appears to increase longevity.

Protein

Protein requirements are highest in the youngest puppies and decrease with age. Arginine is an essential amino acid in puppies, but the arginine requirement decreases with age. Previously, it was thought that high-protein diets contributed to skeletal problems in giant-breed dogs. However, it has been shown that diets containing higher levels of protein (up to 32% DM) do not cause skeletal problems as long as the calcium and phosphorus content of the diet is adequate. Recommended protein content in diets is 22%–32% DM for dogs with an adult body weight less than 55 lb and 20%–32% DM for dogs with an adult body weight greater than 55 lb (Table 6.1).

Table 6.1. Dietary recommendations for the growing puppy.

Nutrient	Dietary Recommendation	
	Dogs with an adult BW less than 55 lb	Dogs with an adult BW greater than 55 lb
Protein	22%–32% DM	20%–32% DM
Fat	10%–25% DM	8%–14% DM
Calcium	0.7%–1.7% DM	0.7%–1.4% DM
Phosphorus	0.6%–1.3% DM	0.6%–1.1% DM
Calcium/phosphorus ratio	1:1–1.8:1	1:1–1.5:1

BW, body weight; DM, dry matter.

Carbohydrate

Puppies should be fed about 20% DM carbohydrate until at least 4 months of age. With a low-carbohydrate diet, puppies may exhibit diarrhea, poor appetite, and lethargy.

Fat

Growing puppies require about 250 mg/kg body weight of linoleic acid. Fat contents of diets for puppies whose adult body weight is less than 55 lb should be 10%–25% DM. For puppies with an adult body weight greater than 55 lb, the dietary fat content should be 8%–12% DM. Fat is energy dense, contributing considerable energy to the diet. Excessive fat can affect bone formation in large-breed and giant-breed dogs. Therefore, the fat content of diets for large- and giant-breed dogs should be carefully controlled to avoid excessive energy intake.

Minerals

Calcium and phosphorus are critical minerals for the growing puppy. Calcium absorption in the intestine is high when the puppies are between 2 and 6 months of age, and overall there is less control of calcium homeostasis at this age. Even when the calcium content of the diet is high, and there is danger of excess calcium absorption, intestinal calcium absorption remains at about 40%. After about 10 months of age, calcium homeostasis becomes better regulated, and puppies become less sensitive to an excess of dietary calcium. For large- and giant-breed puppies, the diet should contain 0.7%–1.2% DM calcium. For small- to medium-breed puppies, the diet can contain 0.7%–1.7% DM calcium.

Nutrition of the Growing Kitten

■ Nursing Period

Newborn kittens should be closely monitored for warmth and weight gain. As in newborn puppies, newborn kittens poorly regulate their body temperature during the first month of life. Kittens should be weighed at birth and then at least weekly. The average kitten birth weight is about 100 g, and kittens should gain about 100 g/week for the first 6 months of life. Poor weight gain or a weight loss suggests inadequate milk production by the queen, inadequate milk intake by the kitten (inability to suckle), or illness of the kitten or queen.

The energy content of colostrum is very high on day 1 of production and decreases by day 3. The energy of queen's milk then increases throughout lactation. The calcium and phosphorus concentration of milk increases through day 14 of lactation, and iron, copper, and magnesium concentrations decrease during this period. Taurine is important for normal development, and queen's milk is rich in taurine. Cow and goat milk are low in taurine and are not acceptable replacements for queen's milk. Lactose is the primary carbohydrate in queen's milk, but the concentration is lower than in cow's milk. The nutrient composition of queen's milk is ideal for growth, and milk from other species does not provide the same nutrient levels. If milk production is inadequate, a milk replacer especially formulated for kittens should be fed.

■ Postweaning Period

Energy
Kittens have a high energy requirement due to their rapid growth rate. Diets should be high in energy so that small amounts of food will meet the energy needs. The daily energy requirement decreases until about 10 months of age. Neutering at any age decreases the energy requirement by about 30%. Kittens should be monitored for the development of obesity, especially those that have been neutered. Energy requirements for growing kittens can be found in Chapter 4.

Protein
The protein requirement of kittens is high and declines gradually to adult levels. Kittens especially require high levels of sulfur-containing amino acids. To provide adequate sulfur-containing amino acids, at least 19% DM of protein must come from an animal source.

Table 6.2. Dietary recommendations for the growing kitten.

Nutrient	Dietary Recommendation
Protein	35%–50% DM
Fat	18%–35% DM
Fiber	<5% DM
Calcium	0.8%–1.6% DM
Phosphorus	0.6%–1.4% DM
Calcium/phosphorus ratio	1:1–1.5:1
Potassium	0.6%–1.2% DM
Magnesium	0.08%–0.15% DM

DM, dry matter.

Protein concentrations in kitten diets are usually between 35% and 50% DM and provide a maximum of 26% of the total kilocalories in the diet (Table 6.2).

Carbohydrates

Kittens do not have a requirement for carbohydrates, but they can be readily digestible. Lactose in cow's milk is not very digestible by the kitten and can cause diarrhea and gas.

Fat

Body fat rapidly increases in growing kittens. Kittens require linoleic acid, linolenic acid, and arachidonic acid, as do adult cats; they also require long-chain omega-3 fatty acids (such as docosahexaenoic acid) for proper neural development. The fat content in kitten diets is typically 18%–35% DM to provide adequate fatty acids and enhance palatability.

Minerals

The calcium concentration of kitten diets should be 0.8%–1.6% DM. Excess dietary calcium does not lead to developmental skeletal disease in kittens as it does in dogs, but excessive dietary calcium can restrict magnesium availability. Calcium deficiency is a significant problem in kittens that are fed all-meat diets. Meat is high in phosphorus and low in calcium, and an all-meat diet can lead to the development of nutritional secondary hyperparathyroidism, which causes decreased bone density, lameness, and fractures. Potassium losses can be high when a high-protein diet is fed. Dietary potassium should be present at 0.6%–1.2% DM to provide adequate potassium. Diets fed to kittens should not cause an extremely acidic urine; urinary pH should be 6.2–6.5.

Puppy Recipes

Chicken and Rice   311
Chicken and Rice   312
Chicken and Pasta   313
Chicken and Potato   314
Chicken and Quinoa   315
Ground Beef and Rice   316
Ground Beef and Pasta   317
Ground Beef and Pasta   318
Ground Beef and Potato   319
Lamb and Rice   320
Eggs and Rice   321
Eggs and Pasta   322
Eggs and Potato   323
Tofu and Rice   324
Tofu, Black Beans, and Rice   325
Chicken and Rice   326
Chicken and Pasta   327
Chicken and Potato   328
Ground Beef and Rice   329
Ground Beef and Pasta   330
Pork and Pasta   331
Tuna and Pasta   332
Rabbit and Quinoa   347
Venison and Quinoa   349
Tofu and Quinoa   351
Chicken and Potato   368

Large Breed Puppy Recipes

Chicken and Rice   326
Chicken and Pasta   327
Chicken and Potato   328
Ground Beef and Rice   329
Ground Beef and Pasta   330
Pork and Pasta   331
Tuna and Pasta   332

Kitten Recipes

Additional Reading

AAFCO. 2009 Official Publication. Association of American Feed Control Officials Inc. Available from: http://www.aafco.org.

Case LP, Carey DP, Hirakawa DA, Daristotle L (Eds). 2000. Growth. In *Canine and Feline Nutrition: A Resource for Companion Animal Professionals*, 2nd edition. Mosby, St. Louis, pp. 245–254.

Case LP, Carey DP, Hirakawa DA, Daristotle L (Eds). 2000. Overnutrition and supplementation. In *Canine and Feline Nutrition: A Resource for Companion Animal Professionals*. 2nd edition. Mosby, St. Louis, pp 331–344.

Debraekeleer J, Gross KL, Zicker SC. 2000. Normal dogs. In *Small Animal Clinical Nutrition*, 4th edition. Hand MS, Thatcher CD, Remillard RL, Roudebush P (Eds). Mark Morris Institute, Topeka, KS, pp. 211–260.

Elliot DA. 2006. Nutritional management of chronic renal disease in dogs and cats. Vet Clin North Am Small Anim Pract 36(6):1377–1384.

Kirk CA, Debraekeleer J, Armstrong PJ. 2000. Normal cats. In *Small Animal Clinical Nutrition*, 4th edition. Hand MS, Thatcher CD, Remillard RL, Roudebush P (Eds). Mark Morris Institute, Topeka, KS, pp. 291–350.

Lauten SD. 2006. Nutritional risks to large-breed dogs: From weaning to the geriatric years. Vet Clin Small Anim 36:1345–1359.

Lawler DF, Ballam JM, Meadows R, Larson BT, Li Q, Stowe HD, et al. 2007. Influence of lifetime food restriction on physiological variable in Labrador retriever dogs. Exp Gerontol 42(3):204–214.

CHAPTER 7
Feeding the Pregnant or Lactating Dog or Cat

The goal of proper nutrition during gestation and lactation is to produce an optimal number of healthy puppies or kittens. For optimal reproduction, proper nutrition should begin during the growth phase of the dam or queen, while they are young, and should continue during adulthood, breeding, gestation, and lactation.

The Impact of Improperly Formulated Diets

Special care needs to be taken to ensure that the diet of the pregnant dog or cat is properly balanced and meets energy needs. Diets deficient in protein can result in low birth weights and increased illness or death of newborns. Carbohydrate-free diets are associated with low birth weights, increased stillbirths, and increased illness of newborns. Carbohydrate-free diets may also predispose the bitch to periparturient hypoglycemia. Deficiency of dietary zinc can result in fatal resorption and small litter size. Deficiencies in iron, pyridoxine, or biotin can lead to decreased immunity of the puppies. Excess dietary vitamin A can result in small litters and congenital abnormalities. Excess dietary vitamin D can lead to calcification of soft tissues.

Prior to Breeding

Breeding animals should be chosen based on their conformation, temperament, and overall health. All breeding animals should be screened for any genetic abnormalities. In addition, a thorough physical exam should be performed just prior to breeding and should include a check for fecal parasites and serum testing for brucellosis.

The dam or queen should be at a good body weight prior to breeding and should not be underweight or overweight (body condition score of 3 out of 5). If the dam or queen is underweight, she may not be able to consume enough calories during gestation to meet her nutritional needs, which can impact conception, litter size, and puppy or kitten viability. Obese animals may have smaller litters, a decreased rate of conception, and may not produce adequate milk. Obese dogs may also have irregular heat cycles, which makes conception more difficult, and can have a higher incidence of difficult delivery.

During estrus, there are no special nutritional requirements other than that for adult maintenance. Some bitches may decrease their food intake during estrus, with the lowest intake at the time of ovulation. The short-term decrease in caloric intake does not appear to have an impact on fertility or litter size, but it may be helpful to feed multiple small meals to promote intake.

Gestation in Dogs

In dogs gestation averages 63 days. Prior to whelping, bitches gain about 15%–25% of their prebreeding body weight; after whelping, dams should weigh about 5%–10% more than their prebreeding weight.

Fetal growth is very slow during the first 40 days of pregnancy, with only 5.5% of fetal mass developed by day 40. No increase in food intake is necessary early in pregnancy. After day 40, there is rapid fetal growth, with peak growth in weeks 6–8 of pregnancy. During the rapid fetal growth phase, the energy requirement in bitches is about 30% higher than during maintenance; if the bitch is carrying a large litter, the energy required may be up to 60% higher than during prebreeding. Unfortunately, during the last week of pregnancy when the energy requirement is highest, food intake is somewhat limited by the space-occupying uterus and fetuses. Large breeds carrying large litters may not be able to consume enough calories to meet their caloric needs. Diets should be highly digestible and high in energy density to provide maximum calories and fed in multiple smaller portions to promote intake.

The protein requirement of pregnant dogs increases during late gestation to about 40%–70% above that of normal maintenance.

Table 7.1. Dietary recommendations for the reproducing dog.

Nutrient	Dietary Recommendation	
	Gestation	Lactation
Protein	22%–32% DM	25%–35% DM
Fat	10%–25% DM	≥18% DM
Carbohydrate	≥23% DM	≥23% DM
Fiber	≤5% DM	≤5% DM
Calcium	0.75%–1.5% DM	0.75%–1.7% DM
Phosphorus	0.6%–1.3% DM	0.6%–1.3% DM

DM, dry matter.

Homemade diets for late gestation should provide about 20%–25% protein on a dry matter (DM) basis, with about 4 kcal metabolizable energy (ME)/g DM (or about 4 g of protein per 100 kcal ME). To obtain a diet with a density of 4 kcal/g, 10%–25% fat is typically provided in the diet. Bitches also have a high requirement for glucose during the last weeks of gestation; about 20% energy from carbohydrate is sufficient. Calcium and phosphorus requirements increase by about 60% during the last month of gestation due to the rapid growth of fetuses. Excess calcium should be avoided though, and diets should provide a calcium-to-phosphorus ratio of 1:1–1.5:1 (Table 7.1).

Gestation in Cats

In cats gestation usually lasts 63–65 days. The pattern of weight gain is different in cats as compared to dogs. The queen will start to gain weight during the second week of pregnancy. This early weight gain is not associated with fetal growth, but rather is stored energy for lactation. After giving birth, the queen will only lose about 40% of the weight that was gained during pregnancy. The 60% of weight gained during pregnancy that is not lost will be used to support milk production. Queens need to be in good body condition at the time of mating and during pregnancy. Underweight queens have an increased incidence of conception failure, fetal malformations or death, and underweight kittens. In addition they may be unable to support adequate milk production. Obesity also leads to reproductive problems, with an increase in stillbirths and dystocia; thus, it is recommended that the queen be in ideal body condition at the time of mating.

Table 7.2. Dietary recommendation for the reproducing cat.

Nutrient	Dietary Recommendation for Gestation/Lactation
Protein	35%–50% DM
Fat	18%–35% DM
Fiber	<5% DM
Calcium	1.0%–1.6% DM
Phosphorus	0.8%–1.4% DM
Potassium	0.6%–1.2% DM
Magnesium	0.08%–0.15% DM

DM, dry matter.

Energy requirements increase throughout gestation in the cat. Food intake in the queen may actually decrease about 2 weeks after mating when fetal implantation occurs. Food intake may also decrease in the last week of gestation. The energy needed during gestation is about 25%–50% greater (approximately 90–110 kcal/kg BW/day) than that needed for adult maintenance. Energy requirements are typically met by foods containing 35%–50% protein, 18%–35% fat, and 10% carbohydrate (Table 7.2). Free-choice feeding of an energy-dense food is recommended during gestation to ensure adequate energy intake.

Copper deficiency during gestation can lead to fetal death, abortions, and deformities. Copper should be present in the diet at 15 mg/kg food DM and should come from a digestible source. Foods for the reproducing cat should also produce a urinary pH between 6.2 and 6.5 to prevent metabolic acidosis, which can lead to poor bone development in kittens.

Lactation in the Dog

Lactation requires a considerable amount of energy, more than during any other life stage. The amount of milk produced by the dam equates to the dairy cow; dogs in peak lactation can produce an average of greater than 8% of their body weight in milk per day. For example, a German Shepherd dam may produce 1700 mL milk/day during peak lactation, as compared to the average human producing 750 mL/day. Dam's milk contains twice the protein and fat as compared to cow's milk due to the rapid rate of growth of puppies compared to calories.

Water intake is very important for milk production; a large dog may drink 5–6 liters of water per day during peak lactation. Fresh, clean water should be available at all times during lactation.

The energy requirement increases after whelping and reaches a peak between 3 and 5 weeks at approximately two to four times that of maintenance requirements. The limiting factor for energy intake is typically the energy density of the food; if the diet provided is low in energy density, it may be impossible for the dam to consume enough calories to meet the puppies' energy needs. Thus, it is recommended to feed a diet during lactation that is highly digestible and high in energy density. Free-choice feeding is the best option for the lactating dam. The stress of caring for puppies increases the energy requirement, but most energy is used for milk production. Approximately 180 kcal is used to produce 100 g of milk. The amount of milk produced is dependent on the number and size of the puppies; the greatest quantity of milk is produced during midlactation when puppies are rapidly growing but are not yet eating any solid food.

The protein requirement increases greatly during lactation. Dams require about 6 g digestible protein/100 kcal ME, which corresponds to about 19%–27% protein in a diet. In a homemade diet, the protein intake is calculated at 20 g protein/kg$^{0.75}$. Increasing the fat content of the diet will greatly increase the energy in the diet. A diet between 12% and 20% fat can increase the fat calories for the puppies. It may be beneficial to increase the long-chain omega-3 fatty acid content in the diet of dams to increase the omega-3 fatty acid content in the milk. Puppies require docosahexaenoic acid (DHA; a long-chain omega-3 fatty acid) for proper retinal and nervous system development, and this is obtained through milk. Carbohydrates in the diet should provide 10%–20% of the energy. Calcium and phosphorus requirements also increase during lactation, but the calcium-to-phosphorus ratio should be maintained at 1.3:1 in the diet. During peak lactation, dams require about two to five times more calcium than during maintenance. Diets for lactation should contain 0.8%–1.1% calcium and 0.6%–0.8% phosphorus.

Lactation in the Cat

In the queen, peak lactation occurs at 3–4 weeks of lactation. The energy requirement during lactation can be two to six times that during maintenance. The energy density of the diet for a lactating queen should be approximately 4–5 kcal ME/g diet, and free-choice feeding is recommended. The protein requirement also greatly increases during lactation to provide essential amino acids. A queen with a large litter may lose 19 g protein/day in the milk. Protein levels at 30%–35% are recommended to meet protein needs. Animal-based protein sources are preferred because they are more digestible and provide better amino acid profiles as compared to vegetable sources of protein. The taurine requirement during lactation is similar to that during maintenance, so a specific increase in taurine is not necessary during lactation.

Fat is an important source of calories because it provides more calories than does protein or carbohydrate. The diet should provide approximately 20% fat for best reproductive performance. Providing a higher fat content in the diet increases the number of kittens per litter, decreases kitten mortality, and improves reproductive efficiency of the queen. Linoleic, linolenic, and arachidonic acid are required fatty acids for the cat and must be provided in the diet. Dietary deficiencies of linoleic and arachidonic acid can result in reproductive failure in which queens do not bear live kittens. Male cats, however, can maintain spermatogenesis even on an arachidonic acid–deficient diet. DHA is also required by kittens for proper retinal and nervous system development, as it is in puppies. Thus, it is beneficial to add long-chain omega-3 fatty acids to the diet of the lactating queen.

Dietary carbohydrates are important to help prevent weight loss during lactation and provide a substrate for lactose. Carbohydrate should be included at about 10% DM in the diet.

Calcium and phosphorus requirements also increase during lactation, but the calcium-to-phosphorus ratio should be maintained at 1:1–1.5:1. The recommended dietary level of calcium is 1.0%–1.6% DM in the diet. Magnesium should not be restricted during lactation, and levels of 0.08%–0.15% DM are recommended in the diet.

Weaning Puppies

Weaning begins as puppies start eating some solid food, usually between 3 and 4 weeks of age. As puppies start consuming more and more solid food, there is less nursing, which decreases the amount of milk produced. However, some dams continue to produce a large quantity of milk, which increases the risk for mastitis. Food intake should be restricted for a few days prior to weaning to decrease nutrients available for milk production. This will decrease the amount of milk produced and help prevent mammary gland engorgement.

Weaning Kittens

In kittens, weaning is a gradual process that usually starts at about 3–4 weeks of age and continues until kittens are 6–10 weeks of age when kittens are typically completely weaned. Allowing kittens to nurse until 9 or 10 weeks of age decreases the stress of weaning and allows more kitten growth and immune system maturation. As kittens are being weaned, the energy requirement of the queen's diet will decrease because less milk is being produced. In queens that are heavy milk producers, it may be best to restrict the energy intake of the queen for a few days prior to complete weaning to prevent mammary gland engorgement.

Disorders Occurring during Gestation/Lactation

■ Eclampsia (Puerperal Tetany)

Dams are most likely to develop eclampsia at the point of peak lactation (about 3–4 weeks postparturition). At this time, there is a tremendous amount of calcium lost in the milk. Eclampsia is usually seen in dams with large litters, especially small-breed dams. With the large loss of calcium in the milk, the serum concentration of calcium decreases, causing hypocalcemia. Signs of hypocalcemia include a stiff gait, restlessness, agitation, uncoordination, muscular tremors, and seizures; death can occur if the low calcium level is not treated. If clinical signs appear, prompt veterinary treatment is required and usually entails intravenous administration of solutions containing calcium. Since this condition usually occurs just prior to weaning, puppies are separated from the dam and are typically weaned at this time. Occasionally, eclampsia will occur during whelping; this is usually due to excessive panting during a difficult whelping, which can alter the serum pH and cause hypocalcemia. Cats more commonly exhibit signs of eclampsia during the last 3 weeks of pregnancy. Signs include weakness, muscle tremors, anorexia, vomiting, flaccid paralysis, and malaise.

Prevention of eclampsia involves feeding adequate amounts of a properly balanced diet during pregnancy and lactation. The dietary calcium-to-phosphorus ratio should be maintained close to 1:1. Some breeders will supplement with additional calcium during pregnancy to prevent this problem, but this is not recommended and can actually potentiate the occurrence of eclampsia.

■ **Periparturient Hypoglycemia**

Periparturient hypoglycemia (low concentration of glucose in the serum) occurs infrequently in bitches, but it can occur during the last few weeks of gestation. Clinical signs may appear to be similar to those of eclampsia and include nervousness, twitching, and seizures. Hypoglycemia usually occurs in bitches that are in poor body condition, are malnourished, or are fed a high-fat, low-carbohydrate diet. Veterinary treatment is required and involves intravenous administration of a glucose solution. The condition is typically prevented by keeping the bitch in good body condition during pregnancy and feeding her a highly digestible diet.

Dog Recipes for Gestation

Dog Recipes for Lactation

Cat Recipes for Gestation

Cat Recipes for Lactation

Additional Reading

Case LP, Carey DP, Hirakawa DA, Daristotle L (Eds). 2000. Pregnancy and lactation. In *Canine and Feline Nutrition: A Resource for Companion Animal Professionals*, 2nd edition. Mosby, St. Louis, pp. 225–232.

Debraekeleer J, Gross KL, Zicker SC. 2000. Normal dogs. In *Small Animal Clinical Nutrition*, 4th edition. Hand MS, Thatcher CD, Remillard RL, Roudebush P (Eds). Mark Morris Institute, Topeka, KS, pp. 211–260.

Greco DS. 2008. Nutritional supplements for pregnant and lactating bitches. Theriogenology 70:393–396.

Kirk CA, Debraekeleer J, Armstrong PJ. 2000. Normal cats. In *Small Animal Clinical Nutrition*, 4th edition. Hand MS, Thatcher CD, Remillard RL, Roudebush P (Eds). Mark Morris Institute, Topeka, KS, pp. 291–350.

CHAPTER 8
Feeding the Senior Pet

Better health care, nutrition, and genetic background of pets have contributed to an increasing life span in both dogs and cats. Greater than 40% of dogs and 30% of cats in the United States are 6 years of age, and more than 30% of those are over 11 years of age. The goals of nutrition in the senior pet are to minimize the signs of aging, slow metabolic processes associated with aging, enhance the quality of life, and increase life span, if possible. Older pets can have a large variation in health status, so it is important to evaluate each pet on an individual basis.

The Senior Dog

Dogs of different breeds mature at different rates. The overall average life span is about 13 years, but small breeds of dogs can live significantly longer than large or giant breeds of dogs. Thus, dogs are considered to be senior at different ages based on size. Small to medium dogs weighing less than 50 lb are considered to be senior at 11–15 years of age; those 50–90 lb are senior at about 9 years of age, and very large dogs greater than 90 lb are senior at about 7.5 years of age.

Older dogs can suffer from a number of health problems. The leading causes of death in the older dog are cancer, kidney disease, and heart disease, and all older pets should be routinely screened for these disorders.

■ Nutritional Needs of the Senior Dog

Because of the incidence of decreased kidney function, a fresh, clean source of water should be available at all times. Water intake should be monitored to identify increases in intake, which could be an early indication of changes in renal function or the presence of other disorders.

The resting metabolic rate gradually slows with age. This decrease is due to a loss of lean body tissue and an increase in body fat. By the age of 7 years, there is an approximate 13% decrease in the daily energy requirement in most dogs. This decrease can lead to weight gain in the senior pet. As dogs get very old, however, they may become underweight due to decreasing food intake. The very old dog may benefit from being fed a highly digestible, energy-dense diet.

Senior dogs have a tendency to become overweight, so the fat content of the diet should be adequate but not excessive. For very old dogs that lose weight due to decreased food intake, increasing the fat content in the diet helps improve palatability, which helps increase intake. Increased fat content also increases the energy density of the diet so less needs to be consumed to meet energy needs. Fat contents in diets for senior dogs will vary from 7% to 15%, depending on body condition (Table 8.1).

The protein requirement for older dogs is debated. Due to the decrease in lean body mass and decrease in protein synthesis, the recommended level of protein in the diet may be higher than that for the younger dog. Diets providing 15%–23% dry matter (DM) high-quality protein are adequate for most senior dogs. It has been suggested to decrease the level of dietary protein in senior dogs to prevent the occurrence of kidney disease. However, it has been shown that a higher protein intake does not contribute to the occurrence of kidney

Table 8.1. Dietary recommendations for senior dogs.

Nutrient	Dietary Recommendation
Protein	15%–23% DM
Fat	7%–15% DM
Fiber	≥2.0% DM
Calcium	0.5%–1.0% DM
Phosphorus	0.25%–0.75% DM

DM, dry matter.

disease in healthy dogs. Once kidney disease is present, it then may be beneficial to decrease dietary protein.

Excessive phosphorus in diets should be avoided because of the increased incidence of renal disease. For senior dogs, diets providing 0.25%–0.75% DM phosphorus are recommended. The calcium-to-phosphorus ratio should be maintained, and diets should provide 0.5%–1.0% DM calcium. Osteoporosis is not a problem in older dogs as it is in people, and thus excess calcium supplementation is not required or recommended.

Sodium and chloride do not necessarily need to be restricted in the healthy senior dog, but there is no reason to feed excessive levels either. Diets for senior dogs should provide 0.2%–0.35% DM sodium.

The Senior Cat

Cats are considered senior at about 7 years of age, and geriatric at about 12 years of age. As in dogs, the older cat is more susceptible to a variety of diseases. Senior cats are less active and have a decreased basal metabolic rate due to a decrease in lean body mass. They are also less adaptable, and are not able to withstand changes in their environment and diet as well as do younger cats. Older cats may have decreased senses of smell or taste, and diets should be highly palatable to avoid a reduction in food intake.

■ Nutritional Needs of the Senior Cat

The nutrient requirements of older cats are similar to those of young to middle-aged cats. Dehydration is a common problem in older cats as thirst sensitivity decreases with aging. Clean, fresh water should be available at all times, and water intake should be about 200–250 mL/day.

Even though energy needs decrease in the older cat, the prevalence of obesity decreases after 7 years of age, and the prevalence of underweight cats increases after 11 years of age. Old cats can become underweight due to concurrent disease, decreases in appetite or sensory function, and decreased digestion and absorption of food. Decreased pancreatic enzyme secretion reduces fat digestion in older cats, and changes in liver function can affect nutrient absorption. Thus, older cats need to be monitored closely to maintain an optimal body condition. Diets for the very old cat should be highly digestible and energy-dense to promote caloric intake.

Table 8.2. Dietary recommendations for senior cats.

Nutrient	Dietary Recommendation
Protein	30%–45% DM
Fat	10%–25% DM
Fiber	<10% DM
Calcium	0.6%–1.0% DM
Phosphorus	0.5%–0.7% DM

DM, dry matter.

Protein intake should not be restricted in the older cat. In elderly humans, the protein requirement is increased by 25% over that of adult maintenance. A benefit of increasing the protein content of diets is an increase in palatability, which promotes food intake. An optimal range of protein for the older cat has not been determined; dietary protein between 30% and 45% DM are recommended for healthy older cats (Table 8.2).

Obesity should be avoided in the older cat as diseases associated with obesity (diabetes mellitus, hypertension, and heart disease) are common. However, older cats have a high requirement for the essential fatty acids (linoleic, linolenic, and arachidonic acid) to maintain skin and coat condition. Fat digestion decreases with age, so dietary fat should not be restricted unless the cat is obese. Dietary fat content should be 10%–25% DM for older cats.

Dietary fiber for the older cat should be less than 10% DM. Some dietary fiber is important because constipation is a common problem in older cats, and fiber promotes intestinal motility. High-fiber diets are not recommended for older cats as they decrease the energy density of the diet and decrease digestibility.

Reduced dietary phosphorus is usually recommended for older cats due to the incidence of kidney disease. Diets providing 0.5%–0.7% DM phosphorus are adequate. As in dogs, osteoporosis is not a common problem in old cats, although there may be some decrease in bone mass due to the decrease in lean body mass. Dietary calcium should be provided at 0.6%–1.0% DM.

Potassium may be required at a slightly higher level in the older cat due to loss of potassium in the urine, decreased intake of food, and increased intestinal loss. Decreased potassium levels may lead to lethargy or muscle weakness. Dietary potassium should be provided at 0.6%–1.0% DM. Older cats may also have increased loss of magnesium, and severe dietary magnesium restriction should be avoided.

Dietary magnesium should be provided at 0.05%–0.1% DM. Excessive dietary sodium should be avoided in older cats due to the increased incidence of hypertension, renal disease, hyperthyroidism, and heart disease. Sodium intake, however, must be adequate to maintain acid-base status. Dietary sodium should be provided at 0.2%–0.6% DM, and chloride levels are typically 1.5 times the sodium concentration.

The pH of the urine is important in older cats as kidney disease is more prevalent. Diets that produce a highly acidic urine should not be fed to older cats due to the increased systemic acidic load and the potential for metabolic acidosis. Urinary pH values in older cats should be maintained between 6.2 and 6.5.

Senior Dog Recipes

Chicken and Pasta   333
Ground Beef and Potato   334
Whitefish and Rice   335
Lamb and Rice   336
Cottage Cheese and Rice   337
Tofu and Barley   338

Senior Cat Recipes

Chicken and Rice   455
Ground Beef and Rice   456
Tuna and Rice   457
Whitefish and Rice   458
Salmon and Rice   459

Additional Reading

Bailoni L, Cerchiaro I. 2005. The role of feeding in the maintenance of well-being and health of geriatric dogs. Vet Res Commun 29(Suppl 2):51–55.

Case LP, Carey DP, Hirakawa DA, Daristotle L (Eds). 2000. Geriatrics. In *Canine and Feline Nutrition: A Resource for Companion Animal Professionals*, 2nd edition. Mosby, St. Louis, pp. 275–287.

Debraekeleer J, Gross KL, Zicker SC. 2000. Normal dogs. In *Small Animal Clinical Nutrition*, 4th edition. Hand MS, Thatcher CD, Remillard RL, Roudebush P (Eds). Mark Morris Institute, Topeka, KS, pp. 211–260.

Hall JA, Tooley KA, Gradin JL, Jewell DE, Wander RC. 2003. Effects of dietary n-6 and n-3 fatty acids and vitamin E on the immune response of healthy geriatric dogs. Am J Vet Res 64(6):762–772.

Kirk CA, Debraekeleer J, Armstrong PJ. 2000. Normal cats. In *Small Animal Clinical Nutrition*, 4th edition. Hand MS, Thatcher CD, Remillard RL, Roudebush P (Eds). Mark Morris Institute, Topeka, KS, pp. 291–350.

Laflamme DP. 2005. Nutrition for aging cats and dogs and the importance of body condition. Vet Clinics Small Anim 35:713–742.

Laflamme DP. 2008. Pet food safety: Dietary protein. Top Companion Anim Med 23(3):154–157.

CHAPTER 9
Feeding the
Performance Dog

Many more dogs are taking part in performance activities than ever before. There is a wide variety of formal activities in which dogs and owners can participate, such as racing, hunting/field trials, herding, coursing, earthdog events, agility competitions, Frisbee events, and weight pulls. In addition, many dogs are used for informal hunting or herding, sledding, service work (guide dogs, therapy dogs), police work, guarding, drug detection, and search and response. Proper training is important for conditioning and maximal performance. Nutrition is also important. By matching proper nutrients to the level and type of exercise, performance can be enhanced.

Exercise Physiology

Exercise requires changes in metabolic processes and in a number of organ systems. Muscular physiology is most impacted by training and exercise. Muscle fibers can be either type 1 or type 2. Type 1 fibers are "slow twitch" and have a high oxidative capacity and endurance. Type 2 fibers are "fast twitch," are larger, and have greater strength. Racing dogs have a higher proportion of type 2 fibers, and those performing in endurance events have a higher proportion of type 1 fibers. With intermediate types of exercise, there is a higher proportion of type 1 fibers as well, since the exercise more closely resembles that of endurance events, only shorter in duration.

Energy used for muscle contraction is stored as ATP (adenosine triphosphate), and the amount used is proportional to the amount of work done. ATP is also used for maintenance of the electrolyte concentration gradient across membranes. The amount of ATP stored in muscle is low, so it must be replenished rapidly during exercise. Creatine phosphate is stored in muscle and can rapidly convert to ATP for energy. Glucose stored as muscle glycogen can also regenerate ATP via anaerobic and aerobic pathways. Anaerobic metabolism is rapid, but generates little ATP, whereas aerobic metabolism is slower, but can generate a much higher amount of ATP. Fatty acids are plentiful in adipose tissue and in muscle and serve as the primary energy source for longer-duration exercise. Amino acids do not serve as a primary energy source, but can provide about 5%–15% of the energy used during exercise.

The major by-product of muscle contraction is heat, which must be removed. In dogs, most heat is dissipated through the respiratory tract through evaporation. Therefore, an adequate supply of water must be maintained to prevent dehydration due to water loss from the respiratory tract. Lactic acid and carbon dioxide are also produced by anaerobic metabolism and can increase the pH, thereby decreasing muscle performance. Carbon dioxide can be eliminated by the respiratory tract or by renal excretion of bicarbonate. Lactate can be used for energy or converted back to glucose.

Metabolism in general increases during exercise, and muscle metabolism can increase more than 20-fold. Cardiac output increases with exercise, along with stroke volume and heart rate. Circulating blood is important for removal of carbon dioxide from muscle and for transporting oxygen to muscle. The number of blood cells increases during exercise due to contraction of the spleen, and plasma volume decreases. Urine output decreases to conserve plasma volume, and more concentrated urine is produced. It is important to maintain adequate hydration during exercise to help maintain plasma volume.

Nutrition of the Performance Dog

■ Energy

The energy required increases with exercise and is dependent upon its type and duration. For long-duration exercise, fat is primarily used for energy; sprinting types of exercise use primarily carbohydrates. Sprinting exercise is typically of short duration and not very frequent, therefore the energy requirement is not much higher than that of a normal dog. Thus, diets formulated for sprinting dogs are higher in carbohydrate and lower in fat. Diets for dogs participating in endurance activities are high in fat and lower in carbohydrates. Energy requirements during exercise can be found in Chapter 4.

■ Protein

Protein is not usually used for energy during exercise; carbohydrate and fat sources are preferred fuels. However, protein is used as an energy source when the intensity and duration of exercise exceeds the level of conditioning of the animal. This can happen early in the training period or during performance events. Carbohydrate stores become depleted, and there is a shift to the use of branded-chain amino acids for gluconeogenesis to maintain blood glucose concentration. The branched-chain amino acids (leucine, isoleucine, and valine) are all essential amino acids because they cannot be adequately synthesized from other amino acids. Thus, when protein is used for energy, the essential amino acids must be replaced by the diet. Using protein for energy is not advantageous because there are essentially no "spare" protein stores in the body, and protein provides much less energy per gram as compared to fat.

Diets for the performance dog should contain adequate high-quality protein, but the protein level should not be excessive. When excess proteins are ingested, amino acid breakdown increases because they are not stored. This increase in breakdown produces ketoacids, and the urea produced is excreted in the urine with a loss of body water.

Protein requirements with exercise do not increase to the same degree as do the energy needs. With sprinting activities (racing, coursing), foods should contain 22%–28% protein dry matter (DM), or 20%–25% of calories from protein (Table 9.1). For intermediate levels of exercise (hunting, field trials, tracking, dogs working livestock, etc.) with low to moderate duration and frequency, diets should contain 22%–32% protein DM, or 20%–25% of calories from protein. For intermediate levels of exercise with high duration and frequency, diets should contain 22%–30% protein DM, or 18%–25% of calories from protein. Dogs participating in endurance activities (sled pulling) should be fed diets containing 28%–34% protein DM, or 18%–22% of calories from protein.

Dogs in sprinting events are fed a diet that is highly digestible, high in carbohydrates, low in fat, and moderate in protein. The energy necessary for a sprinting dog is about 1.6 to 2 times the resting energy

Table 9.1. Dietary recommendations for the performance dog.

Nutrient	Dietary Recommendation		
	Sprinting	Intermediate Exercise	Endurance
Protein	22%–28% DM; 20%–25% total kcal	Low to moderate work: 22%–32% DM; 20%–25% total kcal Strenuous work: 22%–30% DM; 18%–25% total kcal	28%–34% DM; 18%–22% total kcal
Carbohydrate	50%–70% total kcal	Moderate work: ≤45% total kcal Strenuous work: ≤50% total kcal	≤15% total kcal
Fat	8%–10% DM; 20%–24% total kcal	Moderate work: 15%–30% DM; 30%–55% total kcal Strenuous work: 25%–40% DM; 45%–65% total kcal	≥50% DM; 75% total kcal
Calcium	1.2%–2.0% DM	1.2%–2.0% DM	1.2%–2.0% DM
Magnesium	0.12% DM	0.12% DM	0.12% DM

DM, dry matter.

required. A small amount of food should be provided more than 4 hours before the event, and a small high-carbohydrate meal should be fed within 30 minutes after the event to replenish glycogen stores. Frequent access to water should be provided, except just before racing.

For dogs participating in intermediate-level events, the diet depends on the stage of training and work. If the dog is not working or training, then feed as an adult dog. Training should start approximately 6 weeks prior to working. At this time, a highly digestible, moderate-carbohydrate, moderate-protein, and moderate- to high-fat diet should be fed. While working, the energy requirements may be two to five times the resting energy required, depending on the duration, frequency, and intensity of the work. Feeding should occur either after exercise or more than 4 hours prior to exercise. A small amount of food should be given either during exercise or at the end of breaks, less than 15 minutes before returning to exercise. There should be free access to water, and hydration status should be monitored frequently.

Dogs participating in endurance events can have very high energy requirements, from 5 to 11 times the resting energy normally required. Thus, a very energy-dense diet should be fed to meet the caloric needs. The diet should be highly digestible, high in fat, low in carbohydrate, and moderate in protein. Dogs should be fed after exercise or more than 4 hours before exercise. Small amounts of food can be given during exercise or after exercise. Dogs should have free access to water.

■ Carbohydrate

Carbohydrates are an important source of energy for sprinting dogs such as racing greyhounds. Energy must be quickly metabolized to run a race, and greyhounds rapidly use muscle glycogen as a source of energy. This ratio of energy production depends upon the amount of glycogen in muscle, and muscle glycogen can be altered by diet and training. Diets high in carbohydrates should provide about 50%–70% of the total calories in the diet to maximize glycogen stores in muscle. Moderate amounts of carbohydrate should be given to sprinting dogs within 30 minutes after exercise to allow rapid repletion of glycogen. A glucose solution is usually given during this period.

For intermediate levels of exercise, the optimal amount of dietary carbohydrates is quite variable. If a dog is performing high-intensity work in short bursts, then carbohydrates should provide up to 50% of the dietary calories. Dogs performing longer periods of moderate-intensity work should be fed approximately 45% of their dietary calories from carbohydrates.

Dogs participating in endurance events require very little carbohydrate in the diet. Diets for endurance dogs should provide less than 15% of calories from carbohydrate. Small amounts of carbohydrate need to be provided to maintain good stool quality and avoid diarrhea.

Ingredients providing carbohydrates should be highly digestible to decrease stool volume. Increased amounts of carbohydrate present in the colon increase fecal water loss, and "stress" diarrhea can occur. Increased stool volume also results in extra weight, which can hinder performance.

■ **Fat**

Fat is more energy dense than either protein or carbohydrates and therefore is important in increasing the energy density of the diet. Increasing the fat content helps to increase palatability, which is also important for the performance dog. Hard-working dogs may require a very high amount of calories to meet their energy needs; in some cases, sled dogs may require as many as 10,000 kcal per day. Diets designed for these dogs must be highly digestible, be highly palatable, and contain high amounts of fat. Even with intermediate exercise, increased dietary fat provides increased dietary energy.

High levels of dietary fat can increase endurance. In trained athletes, free fatty acid (FFA) oxidation provides an increased amount of energy. When dogs are fed high-fat diets, FFA concentrations are increased and thus are more available for oxidation and energy production. Insulin concentrations are also lower in dogs fed high-fat diets, which decreases FFA release from adipose tissue. Performance dogs fed high-fat diets have better endurance. High-fat diets can be tolerated if they are introduced gradually.

For the performance dog, about 2% DM should be essential fatty acids. A combination of both saturated and unsaturated fats should be fed. Unsaturated fatty acids are important for membrane fluidity and are required for hormone synthesis and the integrity of the skin. Long-chain omega-3 fatty acids may enhance oxygen uptake. However, a high intake of unsaturated fatty acids may increase lipid peroxidation of membranes, which can damage cell membranes. If a high concentration of unsaturated fatty acids is fed, then an increased level of vitamin E should be provided as an antioxidant. Medium-chain triglyceride (MCT) supplementation may enhance performance because it may increase the rate of FFA oxidation. MCTs are not very palatable, and further research is needed to evaluate the affect of MCT on performance.

For sprinting dogs, fat content should be 8%–10% DM or should provide 20%–24% of dietary calories. For intermediate-level work, dietary fat content depends on the intensity and duration of work. Dogs in the off-season should be fed as a normal adult dog, but fat content should increase as work increases. With moderate work, fat should provide 15%–30% DM, or 30%–55% of total dietary calories. With more strenuous work, 25%–40% DM, or 45%–65% of total calories, should be provided by dietary fat. Endurance athletes should be fed a level of fat greater than 50% DM, or 75% of total calories.

■ Water

Water is the most important of all nutrients. About 64% of body water is located in cells and 7% in the plasma. Water balance is increased by water intake and water production during metabolism and decreased by water loss in urine, feces, and sweat. During exercise, muscles need to have an increase in nutrients and waste removal. Blood flow and cardiac output will increase in exercise, which helps to get rid of the heat generated by muscles; about 75% of muscles' work produces heat. With exercise, especially in warm and humid climates, there is a decrease in total body water due to heat dissipation, primarily through evaporation in the respiratory tract. This loss of body water can lead to dehydration, which has a significant impact on performance and endurance. Under most circumstances, the performance dog loses more water than electrolytes, which decreases plasma volume. To prevent dehydration, fresh, clean water should be available at all times; if this is not possible, water should be offered at least three times daily. Flavoring may be added to water to promote intake.

■ Vitamins and Minerals

The requirement for some vitamins and minerals increase with exercise. B-complex vitamins and vitamin C requirements increase because they are used as cofactors for enzymes and for collagen synthesis. There may also be an increased loss of water-soluble vitamins due to loss of body water. Even though there is no concrete evidence showing the necessity for increase in water-soluble vitamins during exercise, it is generally safe to supplement these vitamins because excesses are typically excreted in urine. Fat-soluble vitamins, especially vitamins A and D, on the other hand, should not be supplemented, since excesses of these vitamins are stored in fat and can lead to toxicity. However, supplementation with vitamin E may be beneficial as an antioxidant, especially when diets high in polyunsaturated fatty acids are fed.

The calcium/phosphorus ratio is important in diets for the performance dog. A high dietary fat content decreases the amount of digestible calcium. Dietary calcium should be 1.2%–2.0% of the diet. Excess calcium should be avoided since this can inhibit the absorption of zinc. Magnesium should also be fed at 0.12% of the diet.

Sodium may also be lost via saliva in exercising dogs, especially in hot and humid climates. The loss of sodium should stimulate thirst and cause conservation of water by the kidneys. Electrolyte solutions may be popular, but there is debate as to their usefulness. Some electrolyte solutions may actually lead to GI discomfort, diarrhea, and further dehydration.

Feeding Strategies—When to Feed

Diets need to be fed at a time that allows maximal absorption to occur, yet doesn't interfere with performance. Dogs should be fed more than 4 hours prior to exercise. Dogs fed closer to exercise have a higher body temperature during exercise, which is caused by heat released by digestion. This decreases circulation to the skin and can lower heat dissipation during exercise. Dogs fed within a few hours of exercise also use more glucose and less fat. The insulin release caused by a meal decreases the use of fat and promotes carbohydrate use, leading to depletion of glycogen stores. When food is given more than 4 hours before exercise, emptying of the bowel is also promoted. This helps prevent the development of stress-induced diarrhea.

Feeding should also occur within 2 hours after exercise. Glycogen synthesis is more rapid in the immediate postexercise period. Feeding during this time period helps to replete glycogen stores, especially in those undergoing strenuous exercise on consecutive days.

Poorly conditioned hunting dogs can experience "hunting dog hypoglycemia." In this condition, dogs begin working normally, but become weak and have tremors that can progress to injuries or death. Feeding more than 4 hours prior to the start of hunting helps to lower the insulin level by the time exercise starts. Feeding a small amount of food during exercise may also help to better maintain glucose homeostasis in these dogs.

When switching to a diet designed for performance, it can take 6 weeks of feeding to maximize the effects of these diets. Changes in muscle and oxidative capacity take time; training and the change to a performance diet should occur 6 weeks before the exercise event.

For dogs in sprinting events, feed a diet that is highly digestible, high in carbohydrate, low in fat, and moderate in protein. The energy recovery requirements for a sprinting dog are about 1.6–2 times the resting energy required. A small amount of food should be provided more than 4 hours before the event, and a small high-carbohydrate meal should be fed within 30 minutes after the event to replenish glycogen stores. Free access to water should be provided, except just before racing.

For dogs participating in intermediate-level events, the diet depends on the stage of training and work. If the dog is not working or training, then feed as an adult dog. Training should start approximately 6 weeks prior to working. At this time, a highly digestible, moderate-carbohydrate, moderate-protein, and moderate- to high-fat diet should be fed. While working, the energy requirements may be two to five times the resting energy required, depending on the duration, frequency, and intensity of the work. Feeding should occur either after exercise or more than 4 hours prior to exercise. A small amount of food should be given either during exercise or at the end of breaks less than 15 minutes before returning to exercise. There should be free access to water, and hydration status should be monitored frequently.

Dogs participating in endurance events can have very high energy requirements, from 5 to 11 times the resting energy required. Thus, a very energy-dense diet should be fed to meet the caloric needs. The diet should be highly digestible, and high in fat, low in carbohydrate, and moderate in protein. Dogs should be fed after exercise or more than 4 hours before exercise. Small amounts of food can be given during exercise or after exercise. Dogs should have free access to water.

Recipes for Sprinting Dogs

Pork and Potato   304
Chicken and Pasta   305

Recipes for Dogs Doing Moderate Work

Ground Beef and Potato   306
Chicken and Barley   307

Recipes for Dogs Doing Strenuous Work

Salmon and Pasta   308
Ground Beef and Rice   309

Recipes for Dogs in Endurance Events

Ground Beef and Rice   310

Additional Reading

Case LP, Carey DP, Hirakawa DA, Daristotle L (Eds). 2000. Performance and stress. In *Canine and Feline Nutrition: A Resource for Companion Animal Professionals*, 2nd edition. Mosby, St. Louis, pp. 259–274.

Toll PW, Reynolds AJ. 2000. The canine athlete. In *Small Animal Clinical Nutrition*, 4th edition. Hand MS, Thatcher CD, Remillard RL, Roudebush P (Eds). Mark Morris Institute, Topeka, KS, pp. 261–290.

CHAPTER 10
Food Intolerance and Allergy

An abnormal response to an ingested food is termed an *adverse reaction* to food. Adverse reactions to food can have an immunological or a nonimmunological cause. Immunological causes of adverse reactions include food anaphylaxis and food allergy. Nonimmunological causes include dietary indiscretion and food intolerance (metabolic food reaction, food poisoning, food idiosyncrasy, pharmacological reaction to food).

The incidence of adverse reactions to food is unknown but probably accounts for about 62% of all skin diseases seen in a general veterinary practice. Approximately 23% of all dogs with allergic skin disease are actually allergic to some ingredient in the diet. About 25% of those dogs are also allergic to substances other than food, such as ragweed or fleas. Adverse food reactions appear to be more common in cats, and food allergy is the third most common allergic skin disease in dogs and cats after flea hypersensitivity and atopy.

Clinical Signs of Food Allergy

Food allergy may occur at any age, but most cases occur after the pet has been exposed to the particular food for 2 or more years. It is not uncommon for a pet to suddenly become allergic to the food it has been eating routinely for several years. Up to one third of food allergy cases may occur in dogs under 1 year of age. Dog breeds that appear to be at increased risk for development of food allergy include cocker spaniels, springer spaniels, Labrador retrievers, golden retrievers, collies, miniature schnauzers, Chinese Shar-Pei, West Highland white terriers, soft-coated wheaten terriers, boxers, dachshunds, Dalmatians, Lhasa apsos, and German shepherd dogs.

Dogs with food allergies can start showing clinical signs at any time of year, and it is usually a constant problem. However, food allergy can be episodic when the pet eats the offending food only periodically, such as a particular type of treat or rawhide chew. Food allergies typically cause itching (pruritus), which can vary in severity. Pruritus may be accompanied by gastrointestinal (GI) signs. Signs of itchy skin will appear within several hours after eating the offending food. Dogs fed in the morning may tend to scratch more in the afternoon or early evening. Dogs fed in the early evening may scratch all night. Pruritus is most common on the feet, face, armpits, inguinal region, rump, and ears. About 25% of dogs with food allergy will only have signs of itchy ears.

Food anaphylaxis is an acute reaction to ingestion of food. Swelling of the lips, face, eyelids, ears, conjunctiva, and tongue occurs (angioedema) and may or may not be pruritic. Hives can also occur within minutes of food ingestion.

Cats usually develop food allergies by 2 years of age, although onset ranges from 6 months to 12 years. Siamese cats are at increased risk. Pruritus is most common, although up to 33% of cats with food allergy have angioedema. Lymph nodes are enlarged in about 33% of cats with food allergy, and an increase in circulating eosinophils is seen in 20%–50% of feline cases.

Chinese Shar-Peis and German shepherd dogs are at increased risk for the development of GI signs with food allergy. Food allergy can affect all segments of the GI tract, including the stomach, small intestine, and large intestine. Vomiting and diarrhea are common, and the diarrhea may be profuse and watery, mucoid, or bloody. Abdominal pain may also be present. About 15% of dogs and cats with skin signs also have GI signs. Inflammatory bowel disease (IBD) may in part be associated with food allergy. Inflammation of the intestinal mucosa may predispose the pet to development of food allergy.

Causes of Food Allergy

The GI tract of the dog and cat is essentially a large tube lined with cells that control the absorption of nutrients from food. These cells also protect the body against injury from a number of harmful substances. This defense system includes an effective mucosal barrier and the immune system of the gut-associated lymphoid tissue (GALT). The gut is one of the largest immune organs in the body. Certain immune cells (B lymphocytes) produce antibodies such as IgG and IgE. These immunoglobulins protect against invasion by bacteria and parasites and control the absorption of antigens that can stimulate antibody production.

In the normal dog, the ingestion of a particular food causes a very small amount of IgE to be released. This small amount of IgE is quickly controlled by other cells of the immune system. However, in the allergic dog, a much larger amount of IgE is produced in response to a particular food. The immune system cannot control this large amount of produced IgE, and clinical signs of food allergy occur. The amount of IgE produced depends on a number of factors, including the genetic predisposition to allergy and the length of time the dog has been exposed to the offending food. The large quantity of IgE produced stimulates the breakdown of mast cells, which are present in the skin and gut. These mast cells release a number of irritating substances that can cause itchy skin and diarrhea.

Food Allergens

Almost any diet ingredient can cause an allergic response. The most common allergen is a protein with a molecular weight between 10,000 and 60,000 daltons. In dogs, allergies to beef, dairy products, or fish account for about 89% of food allergies.

■ Gluten (Gliadin) Enteropathy

Gluten intolerance affects Irish setters and possibly other breeds of dogs. Cereal grains contain some proteins; in wheat, two of these proteins are gliadin and glutenin. Gluten is a mixture of gliadin and glutenin. Normally, pancreatic enzymes digest gluten, rendering it nontoxic. In gluten-sensitive dogs, increased intestinal permeability occurs prior to development of gluten sensitivity. Macrophages can be activated by gliadin and cause a delayed hypersensitivity reaction.

Food Intolerance

Food intolerance includes food poisoning, reactions to vasoactive amines, and carbohydrate intolerance. Food poisoning and reactions to vasoactive amines such as histamine have been discussed in Chapter 2.

Carbohydrate intolerance is typically due to lactose intolerance. When pets with lactose intolerance consume milk products, diarrhea, bloating, and abdominal discomfort can occur. Puppies and kittens usually have adequate levels of intestinal lactose so that lactose can be digested. After weaning, these levels of lactose greatly decrease, and lactose may not be able to be digested. Goat and cow milk contain a much higher level of lactose than does milk from dams or queens, thus puppies fed cow or goat milk can also exhibit diarrhea due to the excess lactose that cannot be digested. There are most likely a small number of puppies and kittens that are born with metabolic defects in lactose digestion. These puppies and kittens have diarrhea during the neonatal period and typically fail to survive.

Some pets may be intolerant of disaccharides, especially secondary to enteritis. With enteritis, the intestinal brush border is altered, and loss of disaccharidase activity contributes to the diarrhea. Disaccharidase activity can take several days to increase after a change in ingested carbohydrate. Thus, pets can have acute diarrhea for several days if a rapid change to a high-carbohydrate diet is made.

Dietary Modification in Food Allergy

To determine the offending allergen, elimination trials are conducted. An elimination diet should include only one or two sources of novel proteins and should be nutritionally balanced and complete. Excess protein should be avoided, and the protein should be highly digestible. Digestibility is important as complete digestion of a protein results in amino acids that are poor antigens. The protein sources should be proteins to which the pet has not previously been exposed. Ingredients typically recommended for homemade dog foods include lamb, rice, potato, fish, rabbit, venison, or tofu. Ingredients recommended for cats include lamb, rice, rabbit, or venison.

Prior to starting an elimination trial, the pet should be fed the usual diet for 7–14 days, during which time a record should be kept detailing all foods and treats fed and the occurrence of adverse reactions. Then the elimination diet is fed for 4–12 weeks. During this time, no other foods or treats should be fed. If clinical signs of skin allergy decrease, then a diagnosis of food allergy is made. At this time, single ingredients fed previously can be reintroduced into the diet to see whether clinical signs of allergy recur. In cases where GI signs are the predominant allergic signs, an elimination diet can be fed for a shorter period of time (2–4 weeks).

Fatty Acids and Inflammatory Skin Disease

Macrophages are present in the skin and are the most significant source of inflammatory mediators. Alteration of the inflammatory mediators produced can modify the inflammatory response. Arachidonic acid (an omega-6 fatty acid) is the predominant polyunsaturated fatty acid (PUFA) present in macrophages. Certain leukotrienes and prostaglandins are produced from arachidonic acid in macrophages, and these substances are very strong inflammatory mediators. Consumption of omega-3 fatty acids (such as found in fish oil) can partially replace the arachidonic acid in macrophages with long-chain omega-3 fatty acids such as eicosapentaenoic acid (EPA). Other leukotrienes and prostaglandins are produced from EPA, and these substances are less inflammatory than those produced from arachidonic acid. During an inflammatory episode, fewer strong inflammatory mediators are produced. Thus, the inflammatory response is reduced. There are limited studies evaluating dose and effect, but a dose of 1 g fish oil/10 lb body weight appears to be safe for dogs and cats. About 50% of dogs and cats with allergic skin disease will improve with omega-3 fatty acid supplementation if other contributing diseases, such as flea allergy or bacterial skin disease, is controlled.

Dog Recipes for Allergies

Cat Recipes for Allergies

Additional Reading

Biourge VC, Fontaine J, Vroom MW. 2004. Diagnosis of adverse reactions to food in dogs: Efficacy of a soy-isolate hydrolyzate-based diet. J Nutr 134:2062S–2064S.

Case LP, Carey DP, Hirakawa DA, Daristotle L (Eds). 2000. Nutritionally responsive dermatoses. In *Canine and Feline Nutrition: A Resource for Companion Animal Professionals*, 2nd edition. Mosby, St. Louis, pp. 429–450.

Cave NJ. 2008. Nutrition and immunity. In *Encyclopedia of Feline Clinical Nutrition*. Pibot P, Biourge V, Elliott D (Eds.). Aniwa SAS, Aimargues France, pp. 480–509.

Cave NJ. 2006. Hydrolyzed protein diets for dogs and cats. Vet Clin Small Anim 36: 1251–1268.

Guilford WG, Jones BR, Markwell PJ, Arthur DG, Collett MG, Harte JG. 2001. Food sensitivity in cats with chronic idiopathic gastrointestinal problems. J Vet Intern Med 15:7–13.

Leistra MHG, Markwell PJ, Willemse T. 2001. Evaluation of selected-protein-source diets for management of dogs with adverse reactions to foods. J Am Vet Med Assoc 219:1411–1414.

Roudebush P, Guilford WG, Shanley KJ. 2000. Adverse reactions to food. In *Small Animal Clinical Nutrition*, 4th edition. Hand MS, Thatcher CD, Remillard RL, Roudebush P (Eds). Mark Morris Institute, Topeka, KS, pp. 431–454.

Saker KE. 2006. Nutrition and immune function. Vet Clin Small Anim 36:1199–1224.

Verlinden A, Hesta M, Millet S, Janssens GP. 2006. Food allergy in dogs and cats: A review. Crit Rev Food Sci Nutr 46(3):259–273.

CHAPTER 11
Obesity

Obesity is a common problem in pets. It has been estimated that 40% of dogs and 30% of cats are obese. Pets that are less than 10% above ideal weight are considered to be "above optimal" weight, pets between 10% and 20% above ideal weight are considered overweight, and those 20% or more above ideal body weight are obese. Overweight and obese pets typically have an increase in body fat. Pets in optimal body condition have 15%–20% body fat.

Health Risks of Obesity

There are a number of conditions associated with or exacerbated by obesity. Obese dogs have a reduction in longevity. In a group of Labrador retrievers, energy restriction prolonged life to an average of 13 years compared to 11 years in the group that was not energy restricted. The energy-restricted group weighed an average of 26% less than the nonrestricted group.

Orthopedic disorders are common in obese pets. Obesity in large-breed puppies during growth promotes the development of orthopedic problems and can exacerbate hip dysplasia. Torn cruciate ligaments are more common in overweight dogs, and overweight cats are five times more likely to limp compared to cats of normal body weight.

The frequency of cardiovascular disorders increases with obesity; heart rhythm, ventricle volume, and plasma volume increase. The correlation between hypertension and obesity is controversial. In dogs there is a correlation between obesity and tracheal collapse.

Obesity is a major risk factor for diabetes mellitus in cats. Insulin controls the uptake of glucose by cells, and obese cats have significantly reduced sensitivity to insulin. Insulin resistance may also occur in obese dogs fed diets high in fats.

In humans there are correlations between obesity and certain types of cancer (breast, uterus, colon, and prostate). However, in dogs and cats there have been no clear associations between obesity and any type of cancer.

Obese cats may be more likely to suffer from diarrhea. In cats there is a strong association between hepatic lipidosis and obesity. Obese cats that undergo rapid weight loss are at risk for development of hepatic lipidosis. Hepatic lipidosis is characterized by accumulation of fat in the liver, which leads to cholestasis and liver dysfunction. Hepatic lipidosis is further discussed in Chapter 20, Diet and Hepatic Disease.

Risk Factors

The prevalence of obesity is influenced by a number of factors. Dog breeds that appear to be at higher risk for the development of obesity include the Saint Bernard, Bernese mountain dog, Newfoundland, Labrador retriever, collie, golden retriever, Rottweiler, beagle, cocker spaniel, basset hound, Cairn terrier, dachshund, Cavalier King Charles spaniel, and Scottish terrier. Dogs at decreased risk of obesity include Doberman pinscher, German shepherd, greyhound, and Yorkshire terrier. Mixed-breed cats are predisposed to obesity. Genetic factors in the development of obesity are poorly understood.

In dogs, the frequency of obesity increases with age; however, the frequency of obese dogs decreases in dogs over 12 years of age. The prevalence of obesity in cats is highest in cats between 5 and 11 years of age. Cats over 13 years of age have a decreased incidence of obesity.

In dogs, intact females are more predisposed to obesity than are intact males. In cats, intact males appear to have a higher incidence as compared to intact females. In both cats and dogs, neutering increases the frequency of obesity. The increase in obesity after neutering may be due to a combination of factors, including a decrease in activity and an increase in food intake due to a change in circulating hormone concentrations.

Decreased activity is also a primary factor in the development of obesity. The duration of daily exercise is directly correlated to the incidence of obesity. Dogs living in apartments have a higher risk of obesity than do those living outdoors.

Interactions with owners also have an impact on the incidence of obesity. Owners of obese pets tend to humanize their pets more, spend more time talking to their pets, allow them to sleep on the bed, and spend more time watching their pet eat. Obese pets also tend to receive more treats than do pets of normal body weight.

Regulation of Body Weight

There are a number of hormones that regulate appetite, food consumption, and energy expenditure. These hormones are currently the focus of many research studies and include leptin, adiponectin, ghrelin, and cholecystokinin. Results of many of these studies have been confusing, and considerably more research is needed.

Leptin is secreted by fat cells and plays a role in the regulation of food consumption. Leptin decreases food consumption and was initially thought to be a miracle cure for obesity. However, obese individuals do not have a deficiency in leptin; obese individuals actually have higher levels of leptin due to increased secretion by fat. Obese individuals appear to be resistant to the effects of leptin.

Ghrelin (GH-releasing hormone) stimulates the secretion of growth hormone (GH), which increases food consumption. However, the concentration of ghrelin is actually lower in obese animals as compared to animals of normal body weight.

Adiponectin is also secreted by fat cells and plays a role in carbohydrate metabolism, insulin sensitivity, and energy homeostasis. Adiponectin expression is decreased in obese animals.

Cholecystokinin (CCK) is released in response to protein and fat in the diet and acts to decrease the appetite. However, when CCK is administered to patients, it does not appear to decrease appetite over time.

Evaluation of Obesity

Objective measurement of obesity is challenging, especially in dogs with their tremendous range of normal body size, depending on breed. The first step is to obtain the current body weight and then to determine an optimal body weight. A relative body weight can be calculated by dividing the current body weight by the optimal body weight. This can give an estimate of the level of obesity.

Body condition scoring is a subjective assessment of body fat composition. Body condition scoring can be assessed using a 5-point or a 9-point scale. Body condition scoring is discussed in more detail in Chapter 4. Briefly, on a 5-point scale, a body condition score (BCS) of 3 represents the middle of the optimal range, with BCS of 1 or 2 representing underweight pets, and BCS of 4 or 5 representing overweight or obese pets. On a 9-point scale, BCS of 5 is the middle of the optimal body weight range, with BCS of 1–4 representing varying degrees of underweight pets, and BCS of 6–9 representing overweight/obese pets. A pet with a BCS of 3 on a 5-point scale has about 20% body fat, and a BCS of 4 suggests about 30% body fat.

Body measurements can also be used to calculate the percentage of body fat. In the dog, the hock-to-stifle length is measured, along with the pelvic circumference. In the cat, the body length from nose to pelvis is measured, along with the right forelimb length, right hindlimb length, pelvic circumference, and thoracic circumference. These measurements are then used in complicated formulas to calculate the estimated percentage of body fat. The measurements must be made in exact positions, which can be difficult, especially in cats or uncooperative pets.

Weight-Reduction Plan

For obesity to develop, the caloric intake has to exceed the daily calorie expenditure over a period of time. A weight-reduction program includes determining the amount of weight to lose, determining daily caloric intake for weight loss, selecting a diet, determining the amount of exercise, monitoring progress, adjusting caloric intake as needed, and preventing regaining of lost weight. An estimate of daily caloric intake for weight loss in dogs can be found in Table 4-3, and the estimate of daily caloric intake for weight loss in cats can be obtained from Table 4-17. The calories estimated for weight loss should be compared with the calories currently being consumed to ensure that the calculated calories are less than what is being eaten.

When feeding for weight loss, treats and snacks should be eliminated. If treats are going to be fed, then low-calorie snacks such as vegetables (broccoli, carrots, cauliflower, etc.), popcorn without butter, or ice cubes could be given. Calories supplied by treats need to be taken into account in the daily calories allowed. Multiple meals should be fed each day rather than one large meal.

Starvation has been used to induce weight loss in dogs, but dogs should be hospitalized and given only water plus vitamin and mineral supplements under the direct supervision of a veterinarian. Starvation cannot be used for weight loss in cats due to the risk of developing hepatic lipidosis. Starvation leads to protein deficiency, with a loss of lean muscle mass. Starvation should *not* be used at home to achieve weight loss in dogs or cats.

After a weight-loss program has begun, the pet should be weighed after 2 weeks. If there has been a loss of 0.5%–2% body weight per week, then the current program can be continued and the pet weighed again in 2–4 weeks. Weight loss should not be more than 2% per week because a greater proportion of lean body mass will be lost if more than that is lost during that time period. If weight loss has been less, continue with the program but reweigh in 1–2 weeks. If the body weight has increased, then decrease the calories fed by 10%–20% or increase exercise and reweigh in 1–2 weeks.

Diets for Weight Loss

Energy restriction cannot be achieved by simply feeding less of the current diet. Some restriction of a particular diet will result in deficiencies of essential nutrients. A diet specifically designed for weight reduction should be fed to limit energy intake and to ensure that essential nutrients are provided.

The energy content of the diet for weight loss should be reduced, and this is typically accomplished by limiting the amount of fat in the diet. Recommendations for energy density and fat content for diets are given in Table 11.1. The protein content of diets for weight loss is typically higher than in diets for maintenance. This is necessary to provide

Table 11.1. Dietary recommendations for weight loss in dogs and cats.

Factor	Dog	Cat
Energy	Food should contain <3.4 kcal ME/g DM	Food should contain <3.6 kcal ME/g DM
Protein	>25% DM	>35% DM
Fat	5%–12% DM	7–14% DM
Fiber	Up to 30% DM	Up to 20% DM
Carbohydrate	<55% DM	<45% DM

DM, dry matter; ME, metabolizable energy.

essential amino acids. High-protein diets help to maintain muscle mass and facilitate the loss of fat. Proteins provide the same amount of metabolizable energy as do carbohydrates, but excess protein is not stored as fat. In addition, proteins do not induce much insulin secretion, thus preventing hypoglycemia and the feeling of hunger.

The use of fiber in weight-reduction diets is debated. The addition of dietary fiber dilutes the energy density of the diet, and fiber at a level of 20% dry matter (DM) will reduce the voluntary intake of the diet. Increasing the fiber content increases the fecal quantity and frequency of defecation. It can also decrease the digestibility of proteins and minerals and decrease the palatability of the diet. Increasing dietary fiber may cause flatulence and diarrhea. Increasing dietary fiber can have some benefits for weight loss but is not necessary for weight loss to occur.

Dog Recipes for Weight Loss

Cat Recipes for Weight Loss

Additional Reading

Bierer TL, Bui LM. 2004. High-protein low-carbohydrate diets enhance weight loss in dogs. J Nutr 134:2087S–2089S.

Burkholder WJ, Toll PW. 2000. Obesity. In *Small Animal Clinical Nutrition*, 4th edition. Hand MS, Thatcher CD, Remillard RL, Roudebush P (Eds). Mark Morris Institute, Topeka, KS, pp. 401–430.

Case LP, Carey DP, Hirakawa DA, Daristotle L (Eds). 2000. Obesity. In *Canine and Feline Nutrition: A Resource for Companion Animal Professionals*, 2nd edition. Mosby, St. Louis, pp. 303–330.

Diez M, Nguyen P. 2006. Obesity: Epidemiology, pathophysiology and management of the obese dog. In *Encyclopedia of Canine Clinical Nutrition*. Pibot P, Biourge V, Elliott D (Eds). Aniwa SAS, Aimargues, France, pp. 2–57.

German A, Martin L. 2008. Feline obesity: Epidemiology, pathophysiology and management. In *Encyclopedia of Feline Clinical Nutrition*. Pibot P, Biourge V, Elliott D (Eds). Aniwa SAS, Aimargues, France, pp. 3–49.

German AJ, Holden SL, Bissot T, Hackett RM, Biourge V. 2007. Dietary energy restriction and successful weight loss in obese client-owned dogs. J Vet Intern Med 21(6):1174–1180.

Laflamme DP. 2006. Understanding and managing obesity in dogs and cats. Vet Clin North Am Small Anim Pract 36(6):1283–1295.

Weber M, Bissot T, Servet E, Sergheraert R, Biourge V, German AJ. 2007. A high-protein, high-fiber diet designed for weight loss improves satiety in dogs. J Vet Intern Med 21(6):1203–1208.

CHAPTER 12
Skeletal and Joint Diseases

Skeletal and joint diseases are common in dogs, affecting about 25% of dogs overall. In young dogs less than 1 year of age, about 22% have skeletal or joint disease. The term *developmental orthopedic disease* (DOD) refers to a number of disorders affecting young, fast-growing large-breed dogs. Hip dysplasia (HD), elbow dysplasia, and osteochondrosis are common skeletal and joint problems potentially caused by excessive nutrition. Nutritional deficiencies can also cause skeletal and joint problems. The most common problems due to deficiencies are nutritional secondary hyperparathyroidism and rickets.

Bone and Cartilage Composition

Bone contains 25% water, 10% cells, and 65% inorganic material. About 99% of total body calcium and 80% of total body phosphorus are present in bone. Even though bone is solid, it is a very dynamic organ, with new bone forming and bone resorbing constantly. Thus, bone can serve as a large reservoir of calcium in the body. Cartilage contains 70% water and 30% cells. The matrix of cartilage includes glycosaminoglycans (GAGs). Keratin sulfate and chondroitin sulfate are the most important glycosaminoglycans.

Impact of Nutrition on Bone and Joints

In young growing animals, excessive energy intake results in a more rapid rate of growth. Overfeeding puppies causes rapid bone length growth and rapid weight gain. The increased weight adds more stress to the skeleton and joints, which can lead to the development of osteochondrosis, hip dysplasia, and elbow dysplasia. Overnutrition is especially problematic in large-breed puppies, which can experience a considerable rate of growth. Restricting the feeding of large-breed puppies does not impact final body size. High-protein diets (30% DM) do not increase the risk of skeletal or joint problems in giant-breed dogs. Thus, high-protein diets can be fed to growing puppies and help supply the necessary energy. In adults, overfeeding leads to excess body fat and obesity. Obesity is common and occurs in about 28%–44% of dogs. Skeletal and joint disorders are commonly found in obese dogs.

Excess calcium intake can also cause skeletal and joint abnormalities. Dietary calcium is absorbed in the small intestine, and puppies less than 6 months of age lack the physiological mechanisms to prevent excess calcium absorption. Thus, young puppies can absorb about 50% of the calcium present in the diet. When dietary calcium is absorbed, the hormone calcitonin is released to prevent a sharp increase in serum calcium. Calcitonin acts on bone to prevent resorption, and remodeling of bone cannot occur. Chronic excesses of dietary calcium cause chronic high levels of calcitonin, with an overall decrease in bone remodeling. Thus, there is a disturbance in the normal mineralization of bone. Safe calcium intake appears to be 260–830 mg calcium/kg/day at 2 months of age and 210–540 mg calcium/kg/day at 5 months of age.

Excess phosphorus intake can impact calcium metabolism and bone development. Excess phosphorus intake is common in pets fed all-meat diets. The increase in phosphorus decreases the calcium/phosphorus ratio and can lead to nutritional secondary hyperparathyroidism and bone fractures. However, in young growing dogs, the absolute intake of calcium appears to be more important than the calcium/phosphorus ratio.

Copper is important for maintenance of connective tissue. Copper deficiency can cause growth deformities, fractures, and widening of joints in young growing dogs. Homemade diets must be formulated with adequate copper since many ingredients are low in this element.

Zinc deficiency in young growing animals can lead to depression of growth, skin defects, and impaired immune function. Diets for growing puppies should contain adequate zinc to prevent zinc deficiency.

Both deficiency and excess of dietary vitamin A can cause severe bone disease in growing dogs. Excess dietary vitamin A leads to thin bones, decreased appetite, and decreased weight gain. Vitamin A deficiency results in weight loss, decreased appetite, and disturbances in bone remodeling.

Vitamin C is important in the formation of cartilage; however, diets deficient in vitamin C do not cause skeletal problems. Excess vitamin C from supplementation can enhance calcium absorption, leading to excess calcium, which could increase the risk for skeletal disorders. Dogs do not require vitamin C, and supplementation is not recommended.

Disorders Due to Nutritional Excesses

■ Hip Dysplasia

Hip dysplasia (HD) is a common disorder that is heritable. Dogs with HD are born with normal hips, but HD develops, usually by 6 months of age, due to different rates of development of bones and the supporting muscles, ligaments, and joint capsule.

Some breeds have an increased incidence of HD, including Rottweilers, St. Bernards, German shepherds, Bernese mountain dogs, Labrador retrievers, and Golden retrievers. Clinical signs of HD include pain when getting up, decreased range of motion, lameness of the hind limbs, and a "bunny-hopping" gait. Clinical signs may be worse at the start of exercise and get better as exercise progresses. Signs may get worse with rest after exercise. Radiographs of the hips are necessary for diagnosis and can identify the joint laxity and bony changes present.

The head of the thigh bone (femur) normally sits into the hip socket (acetabulum). Both the head of the femur and acetabulum are mostly cartilage at birth. If the hip joint is loose, with increased laxity, the head of the femur touches the acetabulum, causing abnormal pressures. This causes small fractures in the acetabulum and improper formation of bone. Excess body weight increases the load on the hip joints and can increase the severity of HD. Excess calcium intake alters the proper maturation of the skeleton and plays a role in the deformation of the hip joint. Electrolyte balance may also be important in the development of HD. Diets creating acidosis have detrimental effects on skeletal formation. Excess vitamin D has a negative impact on ossification of bone and can lead to deformation of the hip joint.

HD may not be preventable, but signs and severity can be minimized. Puppies should be kept lean, and overfeeding and obesity should be avoided. The calcium content of the diet should be appropriate and not excessive. Diets designed and balanced for young growing dogs should not be supplemented with excessive calcium.

Once HD has developed, weight loss and maintenance of proper body weight will help minimize the clinical signs. Surgery may be an option in selected cases.

■ Elbow Dysplasia

There are a number of disorders that comprise elbow dysplasia (ED), including osteochondritis dissecans (OCD), ununited anconeal process, and fragmented coronoid process. Most dogs with ED are less than 1 year of age and have a "turning out" of the affected front leg. There may be pain on motion of the joint, lameness, and a decreased range of motion. Radiographs are necessary for diagnosis. Many cases of ED affect both front legs.

Breeds at increased risk of ED include Rottweilers, Bernese mountain dogs, Labrador retrievers, golden retrievers, Newfoundlands, German shepherds, St. Bernards, bloodhounds, Bouvier des Flandres, and chow chows. Overfeeding and excessive calcium intake can contribute to the severity of ED. Once ED is present, surgery and weight loss may improve ED.

■ Osteochondrosis

With osteochondrosis, there is abnormal maturation of chondrocytes with a delay in the mineralization of cartilage. The cartilage is retained and becomes thick; this cartilage can detach and may fragment or become mineralized. If articular cartilage is involved, osteochondritis dissecans (OCD) may result. OCD is seen primarily in giant breeds. If growth plates are involved, there can be a decreased length of bone and curvature of bones.

If there is no detachment of cartilage, no clinical signs are present. With OCD, clinical signs include lameness and pain on extension and flexion of the joint. The most common joints affected are the shoulder, elbow, stifle, and hock.

Osteochondrosis is most common in large breeds of dogs, especially Great Danes, Newfoundlands, Rottweilers, Labrador retrievers, and golden retrievers. Most dogs with OCD have more than one joint affected. The shoulder and stifle of Great Danes; the elbows of Newfoundlands; the shoulder, elbow and hocks of Labradors and golden retrievers; and shoulder and hocks of Rottweilers are the most common sites of OCD.

Excess energy intake or excess calcium intake play a significant role in the development of osteochondrosis. Energy intake needs to be controlled in young growing puppies to prevent an overweight puppy. Fast-growing puppies should have their body condition monitored closely so that energy intake can be controlled. Calcium should be provided at the proper amount in the diet.

Diseases Due to Decreased Skeletal Remodeling

Canine wobbler syndrome and enostosis are two diseases characterized by a decrease in skeletal remodeling. In canine wobbler syndrome, there is compression of the spinal cord due to changes in the spinal canal. Pain with extension of the neck and uncoordination of the hind limbs are seen in growing large-breed dogs less than 6 months of age. There is an increased incidence in Great Danes, mastiffs, and Irish wolfhounds.

Enostosis (eosinophilic panosteitis) is characterized by shifting lameness in young dogs. Long bones are affected, and pain is noted on palpation of bones. The German shepherd dog is at increased risk of enostosis.

Chronic excessive intake of calcium results in high calcium absorption, and there is a decrease in bone osteoclast activity, with a decrease in bone remodeling. Diets containing the proper amount of calcium should be fed.

Diseases Due to Nutritional Deficiencies

Nutritional secondary hyperparathyroidism and rickets are disorders characterized by loss of bone density that leads to fractures. Deficiency of calcium results in nutritional secondary hyperparathyroidism, and lack of dietary vitamin D causes rickets. Nutritional secondary hyperparathyroidism is discussed in detail in Chapter 17.

Feeding the Growing Puppy

Controlling the growth rate of growing puppies, especially those of larger breeds, helps to decrease the incidence and severity of skeletal and joint problems. Unfortunately, many people feel that a big, roly-poly puppy is ideal. However, this is incompatible with the development of optimal skeletal growth. Feeding to support normal weight gain rather than to support maximum weight gain is essential to proper skeletal and joint development. Puppies should be fed to maintain a lean body condition and should not be allowed to become overweight. Body condition should be checked at least every other week, and the amount of diet fed should be adjusted to prevent excessive weight gain. Keeping a puppy lean does not restrict maximum adult size, but it does help to prevent skeletal issues. Free-choice feeding is discouraged, as many puppies will overeat and consume excess energy. Restricted meal feeding two to three times per day provides an easy method for ensuring that the proper amount of diet is being consumed. Refer to Chapter 4 for general guidelines on the proper amount of energy to feed to growing puppies.

Osteoarthrosis

Osteoarthrosis (osteoarthritis) is a common orthopedic problem in older dogs, and also affects some cats. Clinical signs include decreased weight bearing, pain especially when getting up, decreased range of motion, and swollen joints. Osteoarthrosis is associated with aging, and overloading of the joint either from obesity or excessive use is the common cause. In osteoarthrosis the joint is not lubricated, and the cartilage does not receive enough nutrients, which damages the cartilage. Cartilage damage causes inflammation within the joint, and inflammatory mediators are released. The inflammatory mediators then cause release of certain factors that cause more joint damage.

In osteoarthrosis, both medical and nutritional management is important. Weight loss in overweight dogs is a main goal of therapy. A number of dietary supplements have been used in the treatment of osteoarthrosis. Some of these supplements are classified as nutraceuticals. The North American Veterinary Nutraceutical Council defines a nutraceutical as "a substance that is produced in a purified or extracted form and administered orally to patients to provide agents required for normal body structure and function and administered with the intent of improving the health and well being of animals." Supplements that have been used as treatment include glucosamine, chondroitin sulfate, eicosapentaenoic acid (EPA), docosahexaenoic acid (DHA), antioxidants, and green-lipped mussel.

Chondroitin sulfate is a cartilage-protectant agent (glycosaminogly-can) that is synthesized by cartilage cells. Chondroitin sulfate prevents the synthesis of some inflammatory mediators and helps to prevent cartilage damage. Glucosamine is a precursor to glycosaminoglycans, and cartilage cells in osteoarthrosis are unable to secrete adequate glucosamine. Glucosamine is well absorbed from the gastrointestinal tract; chondroitin sulfate is partly digested before absorption, but still appears effective if given orally. The combination of glucosamine and chondroitin sulfate given together may be beneficial in osteoarthrosis. EPA and DHA are long-chain omega-3 fatty acids. EPA and DHA are incorporated into cell mediators that are less inflammatory than those derived from omega-6 fatty acids. Thus, omega-3 fatty acid supplementation may be helpful in decreasing some of the joint inflammation in osteoarthrosis. Antioxidants such as vitamin C, vitamin E, β-carotene, selenium, or zinc may help to decrease the damage of joint cells by free radicals and reduce the progression of osteoarthrosis. The New Zealand green-lipped mussel (*Perna canaliculus*) may be beneficial in treatment, as it contains EPA, DHA, chondroitin, and glutamine. Further work is needed to evaluate the effectiveness of these supplements.

Recipes for Large Breed Puppies

Chicken and Rice   326
Chicken and Pasta   327
Chicken and Potato   328
Ground Beef and Rice   329
Ground Beef and Pasta   330
Pork and Pasta   331
Tuna and Pasta   332

Additional Reading

Budsberg SC, Bartges JW. 2006. Nutrition and osteoarthritis in dogs. Does it help? Vet Clin Small Anim 36:1307–1323.

Bui LM, Bierer TL. 2003. Influence of green lipped mussels (*Perna canaliculus*) in alleviating signs of arthritis in dogs. Vet Ther 4(4):397–407.

Case LP, Carey DP, Hirakawa DA, Daristotle L (Eds). 2000. Overnutrition and supplementation. In *Canine and Feline Nutrition: A Resource for Companion Animal Professionals*, 2nd edition. Mosby, St. Louis, pp. 331–344.

Hazewinkel H, Mott J. 2006. Main nutritional imbalances implicated in osteoarticular diseases. In *Encyclopedia of Canine Clinical Nutrition*. Pibot P, Biourge V, Elliott D (Eds). Aniwa SAS, Aimargues, France, pp. 348–386.

Lawler DF, Larson BT, Ballam JM, Smith GK, Biery DN, Evans RH, et al. 2008. Diet restriction and ageing in the dog: Major observations over two decades. Br J Nutr 99(4):793–805.

Richardson DC, Zentek J, Hazewinkel HAW, Toll PW, Zicker SC. 2000. Developmental orthopedic disease of dogs. In *Small Animal Clinical Nutrition*, 4th edition. Hand MS, Thatcher CD, Remillard RL, Roudebush P (Eds). Mark Morris Institute, Topeka, KS, pp. 505–528.

Runge JJ, Biery DN, Lawler DF, Gregor TP, Evans RH, Kealy RD, et al. 2008. The effects of lifetime food restriction on the development of osteoarthritis in the canine shoulder. Vet Surg 37(1):102–107.

Sallander MH, Hedhammar A, Trogen ME. 2006. Diet, exercise and weight as risk factors in hip dysplasia and elbow arthrosis in Labrador retrievers. J Nutr 136(Suppl 7):2050S–2052S.

Schoenherr WD, Roudebush P, Swecker WS. 2000. Use of fatty acids in inflammatory disease. In *Small Animal Clinical Nutrition*, 4th edition. Hand MS, Thatcher CD, Remillard RL, Roudebush P (Eds). Mark Morris Institute, Topeka, KS, pp. 907–922.

Smith GK, Paster ER, Powers MY, Lawler DF, Biery DN, Shofer FS, et al. 2006. Lifelong diet restriction and radiographic evidence of osteoarthritis of the hip joint in dogs. J Am Vet Med Assoc 229(5):690–693.

CHAPTER 13
Diet and Gastrointestinal Disease

Gastrointestinal Physiology

The digestive tract is a large organ that provides a protective barrier from the environment and absorbs nutrients. The mucosal barrier of the gastrointestinal (GI) tract protects the body from invasion by bacteria, toxins, and other harmful agents. The gut-associated lymphoid tissue (GALT) plays an important role in mounting an inflammatory response against toxic agents. Damage to any part of the GI tract can result in invasion of harmful substances and a decrease in absorption of nutrients.

The small intestine is the primary site for digestion and nutrient absorption. The small intestine is characterized by the presence of many villi and microvilli, which increase the surface area of the small intestine and provide a greater area for absorption of nutrients. Enterocytes are specialized cells in the mucosa of the small intestine that contain enzymes necessary for absorption of nutrients.

■ Digestion and Absorption

When dietary protein reaches the stomach, the enzyme pepsin starts the digestive process. Once proteins reach the small intestine, pancreatic enzymes and enzymes from the brush border of the small intestine digest the proteins. As a result of digestion, small peptides and amino acids are released and can be absorbed by the small intestine cells.

Ingested fats combine with bile acids in the small intestine and then can be digested by the pancreatic enzymes lipase, phospholipase, and cholesterol esterase. Triglycerides are broken down to monoglycerides and free fatty acids. Bile acids help with the absorption of the mono-glycerides and free fatty acids by forming micelles that can associate with small intestine cells. Once these are absorbed, the bile acids are reabsorbed in the ileum and are transported back to the liver where they can again be released at a later time. Once the free fatty acids and monoglycerides are absorbed, they are re-esterified to triglycerides, become incorporated into chylomicrons within the small intestine cells, and then are secreted into the lymphatic channels.

Ingested carbohydrates are digested by pancreatic amylase, pro-ducing maltose. Maltose, along with sucrose and lactose, are digested by enzymes from the brush border of the small intestine, producing monosaccharides. These monosaccharides can then be transported through the intestinal cell into the portal circulation.

Minerals are absorbed in both the small and large intestine. The absorption of calcium in the small intestine is tightly regulated and is controlled by calcium metabolic hormones. Phosphorus, zinc, iron, and manganese absorption are also regulated. Sodium, potassium, and chloride are about 90% absorbed in the small intestine. Most other minerals are absorbed by passive diffusion. The fat-soluble vitamins (A, D, E, and K) are absorbed in micelles, along with free fatty acids and monoglycerides. The water-soluble vitamins are absorbed by passive diffusion.

■ Intestinal Microflora

There is a population of bacteria that normally lives within the intestinal tract. This bacterial population stimulates the immune system, helps with digestion, and protects against invasion by other pathogens. There is a higher concentration of bacteria in the large intestine as compared to the small intestine. The bacterial flora is dependent on intestinal motility, nutrients present in the intestine, and GI secretions (gastric acid, bile acid, pancreatic enzymes). The proper concentration of bacteria in the intestine is unknown, so it can be dif-ficult to determine when bacteria are present in excess. Diet ingredi-ents influence the bacterial composition in the intestine; high-protein diets favor the growth of clostridial bacteria, whereas fermentable fiber favors the growth of bifidobacteria and lactobacilli.

■ Gastrointestinal Immune System

The GI tract contains the most immune cells in the body. The GALT includes the mesenteric lymph nodes, Peyer's patches, and lymphoid follicles. The immune cells include T lymphocytes, B lymphocytes, plasma cells, macrophages, eosinophils, and mast cells. A good immune response is necessary to prevent invasion of pathogens. The GI tract must also not overreact to dietary ingredients or normal intestinal bacterial flora, so mucosal tolerance is important. If every substance presented to the GI tract was regarded as foreign, there would be a continual state of inflammation. A breakdown in mucosal tolerance is implicated in inflammatory bowel disease. How exactly GALT maintains mucosal tolerance is not clear.

Oral Disorders

Inflammatory conditions of the oral cavity are uncommon and include eosinophilic granuloma complex, granulomas, stomatitis, and inflammation due to radiation therapy of the head and neck. Cleft palate is the most common congenital problem of the oral cavity. Trauma can occur from fighting, falls, burns, vehicle accidents, and foreign bodies. Oral neoplasia is not uncommon and is the fourth most common cause of cancer in dogs and cats.

Clinical signs of oral disease include difficulty eating or a reluctance to eat. Many pets with oral disorders also have difficulty drinking, so dehydration is a common problem. Energy-dense foods should be fed to provide a high number of calories in a small quantity of food. Adding water to the diet to provide a gruel or slurry and feeding multiple small meals during the day may help to promote intake. Growth or performance-type diets may be best to provide an increased energy density.

Swallowing Disorders

Swallowing disorders are uncommon in dogs and rare in cats but can have a profound impact on nutrition. Swallowing problems result from disorders of both the pharynx and esophagus. The most common swallowing disorders are due to problems with motility (megaesophagus), inflammation (esophagitis, gastroesophageal reflux), or obstruction (strictures, foreign bodies).

Clinical signs of swallowing disorders include coughing or gagging when trying to swallow, excessive salivation, pain on swallowing, gurgling noises, and regurgitation of undigested food immediately after eating. Aspiration pneumonia is not uncommon from aspiration during regurgitation.

■ Megaesophagus

Megaesophagus occurs when a motility disorder affecting the esophagus results in a large and flaccid esophagus. Congenital megaesophagus is most common in the Chinese Shar-Pei, fox terrier, German shepherd dog, Great Dane, Irish setter, Labrador retriever, miniature schnauzer, Newfoundland, wire-haired fox terrier, and Siamese cat. Acquired megaesophagus is most common in the German shepherd dog, golden retriever, Great Dane, and Irish setter. The exact reasons that megaesophagus occurs are unknown, but it is related to neuromuscular dysfunction. Regurgitation is the primary clinical sign; weight loss also occurs. Aspiration pneumonia is a common complication.

Diets for pets with megaesophagus should be a slurry or liquid. The more liquid a diet, the easier for the diet to pass through the esophagus and reach the stomach, decreasing the likelihood of regurgitation. Diets should be thoroughly mixed in a blender with added water. Multiple small meals should be fed throughout the day and should be fed with the dog or cat in an upright position. Feeding bowls should not be put on the floor since the pet would have to flex the neck to eat. Bowls can be propped up so that the neck does not need to be flexed, or special elevated feeding platforms can be purchased. Pets should be kept in an upright position for 10–15 minutes after feeding to allow food to flow into the stomach. A diet that is energy dense, containing greater than 25% dry matter (DM) fat is best (Table 13.1).

■ Esophagitis

Esophagitis is an inflammation of the esophagus and can result from foreign bodies, oral medications, heat injuries, or gastroesophageal reflux. In cases of esophagitis from gastroesophageal reflux, the fat content in the diet should be less than 15% DM (Table 13.1). High dietary fat promotes gastroesophageal reflux due to delayed gastric emptying times and should be avoided. Protein content should be

Table 13.1. Dietary recommendations for dogs with swallowing disorders.

Nutrient	Esophagitis	Megaesophagus	Obstructive Disorders
Protein	≥25% DM	≥25% DM	≥25% DM
Fat	<15% DM	≥25% DM	≥25% DM

DM, dry matter.

greater than 25% DM to enhance esophageal sphincter tone. Food should be a gruel consistency, and several small meals should be fed throughout the day.

■ Obstructive Disorders (Strictures, Foreign Body)

Strictures can occur from scarring, or from congenital conditions. Dietary treatment is similar to that for megaesophagus (Table 13.1). An energy-dense food fed in multiple small meals daily is best. Diets should be a slurry or liquid.

Stomach Disorders

■ Vomiting

Vomiting is common and can be associated with both GI and non-GI diseases. Frequent or profuse vomiting can lead to serious metabolic consequences. If vomiting is mild and of short duration, then typically there is not a significant fluid loss or electrolyte abnormalities. However, if vomiting is profuse and frequent, significant fluid loss can result, leading to dehydration. Electrolyte imbalances are common with severe vomiting and include decreased serum potassium (hypokalemia), decreased serum sodium (hyponatremia), and decreased serum chloride (hypochloremia). Aspiration pneumonia and esophagitis can occur as a result of vomiting. Nausea may precede vomiting. Signs of nausea include salivation, licking of the lips, or retching.

The type of vomiting may give an indication as to its cause. If the vomit contains undigested food more than 12 hours after a meal, then a delay in gastric emptying is suspected. Projectile vomiting indicates gastric outflow obstruction or upper small intestine obstruction. The underlying cause of vomiting should be determined and treated.

The oral intake of food should be restricted to minimize vomiting and fluid loss. Food should be withheld for 12–24 hours. If vomiting resolves, then a highly digestible, fat-restricted diet should be fed. After a few days on the fat-restricted diet, the pet's regular diet can be reintroduced over a period of a few days.

■ Hairballs

Hairballs are a common problem in cats because of their grooming behavior. Ingested hair accumulates in the stomach in a loose ball and is occasionally regurgitated. Hairballs typically are not a problem in most cats unless they form a large hard ball in the stomach. There are a number of laxative or lubricant products available on the market for the treatment and prevention of hairballs. Special diets are not typically necessary. If cats exhibit regurgitation daily, or have diarrhea, weight loss, loss of appetite, or abdominal pain, then they should be evaluated for an underlying GI disorder.

■ Gastritis

Acute gastritis is usually a mild condition with acute vomiting that resolves within 24–48 hours. Chronic gastritis can be problematic as vomiting may be more chronic. The chronic inflammation can also interfere with gastric motility, leading to further vomiting. There are many possible causes of gastritis, including dietary indiscretion, foreign body ingestion, ingested plant material, chemical irritants, drugs, viral infections, bacterial infections, parasitic infections, or systemic disorders (liver disease, renal disease, shock, stress, and others). Older pets are more likely to have a metabolic or neoplastic cause of gastritis. Hemorrhagic gastroenteritis is more common in dachshunds, miniature schnauzers, toy poodles, and other small breeds.

Water is an important nutrient for any vomiting patient. Loss of water can lead to dehydration, and water deficits should be replaced using intravenous or subcutaneous fluid therapy if it is severe.

Antigens from proteins may play a role in some cases of chronic gastritis; thus, it may be beneficial to choose a diet with a novel protein source. The protein source should be highly digestible, and excess protein should be avoided (Table 13.2). Fat should be moderately restricted since high-fat diets are retained in the stomach for a longer period of time. Diets for gastritis should contain less than 15% DM fat for dogs and less than 22% DM fat for cats.

Table 13.2. Dietary recommendations for dogs and cats with gastritis.

Factor	Dog	Cat
Protein	16%–20% DM; consider novel source	30%–50% DM; consider novel source
Fat	<15% DM	<22% DM
Sodium	0.35%–0.50% DM	0.35%–0.50% DM
Potassium	0.8%–1.1% DM	0.8%–1.1% DM
Chloride	0.5%–1.3 % DM	0.5%–1.3% DM

DM, dry matter.

Since chronic vomiting can lead to loss of electrolytes, diets should contain potassium, sodium, and chloride in concentrations above the recommended minimums.

With gastritis, food is typically withheld for about 24 hours, and if there is no vomiting, then small amounts of water or ice cubes are offered. If water is tolerated, then the pet is fed the recommended diet about six to eight times per day, so that very small amounts are consumed in one meal. If this is tolerated, then after a few days, the pets' regular diet may be reintroduced over several days.

■ Gastric Dilatation-Volvulus

Gastric dilatation (GD) occurs when the stomach becomes distended with gas, fluid, and air. Gastric dilatation-volvulus (GDV) occurs when the stomach then rotates on its axis and entraps gas and fluid within the stomach. This rotation also twists the blood supply to the stomach, spleen, and pancreas. GDV is a surgical emergency with a high mortality rate. GDV is most common in deep-chested, large-breed dogs. Breeds at risk include Great Danes, Irish setters, Gordon setters, Weimaraners, Saint Bernards, Doberman pinschers and basset hounds. The retriever breeds have a lower risk for GDV. GD and GDV are more common in middle-aged dogs. Male dogs, dogs with a nervous temperament, or dogs that are underweight are at higher risk.

Nausea, belching, and vomiting are clinical signs of GD. Vomiting may not be present, and the dog may just be reluctant to move and make grunting sounds. GDV usually occurs acutely, often at night or in the early morning. A stressful event such as boarding, travel, or participation in dog show events may precipitate GDV. Dogs with GDV are restless, have abdominal distention, increased salivation, abdominal pain, and nonproductive vomiting.

Dietary risk factors have been identified for the occurrence of GD and GDV. Consumption of one large meal per day, rapid eating, overeating, drinking large amounts of water, and postprandial exercise have all been implicated. In one study, the inclusion of moist foods or table foods in the diet decreased the risk of GDV. It had been previously thought that the feeding of commercial dry pet foods increased the risk of GDV; however, in a controlled study comparing dry foods to a wet diet, there was no difference in the incidence of GDV. Soybeans in the diet had once been implicated as a possible cause, but this has also been disproven in long-term feeding studies. Eating behaviors such as rapid food consumption, excitement, and exercise increase the amount of swallowed air, which increases the risk for GDV. Thus, eating behaviors that increase the risk of GDV should be minimized, especially in large-breed, deep-chested dogs. Dogs should be fed two to three meals per day and should be fed in a calm environment with no competition for food. If the dog still eats too fast, the diet can be portioned out into muffin tins to make it more difficult for the dog to eat quickly. Large balls or rocks can also be placed in the food bowl so that the dog must pick the diet from around the obstacles. Limiting the amount of exercise for three to four hours after feeding is advised.

■ Gastric Motility Disorders

Gastric motility disorders are poorly understood and result in weak gastric contractions that cause delayed emptying of food from the stomach. There are many causes of decreased gastric motility, including high-fat diets, drugs, inflammation, pancreatitis, nervous inhibition (stress, trauma, or pain), hypothyroidism, decreased serum potassium, and vagal nerve damage. Abdominal distention, discomfort after eating, vomiting of undigested food more than 12 hours after eating, belching, and loss of appetite are clinical signs of gastric motility disorders. Weight loss and a thin body condition may be present if the condition is chronic. Some may have severe vomiting with dehydration.

Some breeds may be at increased risk of gastric motility disorders depending on the underlying condition. Congenital pyloric stenosis is more common in Siamese cats and brachycephalic breeds of dogs. Chronic hypertrophic pyloric gastropathy is most common in middle-aged Lhasa apsos, Maltese, shih tzu, and Pekingese dogs. Gastric foreign bodies are more common in young dogs, and neoplasia that obstructs gastric outflow is more common in older dogs.

Dehydration is common with gastric motility disorders as a result of the persistent vomiting. Fluid deficits should be corrected with fluid therapy (intravenous or subcutaneous), and water should be available as free choice. Cold water (below room temperature) should be avoided because this can delay gastric emptying.

Pets with gastric motility disorders are often underweight because of inadequate caloric intake over a period of time. However, it is difficult to provide a very energy-dense diet without increasing the dietary fat content. Unfortunately, diets high in fat delay gastric emptying. A high fat content in the duodenum stimulates the release of cholecystokinin, which slows gastric emptying. Thus, the dietary fat content should be less than 15% DM for dogs and less than 22% DM for cats (Table 13.3). Liquid diets are emptied from the stomach faster

Table 13.3. Dietary recommendations for dogs and cats with gastric motility disorders.

Factor	Dog	Cat
Diet	Liquid or semiliquid; temperature of food should be between room temperature and body temperature.	Liquid or semiliquid; temperature of food should be between room temperature and body temperature.
Fat	<15% DM	<22% DM

DM, dry matter.

than solid diets, thus diets should either have a liquid or slurry consistency. Since cold foods delay gastric emptying, the food should be warmed to between room and body temperature.

Diarrhea

Diarrhea is not truly a disease process but rather is a clinical sign of some underlying disorder. Diarrhea can be acute or chronic and can originate from the small intestine or large intestine.

■ Acute Diarrhea

Acute diarrhea is characterized by an abnormal frequency and consistency of the stool, and it is the most common sign of intestinal disease in the dog. Diarrhea occurs when intestinal absorption is decreased, intestinal secretions have increased, or a combination of the two occurs.

Depending on clinical signs, dogs may be categorized as having mild diarrhea or moderate/severe diarrhea. In mild cases, dogs are alert and active, have no evidence of dehydration, and have had less than three to four episodes of diarrhea within 24 hours, with no blood in the stool. Dogs with moderate illness exhibit dehydration, depression, more frequent episodes of diarrhea (more than six per day), and blood in the stool.

Causes of acute diarrhea include dietary indiscretions, dietary intolerance, infectious agents, intestinal parasites, drugs and toxins, and miscellaneous agents. Young dogs are more likely to have diarrhea from dietary indiscretions or from infectious causes. Dietary indiscretions include eating table scraps, eating spoiled food, overeating, sudden changes of diet, ingestion of foreign material, or ingestion of poor-quality water. Dietary intolerances are most commonly to dairy products and fat. Ingestion of milk or cheese in many dogs can cause mild diarrhea.

Infectious causes of diarrhea can be viral, bacterial, rickettsial, or fungal. Viral causes include parvovirus, coronavirus, and rotavirus. Parvovirus is a common cause of severe diarrhea in young, nonvaccinated dogs. Coronavirus is also common in nonvaccinated dogs, but typically the diarrhea is not as severe as that seen in parvovirus. Bacterial causes include *Salmonella*, *Clostridium*, *Campylobacter*, *Escherichia coli*, *Yersinia*, and *Bacillus piliformis*. Rickettsial diarrhea is most often caused by *Neorickettsia*, and fungal agents can cause acute diarrhea but are more commonly associated with chronic diarrheas.

Intestinal parasitism is one of the most common causes of acute diarrhea, and any intestinal parasite can cause diarrhea. The most common causes are *Giardia*, coccidia, and hookworms. Infection with *Giardia* or coccidia may occur in dogs that are on a preventive program for worming, since these programs do not have any effect on these parasites.

Drugs and toxins may also cause diarrhea. Nonsteroidal anti-inflammatory drugs, corticosteroids, anticancer agents, antibiotics, insecticides, heavy metals, and lawn and garden products may all cause acute diarrhea in the dog. In addition, hemorrhagic gastroenteritis, hypoadrenocorticism, liver disease, renal disease, or pancreatitis may all result in diarrhea.

Dogs with mild diarrhea will recover with minimal therapy, and therefore only minimal testing and treatment is necessary. Dogs with moderate diarrhea require more extensive testing and treatment, since they are more likely to have metabolic abnormalities. In mild diarrhea, examining the stool for parasites is the first diagnostic test that should be performed. Multiple fecal samples should be analyzed (at least three), since some parasites such as *Giardia* and coccidia may not appear in every fecal sample. Even if dogs are on a regular worming schedule, fecal examinations are still of value, since a regular worming program is not aimed at prevention of *Giardia* or coccidia. Dogs that have been recently wormed (within the last month) may become reinfected, and depending on the agent used for worming, all parasites may not have been destroyed. So even in these dogs, repeated fecal examination is of benefit. Depending on age and vaccination status, the presence of fecal parvoviral antigen may be tested. Blood work should include a PCV (packed cell volume) and total protein, to assess dehydration and protein loss.

Dogs with moderate to severe diarrhea require more extensive testing. In addition to multiple fecal examinations, a CBC (complete blood count) and blood biochemistry panel should be performed, since dehydration and metabolic abnormalities are common in these patients.

Dogs with mild diarrhea are typically treated as outpatients, whereas those with moderate to severe diarrhea are usually hospitalized for intensive therapy. Any underlying cause of disease (such as parasites) should be treated with the appropriate therapy. In cases of acute diarrhea, dietary modification is an important aspect of treatment, though there are two thoughts on feeding. Traditionally, food intake has been restricted for at least 24 hours, then is gradually returned to normal. A bland diet consisting of highly digestible carbohydrates and protein is offered frequently and in small quantities. Fats and dairy products are avoided. Highly digestible protein sources include cooked chicken (with no skin), lean hamburger, and eggs.

An alternative approach to dietary therapy is to continue to feed even though diarrhea is present. There is evidence that feeding even though clinical signs are present decreases the morbidity in dogs with parvovirus. This is not very practical, however, if vomiting is present. One danger with feeding in the face of clinical signs is that the altered permeability of the intestine may allow increased dietary antigens to be absorbed. Thus, hypersensitivity to dietary protein may develop. It may be prudent to feed a novel dietary protein source if using this alternative approach.

Fluid therapy is an important aspect of diarrhea therapy and is aimed at rehydrating the patient and correcting an electrolyte imbalance. In mild cases, oral fluid therapy is effective and economical. In moderate to severe cases, either subcutaneous or intravenous therapy will be required.

Pharmacological therapy may include motility modulators, antisecretory agents, intestinal protectants, or antibiotics. Motility modulators should be used only in those patients with diarrhea so severe that fluid balance cannot be maintained. Motility modulators cause the transit time of the intestine to increase, allowing more time for water reabsorption. These should not be used for more than a few days due to the side effects that are associated with them. Anticholinergics decrease intestinal tone and reduce intestinal secretions. They may worsen the diarrhea in some dogs, however, and should not be used in cases of intestinal obstruction or in dogs with glaucoma. Narcotic analgesics are potent inhibitors of intestinal secretions. They also increase segmental contractions in the intestine, increasing resistance to passage of intestinal contents and decreasing fluid influx. Narcotic analgesics may cause depression, confusion, gastrointestinal atony, pancreatitis, and loss of appetite. They should not be used in patients with liver disease or bacterial gastrointestinal disease.

Antisecretory agents include anticholinergics, chlorpromazine, opiates, and salicylates. Chlorpromazine inhibits intracellular calmodulin, which increases in dogs with secretory diarrhea. Opiates decrease secretions and increase absorption. This may be due to a slower transit time, which allows for increased absorption. Salicylates inhibit prostaglandins and thereby decrease intestinal secretions that may be caused by enterotoxins.

Intestinal protectants include the bismuth subsalicylate products (Pepto-Bismol) and kaolin- and pectin-type products. Kaolin/pectin products have limited value in pets with severe diarrhea, since they have not been shown to alter fluid and electrolyte losses.

Antibiotics are only indicated in dogs with bacterial causes of intestinal disease or in dogs that are passing blood in the feces due to bacterial invasion of the intestinal mucosa. The use of antibiotics indiscriminately in diarrhea is ineffective and potentially harmful. They may inhibit the normal bacterial flora of the intestine, which is detrimental to recovery. Antibiotics should not be administered in conjunction with intestinal protectants, since they become bound to the protectants and are thus ineffective.

Most dogs with acute diarrhea that have been treated with appropriate therapy recover within 3–5 days. Dogs that fail to respond to therapy within this period need further testing and treatment to pinpoint the cause of diarrhea.

■ Chronic Diarrhea

Chronic diarrhea is defined as a change in frequency, volume, or consistency of the stool that persists for 3 or more weeks. Chronic diarrhea may be episodic and can be due to problems in either the small or large intestine. The mechanisms of chronic diarrhea include increased fluid excretion into the intestine, decreased fluid absorption by the intestine, altered intestinal permeability, or abnormal gastrointestinal motility.

Clinical signs of small intestine and large intestine diarrhea differ. In chronic diarrheas caused by small intestine disease, there is a larger volume of stool than normal, and the frequency of defecation is moderately above normal (two to four stools per day). Weight loss is usual, and there may be dark blood in the stool. Mucus is typically not present in the stool. Usually there is no straining, and some dogs may exhibit vomiting.

In chronic diarrheas caused by large intestine disease, there is a smaller volume of stool than with small intestine diarrheas. The frequency of defecation is increased (more than four times per day), and usually there is no weight loss. Bright red blood or mucus may be present in the stool. Straining is not uncommon, and vomiting is rare.

Pets experiencing chronic diarrhea should be examined by a veterinarian to determine the cause. On physical examination, dogs with small intestine diarrheas usually exhibit poor body condition if they have malabsorption, maldigestion, or protein-losing enteropathies. Abdominal palpation may reveal masses or thickened bowel loops. Rectal palpation is important and may reveal irregularities or thickening of the large bowel, masses, or strictures.

There are many potential causes of small intestine diarrheas. Inflammatory causes such as enteritis, lymphangiectasia, neoplasia, and bacterial or fungal infections from histoplasmosis, *Salmonella*, *Clostridium perfringens*, and phycomycosis, may be causes. Also, parasites such as *Giardia*, ascarids, hookworms, and strongyloides are common causes of small bowel diarrhea. Partial obstruction due to foreign bodies, small intestinal bacterial overgrowth, short bowel syndrome, or duodenal ulcers may be primary causes of this type of diarrhea as well.

In addition to primary small intestinal disease, maldigestion due to exocrine pancreatic insufficiency (EPI; a lack of pancreatic digestive enzymes) or hepatic disease is not uncommon. Dietary sensitivities may be a problem, such as gluten-sensitive enteropathy in Irish setters. Metabolic disorders, such as liver disease and Addison's disease, or uremia, toxins, and drug administration may all cause small intestine diarrheas.

There are also many causes of large intestine diarrheas. Inflammatory causes such as colitis, noninflammatory causes such as intussusception, neoplasia, and bacterial infections from histoplasmosis, *C. perfringens*, *Salmonella*, *Campylobacter jejuni*, and *Prototheca*, may be causes. Also, parasites such as whipworms (*Trichuris*), *Giardia*, *Ancylostoma*, *Entamoeba*, and *Balantidium* are common causes of large bowel diarrheas.

In addition to the above primary causes of large intestine diarrhea, other factors such as the eating of garbage or foreign material (bones, hair), feeding a poorly digestible diet, irritable bowel syndrome, uremia, Addison's disease, toxins, or drugs may cause large bowel diarrheas.

Diagnosis of causes of chronic diarrheas can be difficult, and may require extensive laboratory testing. A CBC and a serum biochemistry panel should be analyze, to determine hydration status and to assess major organ status. Repeated fecal examinations are very important. Routine fecal flotation, along with zinc sulfate centrifugation for the diagnosis of *Giardia*, should be performed. Direct microscopic examination of feces may reveal organisms associated with fungal or inflammatory diseases. Fecal cultures may be indicated if bacterial infections are suspected, and Sudan Black staining of feces for fecal fat may be necessary if malabsorption or maldigestion is suspected.

If exocrine pancreatic insufficiency is suspected, tests such as trypsin-like immunoreactivity (TLI) may be done. If malabsorption is suspected, a xylose absorption test or serum folate or cobalamin levels may be analyzed.

In addition, abdominal radiographs and/or ultrasound may be indicated to assess intestinal thickening, masses, or foreign bodies. If malabsorption, parasites, and infectious causes have been ruled out, then endoscopy and biopsy of the stomach and upper small intestine are usually required for a definitive diagnosis. If diseases of the colon are suspected, a colonoscopy can be performed.

Treatment depends on whether the small or large intestine is affected. With small intestine diarrheas, the underlying disease must be treated. Symptomatic treatments are rarely successful. Resolution of chronic diarrhea is very gradual, and it may take weeks of treatment before a return to normal stool is seen. Even when treating the underlying disease, complete resolution of the diarrhea may not be possible, especially in pets with intestinal neoplasia, lymphangiectasia, or histoplasmosis. With large intestine diarrheas, therapeutic deworming for whipworms is usually performed, since many dogs with whipworm infections appear negative on fecal examination. In addition, a highly digestible diet that is low in fat should be fed for at least 3–4 weeks. If response to treatment is poor, surgery may be indicated to manually examine the intestine for evidence of disease.

■ Pathogenesis of Diarrhea

There are four basic categories of diarrhea: osmotic diarrhea, secretory diarrhea, increased intestinal permeability, or intestinal motility disorders.

Osmotic diarrhea is the most common cause of diarrhea in dogs and cats and occurs when poorly absorbed solutes are present in the intestinal lumen. Ingestion of large amounts of nondigestible fiber or malassimilation of ingested food retard water absorption in the intestine, leading to an increased amount of water present in the stool. Causes of osmotic diarrhea include maldigestion, malabsorption, administration of osmotic laxatives, and overeating. Osmotic diarrhea is characterized by the passage of large amounts of fluid or soft stools. This type of diarrhea usually resolves within 24–36 hours after fasting.

Secretory diarrhea is relatively uncommon and is caused by bacterial enterotoxins, gastrointestinal hormones, prostaglandins, bile acids, and certain laxatives. Large volumes of liquid diarrhea are passed, and dehydration occurs rapidly.

Increased permeability causes an increased flux of liquid into the intestine and can be caused by inflammatory processes. This is a common cause of diarrhea in dogs and cats and can be of small or large intestine origin. Diseases that cause GI erosions, ulceration, or mucosal inflammation can potentially increase the permeability of the gut. Some patients may present with a protein-losing enteropathy, and diarrhea does not always resolve with fasting.

Motility disorders can be either a primary problem or secondary to some other condition. Decreased intestinal motility can result in small intestinal bacterial overgrowth, and the response to dietary management is variable.

Small Intestine Disorders

■ Acute Enteritis

Acute enteritis is common in dogs and cats, characterized by the sudden onset of vomiting and diarrhea. There are a number of potential causes of acute enteritis, including dietary indiscretion, foreign body ingestion, bacterial infection, parasitic infection, viral infection, or ingestion of toxins. Bacterial infectious agents include *Campylobacter*, *Clostridium*, *E. coli*, *Salmonella*, *Staphylococcus*, and *Yersinia*. Parasites causing acute enteritis include roundworms, hookworms, *Giardia*, and coccidia. Viruses that cause acute enteritis include canine distemper, coronavirus, panleukopenia, parvovirus, and rotavirus.

Acute diarrhea is the most common clinical sign and may be accompanied by vomiting. Diarrhea originating from the small intestine has different characteristics than diarrhea originating from the large intestine (Table 13.4).

Diets for acute enteritis should contain moderate fat concentrations. High-fat diets are energy dense, but they slow gastric emptying and

Table 13.4. Characteristics of diarrhea originating from the small intestine or large intestine.

Characteristic	Small Intestine	Large Intestine
Blood in feces	Digested blood	Fresh blood
Stool quality	Watery, "cow-pie" appearance	Loose to semiformed
Stool volume	Increased	Small quantities
Frequency of defecation	Normal to increased	Increased
Mucus in stool	Usually absent	Usually present
Fat in stool	May be present	Absent
Straining to defecate	Absent	Present
Urgency to defecate	Absent	Present
Vomiting	May be present	Uncommon
Weight loss	May be present	Rare

Table 13.5. Dietary recommendations for dogs and cats with acute enteritis.

Factor	Dogs	Cats
Fat	12%–15% DM	15%–22% DM
Crude fiber	<1% DM	<1% DM
Potassium	0.8%–1.1% DM	0.8%–1.1% DM
Chloride	0.5%–1.3% DM	0.5%–1.3% DM
Sodium	0.35%–0.50% DM	0.35%–0.50% DM
Glutamine	0.5 g/kg body weight daily	0.5 g/kg body weight daily

DM, dry matter.

stimulate pancreatic secretion. Fat helps improve palatability, which is useful for patients with nausea. For dogs, the dietary fat content should be 12%–15% DM, and 15%–22% DM for cats (Table 13.5). The energy density of the diet should be moderate so that small meals can be fed. Very low-fiber diets are fed (<1% DM). Potassium, sodium, and chloride concentrations may be low in patients with acute enteritis due to the loss in vomit and feces. Diets should provide above the minimum concentrations for potassium, sodium, and chloride. Glutamine is an energy substrate for intestinal cells and is necessary for maintaining the proper function of the small intestine. Meat ingredients typically provide adequate glutamine. In acute enteritis, glutamine should be supplemented at 0.5 g/kg body weight daily.

■ **Inflammatory Bowel Disease**

Inflammatory bowel disease (IBD) refers to a group of disorders that cause inflammatory cells to invade the GI mucosa. Lymphoplasmacytic-plasmacytic IBD is most common in dogs and cats and is characterized by an invasion of lymphocytes and plasma cells. In most cases the cause of the inflammation cannot be determined, but could be due to allergy, intestinal bacteria, or the intestinal tract itself. Chronic inflammation may self-perpetuate since loss of the mucosal barrier allows more pathogens to enter the mucosal cells, and further inflammation can result. Several breeds are at increased risk for IBD, including German shepherd dogs, basenjis, soft-coated wheaten terriers, and Chinese Shar-Peis.

Vomiting, diarrhea, and weight loss are the common signs of IBD, and all ages are affected. Vomiting occurs more often in cats with IBD. Clinical signs usually occur off and on over the course of months to years.

A dietary elimination trial should be performed to see if food allergy is the possible cause of IBD. This is discussed in further detail in Chapter 10, Food Intolerance and Allergy. Briefly, a diet is chosen that includes a novel protein source (one that the pet has not previously been exposed to). This diet is fed for about 3–4 weeks, and the pet is observed for clinical improvement.

Dehydration is a frequent problem because of the loss of fluid with vomiting. Fluid deficits should be corrected with intravenous or subcutaneous fluid therapy, and fresh water should be available at all times.

Potassium is lost during vomiting. Thus, a diet for pets with IBD should insure an adequate supply of potassium (Table 13.6). Diets should be energy dense, so that a small volume of food can be fed at each meal, which will help minimize GI secretions. However, high-fat diets should be avoided as these can contribute to osmotic diarrhea, with further fluid loss. Cats can tolerate a higher level of dietary fat as compared to dogs. Moderate-fat diets are best for dogs, but the fat content can be higher in cat diets.

With diarrhea, protein may be lost. Thus, diets for dogs and cats with IBD should provide an adequate level of protein without being excessive. Small quantities of soluble or mixed fiber sources can be included in diets for IBD. Adequate intake of vitamins is critical since water-soluble vitamins, especially, can be lost with diarrhea. Zinc deficiency is common in humans with IBD, so zinc should be supplied in adequate levels in the diet.

Table 13.6. Dietary recommendations for dogs and cats with inflammatory bowel disease.

Factor	Dogs	Cats
Protein	16%–24% DM; limit protein to one or two sources and use a protein that the dog has not been exposed to.	30%–50% DM; limit protein to one or two sources and use a protein that the cat has not been exposed to.
Fat	12%–15% DM	15%–22% DM
Crude fiber	0.5%–5.0% DM	0.5%–5.0% DM
Potassium	0.85%–1.1% DM	0.85%–1.1% DM
Zinc	Maintain adequate levels.	Maintain adequate levels.

DM, dry matter.

Supplemental omega-3 fatty acids may be beneficial in helping to modulate the inflammation present in the intestine. Fish oil is the best source for the long-chain omega-3 fatty acids and can be supplemented at 1 g fish oil/10 lb body weight daily. Probiotic administration may also be helpful in IBD. A probiotic is a live microorganism that is fed that can have health benefits for the host. In one study, a combination of 3 *Lactobacillus* strains were fed to dogs with IBD, and dogs receiving the probiotics had changes in inflammatory mediators produced in the intestine. Treatment of diarrhea with probiotics may also be beneficial by decreasing infection with *Clostridium*, *Salmonella*, and *Campylobacter*. The use of probiotics is generally safe, although caution should be exercised when giving probiotics to immunosuppressed or critically ill pets or to those with severely damaged intestinal mucosa.

■ Gluten-Sensitive Enteropathy

Gluten- or wheat-sensitive enteropathy is a chronic condition primarily seen in Irish setters. There is a hypersensitivity to gliadin, which is a glycoprotein found in wheat, barley, rye, buckwheat, and oats. Gliadin is not found in rice or potatoes, so these carbohydrate sources can be used. Dogs usually show clinical signs by 6 months of age. Sensitivity to gliadin is discussed in further detail in Chapter 10.

■ Lymphangiectasia/Protein-Losing Enteropathy

Lymphangiectasia is a chronic condition due to abnormalities within the lymphatic system and can be a primary problem or occur secondary to IBD, enteritis, or lymphosarcoma. Lymphangiectasia is a cause of protein-losing enteropathy (PLE).

Some patients with lymphangiectasia have chronic intermittent diarrhea and vomiting, but many have no GI signs and exhibit progressive weight loss. In lymphangiectasia, lymphatic channels that are important for delivery of nutrients from the intestine to the circulation leak, and protein and other nutrients are lost. Decreased concentrations of serum protein and albumin are common, and pets may develop edema and fluid accumulation in the abdomen and lungs.

Breeds most commonly affected with primary lymphangiectasia include Yorkshire terriers, golden retrievers, and dachshunds. Basenjis and soft-coated wheaten terriers often have secondary lymphangiectasia.

Restriction of dietary fat is the most critical dietary treatment. Ingested long-chain triglycerides stimulate intestinal lymph flow within 4–6 hours after a meal. The protein content of lymph increases as the fat content increases. Thus, by limiting the dietary fat (<10% DM for dogs and <15% DM for cats; Table 13.7), lymph flow is reduced, and less protein is lost. Unfortunately, the restricted dietary fat decreases the energy density of the food, and thus the pet must consume a large portion of diet to meet energy needs. The addition of medium-chain triglycerides (MCTs) has been suggested, as they partially bypass the lymphatic channels for absorption and do not stimulate the flow of lymph. MCTs are 8–10 carbons in length, do not require bile salts for absorption, and are absorbed faster than long-chain triglycerides. MCT oil is made from coconut oil and does not contain the essential fatty acids. One tablespoon of MCT oil provides about 115 kcal and can be added to the diet. However, MCT oil is not very palatable, and it is expensive.

High-protein diets are recommended to increase the caloric density. Multiple small meals are usually fed throughout the day. Fiber is typically kept to a low level since the addition of fiber decreases the energy density of the diet. Fat-soluble vitamins may need to be supplemented

Table 13.7. Dietary recommendations for dogs and cats with lymphangiectasia or protein-losing enteropathy.

Factor	Dogs	Cats
Protein	>25% DM	>35% DM
Fat	<10% DM	<15% DM
Crude fiber	<5% DM	<5% DM

DM, dry matter.

Table 13.8. Dietary recommendations for dogs and cats with short bowel syndrome.

Factor	Dogs	Cats
Fat	10%–15% DM	15%–22% DM
Carbohydrate	No lactose (no dairy products)	No lactose (no dairy products)
Crude fiber	10%–15% DM	10%–15% DM

DM, dry matter.

if there is long-term fat malabsorption and severe dietary fat restriction. The easiest method for fat-soluble vitamin supplementation is to administer them intramuscularly every 3 months.

■ Short Bowel Syndrome

Short bowel syndrome occurs after a major portion (>70%) of the small intestine has been removed for other reasons and is uncommon in dogs and cats. Conditions leading to small intestine resection include foreign body removal, intestinal intussusception, volvulus, fungal infections, or neoplasia. German shepherd dogs are most commonly affected. Weight loss and diarrhea occur secondary to the decreased malabsorption of nutrients in the shortened intestine.

Diets should be energy dense and contain 10%–15% DM fat for dogs and 15%–22% DM fat for cats (Table 13.8). MCT oil can also be added to the diet. Fiber at 10%–15% DM may be beneficial in modulating intestinal motility. Fat-soluble vitamins may need to be given intramuscularly every 3 months, as these are typically malabsorbed. Vitamin B_{12} absorption will be deficient if the distal ileum has been removed, and vitamin B_{12} may also need to be supplied via injection.

■ Small Intestinal Bacterial Overgrowth

Small intestinal bacterial overgrowth (SIBO) is characterized by an increase in the number of bacteria present in the small intestine. Clinical signs include intermittent small intestine diarrhea, flatulence, and weight loss. Breeds at highest risk include German shepherd dogs, beagles, Yorkshire terriers, and poodles. Decreased gastric acid secretion, loss of intestinal peristalsis, and intestinal stasis can all lead to SIBO.

An energy-dense diet should be fed since these pets are typically underweight. Also, with an energy-dense food, multiple small meals can be fed throughout the day, which helps to minimize GI secretions. The fat content of the diet should be moderate and not high to avoid further diarrhea. Diets should contain 10%–15% fat DM for dogs and 15%–22% DM for cats.

Large Intestine Disorders

■ Colitis

Colitis is common in dogs and cats and can be caused by a large number of infectious, toxic, inflammatory, and dietary factors. Acute colitis can be caused by dietary indiscretion, foreign bodies, drugs, *Campylobacter*, *Clostridium*, *Salmonella*, parasites such as *Giardia* or whipworms, panleukopenia, parvovirus, or hemorrhagic gastroenteritis. IBD (discussed previously) is the most common cause of chronic large intestine diarrhea in dogs and cats. Other causes of chronic large intestine diarrhea include parasites, *Campylobacter*, *Salmonella*, feline immunodeficiency virus, feline leukemia virus, fungal infections, food allergy, food intolerance, or neoplasia.

Young animals are more prone to dietary indiscretion and certain bacterial, viral, and parasitic infections. Older immunocompromised pets are at higher risk for contracting viral and bacterial infections. Dogs kept in unsanitary conditions or in an uncontrolled environment are more likely to be affected. Ulcerative colitis is most common in boxers and French bulldogs.

Dietary protein should be sufficient for life stage, unless a higher protein concentration is required due to a protein-losing enteropathy. Novel source proteins may be beneficial (Table 13.9). Fat content is usually moderate (10%–15% DM for dogs, 15%–22% DM for cats), but dogs and cats with colitis can often tolerate higher levels of fat if a greater dietary caloric density is necessary. Potassium depletion is common with colitis, so diets should contain more than adequate potassium. Sodium and chloride may also be low, so these minerals should be adequate in the diet. Dietary fiber helps to normalize colonic motility, buffers toxins in the GI tract, binds water, supports growth of normal intestinal bacterial flora, and alters the consistency of the contents of the GI tract. Some veterinarians have recommended feeding very low-fiber foods, whereas others have recommended moderate or high-dietary fiber concentrations. All levels of dietary fiber have been used to successfully manage colitis. Diets for pets with colitis should produce alkaline

Table 13.9. Dietary recommendations for dogs and cats with colitis.

Factor	Dogs	Cats
Protein	Consider a novel source	Consider a novel source
Fat	10%–15% DM	12%–22% DM
Crude fiber	0.5%–15% DM	0.5%–15% DM
Sodium	0.35%–0.50% DM	0.35%–0.50% DM
Potassium	0.8%–1.1% DM	0.8%–1.1% DM
Chloride	0.5%–1.3% DM	0.5%–1.3% DM

DM, dry matter.

urine. Supplemental omega-3 fatty acids may be beneficial for controlling inflammation.

■ Irritable Bowel Syndrome

Irritable bowel syndrome (IBS) is poorly characterized and may be caused by a decrease in GI motility. IBS has not been observed in cats. Dogs with IBS have intermittent bouts of large intestine–origin diarrhea. There may be explosive diarrhea accompanied by abdominal pain and straining. Stress is typically associated with IBS and can include the stress of boarding, dog showing, or changes in the environment. Dogs with a nervous temperament are more prone to developing IBS. Working breeds and toy breeds are more commonly affected.

Many dogs with IBS improve when the dietary fiber is increased. Crude fiber in the diet should be 10%–15% DM.

■ Constipation/Megacolon

Constipation refers to absent or infrequent defecation, with retention of feces in the colon and rectum. Obstipation occurs when the colon and rectum become impacted with hard, dry feces, and defecation cannot occur. Megacolon is a condition associated with chronic constipation in which the colon becomes extremely dilated with decreased motility. Causes of constipation include painful defecation, foreign bodies, colon obstruction, neuromuscular disorders, dehydration, or medications. Megacolon is most common in middle-aged to older male cats.

Dietary therapy for constipation and megacolon involves increasing the fiber content of the diet. Increased fiber is beneficial to increase colonic motility and intestinal transit rate. Flatulence or abdominal cramping can be side effects of increased dietary fiber. In some cases of megacolon, dietary therapy alone is not sufficient, and other medical therapies or surgery must be performed.

■ Perianal Fistulas

Perianal fistulas are deep fistulous tracts in the tissue surrounding the anus. German shepherd dogs and Irish setters are most commonly affected. The cause is not known but may involve infection of the glands around the anus and cell-mediated immune mechanisms. Clinical signs include constant licking of the anal area, scooting, straining to defecate, and a foul-smelling discharge from the anal area. Surgical therapy is often necessary.

Dietary therapy is to increase the fiber content of the diet. The fiber content of the diet is increased by 5% per week to prevent abdominal discomfort. A novel protein source may be beneficial in some dogs. Supplemental omega-3 fatty acids may help alleviate some of the inflammation.

■ Flatulence

Flatulence is caused by the production, accumulation, and expulsion of excess gas in the GI tract. Gas production in the GI tract is a normal occurrence, but when this is excessive, excess flatulence is a result. Most of the components of intestinal gas are odorless, and only about 1% of gas is composed of odoriferous compounds. The volume and composition of gas are affected by the types of intestinal bacteria present, feeding behaviors, and the composition of the diet. Other signs of excess gas production include borborygmus (growling stomach/intestines), abdominal discomfort, vomiting, diarrhea, and weight loss.

Feeding behaviors, such as nervous or greedy eaters, can lead to excessive flatulence. This is due to swallowing air with gulping of the food. High-fiber diets or diets high in legume content (such as soybeans) are more likely to cause excess gas formation. The ingestion of milk products can cause excessive gas production and abdominal discomfort due to the inability to digest lactose. Diets containing spoiled fat are also likely to lead to excessive flatulence. A few disease conditions can also cause excessive flatulence. Malabsorption, intestinal parasites, exocrine pancreatic insufficiency, small intestinal bacterial overgrowth, gastroenteritis, neoplasia, and lymphangiectasia can all be medical causes.

To determine the cause of flatulence, a complete physical examination should be performed, along with fecal examinations to rule out the presence of intestinal parasites. Any medical condition should be treated and the pet wormed if indicated. If no medical problems are detected, then the diet and feeding behavior should be examined. Air gulping during eating can be managed in a number of ways. Providing small quantities of food several times per day will help decrease the amount of air ingested at one time. If the dog is a greedy eater when other dogs are present, feeding this dog in an isolated area away from others may help to slow down the ingestion of food and amount of air consumed. Changing the diet to a high-quality, low-fiber, highly digestible diet that does not include soybean should result in decreased gas formation in the GI tract. An increase in exercise promotes increased expulsion of gas, resulting in less gas being passed while the dog is at rest.

Management practices are the most effective methods of dealing with excessive flatulence, but in severe cases, medical therapy may be indicated. The antifoaming agent simethicone does not reduce the amount of gas produced, but helps gas to be released easier, preventing accumulation.

Dog Recipes for Megaesophagus

Chicken and Potato   368
Ground Beef and Pasta   369
Eggs and Rice   370
Ground Beef and Rice   301
Tofu and Rice   303

Dog Recipes for Esophagitis

Cottage Cheese and Rice   371
Chicken and Rice   277
Chicken and Pasta   278
Chicken and Potato   279
Ground Beef and Rice   280
Ground Beef and Pasta   281
Ground Beef and Potato   282
Pork and Sweet Potato   394

Dog Recipes for Gastritis

Dog Recipes for Enteritis

Dog Recipes for Inflammatory Bowel Disease

Dog Recipes for Lymphangiectasia

Dog Recipes for Obstructive Swallowing Disorders

Chicken and Potato   368
Ground Beef and Pasta   369
Eggs and Rice   370
Ground Beef and Rice   301
Tofu and Rice   303

Dog Recipes for Protein-Losing Enteropathy

Turkey and Pasta   388
Whitefish and Pasta   389
Pork and Pasta   346
Chicken and Potato   365
Whitefish and Rice   367
Chicken and Rice   409
Cottage Cheese and Rice   410
Pork and Potato   411

Dog Recipes for Short Bowel Syndrome

Chicken and Rice   383
Ground Beef, Red Beans, and Pasta   343
Chicken and Barley   359
Ground Beef and Potato   360
Eggs and Pasta   361
Tofu and Pasta   362

Dog Recipes for Small Intestinal Bacterial Overgrowth

Chicken and Rice   383
Ground Beef, Red Beans, and Pasta   343
Chicken and Barley   359
Ground Beef and Potato   360
Eggs and Pasta   361
Tofu and Pasta   362

Dog Recipes for Colitis

Whitefish and Couscous   379
Chicken and Rice   383

Dog Recipes for Gastric Motility Disorders

Cat Recipes for Gastritis

Cat Recipes for Gastric Motility Disorders

Cat Recipes for Enteritis

Cat Recipes for Inflammatory Bowel Disease

Cat Recipes for Lymphangiectasia

Cat Recipes for Protein-Losing Enteropathy

Cat Recipes for Short Bowel Syndrome

Chicken and Lentils   474
Ground Beef and Lentils   475
Tuna and Lentils   476
Mackerel and Lentils   477

Cat Recipes for Small Intestinal Bacterial Overgrowth

Lamb and Lentils   462
Whitefish and Lentils   463
Chicken and Lentils   474
Ground Beef and Lentils   475
Tuna and Lentils   476
Mackerel and Lentils   477

Cat Recipes for Colitis

Rabbit and Quinoa   482
Venison and Rice   483
Cottage Cheese and Rice   484
Pork and Barley   485

Additional Reading

Buffington CA, Holloway C, Abood SK (Eds). 2004. Clinical dietetics. In *Manual of Veterinary Dietetics*. Elsevier, St. Louis, pp. 49–142.

Case LP, Carey DP, Hirakawa DA, Daristotle L (Eds). 2000. Nutritional management of gastrointestinal disease. In *Canine and Feline Nutrition: A Resource for Companion Animal Professionals*, 2nd edition. Mosby, St. Louis, pp. 489–504.

Davenport DJ, Remillard RL, Simpson KW, Pidgeon GL. 2000. Gastrointestinal and exocrine pancreatic disease. In *Small Animal Clinical Nutrition*, 4th edition. Hand MS, Thatcher CD, Remillard RL, Roudebush P (Eds). Mark Morris Institute, Topeka, KS, pp. 725–810.

Dikeman CL, Murphy MR, Fahey GC Jr. 2007. Diet type affects viscosity of ileal digesta of dogs and simulated gastric and small intestinal digesta. J Anim Physiol Anim Nutr (Berl) 91(3–4):139–147.

Dikeman CL, Murphy MR, Fahey GC Jr. 2007. Food intake and ingredient profile affect viscosity of ileal digesta of dogs. J Anim Physiol Anim Nutr (Berl) 91(3–4):130–138.

German A., Zentek J. 2006. The most common digestive diseases: The role of nutrition. In *Encyclopedia of Canine Clinical Nutrition*. Pibot P, Biourge V, Elliott D (Eds). Aniwa SAS, Aimargues, France, pp. 92–133.

Guilford WG, Matz ME. 2003. The nutritional management of gastrointestinal tract disorders in companion animals. NZ Vet J 51(6):284–291.

Guilford WG, Jones BR, Markwell PJ, Arthur DG, Collett MG, Harte JG. 2001. Food sensitivity in cats with chronic idiopathic gastrointestinal problems. J Vet Intern Med 15:7–13.

Hickman MA. 1998. Interventional nutrition for gastrointestinal disease. Clin Tech in Small Anim Pract 13(4):211–216.

Leib MS. 2000. Treatment of chronic idiopathic large-bowel diarrhea in dogs with a highly digestible diet and soluble fiber: A retrospective review of 37 cases. J Vet Intern Med 14:27–32.

Marks SL. 2000. Diagnostic and therapeutic approach to cats with chronic diarrhoea. J Fel Med and Surg 2:105–109.

Peterson PB, Willard MD. 2003. Protein-losing enteropathies. Vet Clin North Am Small Anim Pract 33(5):1061–1082.

Raghavan M, Glickman N, McCabe G, Lantz G, Glickman LT. 2004. Diet-related risk factors for gastric dilatation-volvulus in dogs of high-risk breeds. J Am Anim Hosp Assoc 40:192–203.

Sauter SN, Benyacoub J, Allenspach K, Gaschen F, Ontsouka E, Reuteler G, et al. 2006. Effects of probiotic bacteria in dogs with food responsive diarrhea treated with an elimination diet. J Anim Physiol Anim Nutr (Berl) 90(7–8):269–277.

Simpson KW, Fyfe J, Cornetta A, Sachs A, Strauss-Ayali D, Lamb SV, et al. 2001. Subnormal concentrations of serum cobalamin (vitamin B_{12}) in cats with gastrointestinal disease. J Vet Intern Med 15:26–32.

Westermarck E, Frias R, Skrzypczak T. 2005. Effect of diet and tylosin on chronic diarrhea in beagles. J Vet Intern Med 19:822–827.

Will K, Nolte I, Zentek J. 2005. Early enteral nutrition in young dogs suffering from haemorrhagic gastroenteritis. J Vet Med A Physiol Pathol Clin Med 52(7):371–376.

Wynn SG. 2009. Probiotics in veterinary practice. J Am Vet Med Assoc 234(5):606–613.

Zentek J, Freiche V. 2008. Digestive diseases in cats: The role of nutrition. In *Encyclopedia of Feline Clinical Nutrition*. Pibot P, Biourge V, Elliott D (Eds). Aniwa SAS, Aimargues, France, pp. 77–137.

CHAPTER 14
Diet and Chronic Renal Disease
P.A. Schenck

D.J. Chew

Chronic renal failure (CRF) is a common problem in dogs and cats, and dogs and cats of any age can be diagnosed with CRF. CRF is the third most common cause of death in dogs and the second leading cause of death in cats. In a study involving primary care practices, renal disease in all ages of cats had a prevalence of 2.2% compared to 0.8% in dogs. Increasing age and decreasing body condition score increase the likelihood for diagnosis of renal disease. In one study of cats affected with CRF, 37% were less than 10 years old, 31% were between 10 and 15 years of age, and 32% were greater than 15 years of age. It appears that old cats develop CRF more frequently than do dogs of similar age. The prevalence of CRF also increases in aging dogs. In one study, the prevalence of CRF in dogs 7 to 10 years of age was 1.3%, 2.4% in dogs between 10 and 15 years old, and 5.7% in dogs over 15 years of age.

Renal disease is a progressive disorder, starting with the loss of renal reserve and leading to renal insufficiency. Renal insufficiency progresses to azotemia, which is characterized by elevations in circulating urea nitrogen and creatinine concentrations. Azotemia progresses to uremia, where there are overt clinical signs. Chronic renal failure occurs when the compensatory mechanisms of chronically diseased kidneys are no longer able to maintain adequate functions to excrete waste products; regulate electrolyte, water, and acid-base homeostasis; degrade hormones; and synthesize endocrine hormones. As a result, nitrogenous solutes are retained, there are derangements of fluid, electrolyte, and acid-base balance, and there is failure of hormone production. Early renal disease can be difficult to diagnose, as azotemia does not develop until 75% or more of kidney function has been lost. The ability to concentrate urine is lost when 66% or more of kidney function has been lost.

The kidney is an important organ with excretory, regulatory, degradative, and endocrine functions. With CRF, there is loss of excretion of compounds such as urea and creatinine, and derangements in the reabsorption and excretion of solutes, which can lead to abnormalities in water, electrolytes, and acid-base balance. Many small peptides (such as gastrin) are normally filtered by the kidney, reabsorbed, and degraded in the proximal tubular cells. Loss of this clearance function can result in metabolic derangements because a number of these small peptides are hormones. The kidney is also responsible for production of erythropoietin and calcitriol, so these important hormones are decreased in CRF.

Acute Renal Failure

With acute renal failure (ARF), the kidneys are suddenly unable to regulate water balance, with rapid deterioration of renal function. ARF can be detected within hours to days after onset. Causes of ARF include hypotension from shock or heart failure, hemorrhage, severe dehydration, severe infections, obstruction of the ureters or urethra, urinary bladder rupture, or nephrotoxic injury from medications, ethylene glycol (antifreeze), organic solvents, heavy metals, pesticides, leptospirosis, or snake venom. Renal damage associated with ARF may be reversible if treated promptly and aggressively. Irreversible progressive renal damage from ARF can lead to CRF.

Causes of Chronic Renal Failure

There are many different causes of CRF in dogs and cats, although a definitive cause is often not determined. Chronic tubulointerstitial nephritis of unknown cause is the most common pathologic diagnosis for CRF in dogs and cats. Other causes of CRF in dogs include chronic pyelonephritis, chronic glomerulonephritis, amyloidosis, hypercalcemic nephropathy, chronic obstructive uropathy causing hydronephrosis, familial renal disease, progression after ARF, chronic toxicity (food-associated, drug administration, environmental toxins), neoplasia, or primary systemic hypertension. Other causes of CRF in cats include chronic pyelonephritis, chronic glomerulonephritis, amyloidosis (especially Abyssinians), polycystic kidney disease (Persians), hypercalcemic nephropathy, progression after ARF, chronic obstructive uropathy, neoplasia, pyogranulomatous nephritis due to feline infectious peritonitis, hypokalemic nephropathy, chronic toxicity, and primary systemic hypertension.

Breeds at Risk of Chronic Renal Failure

There are several conditions that can cause CRF in young dogs and cats, and some have been shown to be hereditary. The term *nephropathy* has been used to describe disorganized nephrogenesis; familial nephropathy is used to describe the occurrence in related individuals, and hereditary nephropathy is used when a hereditary basis has been documented.

Familial nephropathy has been observed in cocker spaniels, Norwegian elkhounds, Lhasa apsos, shih tzus, Doberman pinschers, standard poodles, soft-coated wheaten terriers, bull terriers, Samoyeds, Bernese mountain dogs, Rottweilers, beagles, golden retrievers, and chow chows. Hereditary nephropathy has been observed in Samoyeds, English cocker spaniels, and bull terriers. These dogs are affected with CRF at a young age and may show stunted growth. Renal amyloidosis occurs in young Chinese shar-peis, beagles, and Abyssinian cats, and polycystic kidney disease is familial in Persian cats. Himalayan, Persian, mixed breed, and Siamese cats also appear to be at increased risk for renal disease or renal failure.

Pathophysiology of Chronic Renal Failure

The development of glomerular hyperfiltration and intraglomerular hypertension are considered the most important factors in the progression of CRF. Hyperfiltration increases the movement of protein across the glomerular capillaries, and this increased filtration of proteins into the urine (proteinuria) is toxic to the kidneys. In dogs, renal disease does not become progressive until 85%–95% of the renal mass has been lost. Cats appear to have a slower progression of renal disease. In addition, compounds that have decreased excretion during CRF contribute to the clinical signs of uremia. Urea, guanidine compounds, products of bacterial metabolism, myoinositol, trace elements, parathyroid hormone and other hormones, have been considered as "uremic toxins."

Clinical Findings in Chronic Renal Failure

The first abnormalities that may be noticed by owners is an increase in the urine produced (polyuria) and thirst (polydipsia). Dog owners may notice this earlier if the dog starts to have accidents in the house, especially overnight. Cat owners may not notice increased urination until an increase in the weight of the litterbox is observed. Both the ability to produce concentrated urine (to conserve water) and the ability to excrete water are impaired in CRF. Impairment of concentrating ability develops when about 67% of the kidney is not functional; however, some cats with CRF retain considerable urine-concentrating ability even after the development of azotemia.

Gastrointestinal signs such as vomiting are more common in dogs with CRF than in cats. Vomiting may be stimulated by the presence of uremic toxins. Gastroenteritis with hemorrhage or gastrointestinal ulcers may result due to increased gastrin concentrations. Diarrhea is relatively uncommon, but may occur late in CRF. Anorexia is common due to the effects of uremic toxins on the brain and also due to oral erosions, gastroenteritis, or secondary hyperparathyroidism causing bone loss in the jaw. Weight loss is due to the lack of adequate intake and to increased catabolic processes. The haircoat may be dull and dry. Lean muscle mass is often lost in CRF, most likely due to the chronic metabolic acidosis that is present. Acidosis increases the breakdown of proteins and enhances branched-chain amino acid catabolism. Uremic encephalopathy may occur when the glomerular filtration rate decreases to less than 10% of normal. Clinical signs of uremic encephalopathy include facial twitching, head bobbing, abnormal behavior, tremors, and seizures. Calcium influx in the brain mediated by high parathyroid (PTH) concentrations may play a role in uremic encephalopathy of CRF. Amino acid alterations due to malnutrition or accumulation of uremic toxins may alter neurotransmitter function. Low serum ionized calcium concentrations, systemic hypertension, or aluminum accumulation in the brain may also contribute to the clinical signs.

Oral lesions are more common in dogs than in cats with CRF. There may be a foul oral odor due to accumulation of ammonia and aliphatic amines, and erosions and ulcers of the mouth and tongue may be due to excretion of urea into saliva and breakdown to ammonia by oral bacteria. Tongue tip necrosis may occur as the result of a poor blood supply to the tongue, and the gums may be pale due to anemia.

Dehydration is a common finding in CRF due to the increased fluid loss in urine and from the gastrointestinal tract (vomit), coupled with a lack of fluid intake. There is a loss of skin elasticity, and the gums appear dry. Heart murmurs and abnormal rhythms are relatively common as a consequence of systemic hypertension and anemia. On abdominal palpation, the kidneys are usually small, hard, and irregular, though normal to enlarged kidneys do not rule out CRF, especially in cats. Edema or ascites suggests a severe loss of plasma proteins. A loss of bone mass (fibrous osteodystrophy) is most dramatic in young growing dogs with uremia, especially in the jaw (rubber jaw). The teeth appear loose or may be lost, and the jaw may actually feel rubbery. Blindness can be observed if there are retinal lesions from systemic hypertension. There may also be hemostasis defects and a predisposition to hemorrhage.

Laboratory Findings in Chronic Renal Failure

Results of a complete blood cell count (CBC) demonstrate that nonregenerative anemia is common in CRF but variable in severity. The severity of the anemia is roughly correlated to the severity of the CRF as judged by serum creatinine concentration. The primary cause of anemia in CRF is a decrease in the production of erythropoietin (EPO) by the damaged kidneys. Erythropoietin stimulates the final differentiation of erythroid cells in the bone marrow into mature red blood cells, and with a lack of EPO, mature red blood cells are produced at a much slower rate. The life span of red cells in uremic patients is approximately 50% that of healthy individuals. The decreased life span is thought to be due to a toxic factor (possibly PTH) that promotes hemolysis. In addition, some uremic toxins may impair red blood cell production. An increase in neutrophils and a decrease in lymphocytes may be seen due to the stress of chronic disease. Platelet numbers may be normal, but platelet function is abnormal.

Results of the serum biochemistry profile show that both serum urea nitrogen and creatinine concentrations are elevated in CRF. In animals with substantial muscle wasting, the serum creatinine concentration may not reflect the severity of CRF. Serum sodium is normal in most patients with CRF, although it may be elevated if dehydration is present. Most animals have normal serum potassium concentrations, although a decrease in serum potassium (hypokalemia) can occur in 10%–30% with CRF due to a combination of anorexia, loss of muscle mass, vomiting, and polyuria. Serum potassium levels can underestimate the total body potassium because most of the body's potassium lies within the cells. Thus, a significant body deficit of potassium can exist without the development of hypokalemia. Hypokalemic nephropathy is a specific syndrome in cats as a result of CRF or as a cause of CRF. In the early stages of CRF, the serum phosphorus concentration is often normal due to the corrective effect of renal secondary hyperparathyroidism. Hyperphosphatemia develops with advancing CRF when 85% or more of the kidneys become nonfunctional.

Serum total calcium concentration is normal in most patients with CRF, but can be low or high in some patients. Frequent errors in interpretation of calcium status occur when serum total calcium is measured. Analysis of the ionized calcium concentration is required for an accurate assessment of calcium status. The "mass law" effect decreases serum calcium as a consequence of increased serum phosphorus concentration. The amounts of calcium and phosphorus that can remain in solution together are defined by the calcium multiplied by phosphorus product. Decreased production of calcitriol also results in impaired intestinal absorption of calcium, lowering the circulating calcium concentration. Hypocalcemia in CRF is usually asymptomatic because metabolic acidosis leads to an increase in the ionized calcium concentration. A small percentage of dogs and cats with CRF can have hypercalcemia, which may further damage the kidneys by causing mineralization, especially if the phosphorus is elevated.

Metabolic acidosis is common in patients with CRF. Metabolic acidosis has been documented in 53% of cats with advanced CRF, but in only 15% of cats with mild CRF. The main cause of metabolic acidosis is limitation of renal ammonium excretion. When the glomerular filtration rate falls to 10%–20% of normal, the diseased kidneys cannot excrete ammonia adequately and acidosis occurs.

Urinalysis demonstrates that animals fail to concentrate their urine when 67% of the kidneys become nonfunctional. An increase in protein in the urine suggests an increased severity of disease and progression of CRF.

Systemic Hypertension

The prevalence of systemic hypertension in dogs with CRF ranges from 9% to 93% and from 19% to 65% in cats with CRF. About 20%–30% of dogs and cats with CRF have systemic hypertension at the time of diagnosis, and another 10%–20% will develop hypertension within a year of the initial diagnosis. Systemic hypertension is a major risk factor for the progression of CRF in humans and rats, and recent evidence suggests that this is also true for dogs and cats with CRF. It is likely that high systemic blood pressure is transmitted to the glomerular vessels, which promotes further injury to the kidneys.

A clinical study of dogs with CRF showed that dogs with systemic hypertension at the time of diagnosis progressively lost renal function at greater rates than dogs with intermediate or lower systemic blood pressure. Those in the high blood pressure group had three times an increased risk for uremic crisis than dogs in lower blood pressure groups and had much greater risk for renal-related death. The correlation of unregulated hypertension to the progression of CRF has not been established in cats. Cats that have systemic hypertension from a variety of causes have been shown to survive longest when their blood pressure is well controlled.

Patients with systolic blood pressure readings consistently above 170 mm Hg or those with abnormally high blood pressure readings that also have eye lesions consistent with hypertensive retinopathy (e.g., retinal edema, intraretinal serous exudation, retinal hemorrhages, arterial tortuosity, retinal detachment) are candidates for antihypertensive therapy. Diuretics and dietary salt restriction are not effective treatment for severe hypertension. Therapy using ACE inhibitors (ACE-I: enalapril, benazepril), calcium channel blockers (amlodipine), beta adrenergic antagonists (atenolol, propranolol), or alpha-1 adrenergic antagonists (prazosin) are used to lower blood pressure.

Renal Secondary Hyperparathyroidism

Renal secondary hyperparathyroidism occurs when parathyroid hormone (PTH) synthesis and secretion become excessive as a result of kidney disease. Excess PTH is a major uremic toxin and exerts adverse effects on the brain, heart, bone marrow, and other tissues. Increased secretion of PTH by each parathyroid cell, as well as increased numbers of cells due to parathyroid hyperplasia, leads to increased circulating PTH. Insufficient production of calcitriol in uremic patients is the most important factor leading to the uncontrolled secretion of PTH. The major effects of calcitriol are to increase the intestinal absorption of calcium and phosphate and to increase bone resorption, thereby increasing the serum ionized calcium concentration. In renal disease, there are fewer healthy proximal tubule cells containing the mitochondrial 1α-hydroxylase enzyme necessary to form calcitriol from the precursor 25-hydroxyvitamin D. Nephron loss during CRF is estimated most commonly by the magnitude of increased serum creatinine. An association of increasing serum creatinine with diminished serum calcitriol in dogs has been shown. Decreased blood calcitriol lowers intestinal calcium absorption, leading to hypocalcemia. As the serum ionized calcium concentration falls, the secretion of PTH is stimulated. In early CRF, the increased PTH concentration can restore calcitriol production and ionized calcium concentrations when there are still enough proximal tubular cells remaining that are capable of calcitriol synthesis.

As glomerular filtration rate is further reduced in late chronic renal failure, greater increases of serum phosphorus occur, mass law interactions contribute to a decrease of ionized calcium, and further PTH production is stimulated. A greater reduction in the activity of the 1α-hydroxylase responsible for calcitriol synthesis occurs as a consequence of the markedly increased serum phosphorus. In addition, the absolute loss of most of the proximal tubular cells makes adequate synthesis of calcitriol no longer possible. At this point, the markedly elevated PTH concentration is no longer able to restore calcitriol concentrations to normal. The ionized calcium concentration decreases, stimulating further increases in PTH production. The excess PTH causes continual reabsorption of bone, especially in the face, leading to severe bone loss in the jaw (rubber jaw).Treatment with oral calcitriol is recommended to decrease the PTH levels and to return the serum ionized calcium concentration to normal.

Treatment of Chronic Renal Failure

The goals in treating CRF are to minimize the clinical signs of uremia, retard the progressive loss of renal function, and to preserve the nutritional status of the pet. Any potentially reversible causes of renal disease (such as pyelonephritis, hypercalcemia, or obstructive nephropathy) should be treated, and concurrent systemic or urinary tract bacterial infections should be treated with the appropriate antibiotics. Extensive therapy is recommended to manage fluid balance, to control vomiting and inappetence, to provide hormone replacement (erythropoietin and calcitriol), and to control proteinuria and hypertension. In addition to medical therapies, dietary management is critical in the treatment of chronic renal failure.

■ Dietary Management

"Renal-friendly" diets are generally restricted in protein, phosphorus, calcium, and sodium. Compared to the average grocery or pet store foods, renal-friendly diets are restricted in protein by about

Table 14.1. Dietary recommendations for renal disease in dogs and cats.

Factor	Dogs	Cats
Protein	≤15% DM	≤30% DM
Phosphorus	0.15%–0.3% DM	0.04%–0.60% DM
Sodium	<0.25% DM	<0.35% DM

DM, dry matter.

33%–50%, while phosphorus is restricted by 70%–80%. Treatment should provide adequate nutrient intake to allow a good quality of life with reasonable body condition. Food intake and body condition commonly deteriorate during CRF and may result from physical changes, altered sense of smell and taste, metabolic changes that suppress appetite, and dietary interventions that adversely affect food intake. Free access to water should be provided at all times to prevent dehydration in the pet with polyuria and CRF.

Phosphorus

Dietary phosphorus restriction is the most valuable dietary modification for dogs and cats with CRF. The beneficial effect of phosphorus restriction is independent of protein restriction. Dietary phosphorus restriction in CRF has been shown to blunt or reverse renal secondary hyperparathyroidism. Renal lesions are less severe, glomerular filtration rate is better maintained, and survival time is longer.

When CRF is diagnosed, phosphorus restriction is initiated by feeding a low-phosphorus diet (Table 14.1). Dietary phosphorus restriction alone may be capable of lowering serum phosphorus and PTH levels in some dogs and cats with chronic renal disease or early renal failure. Decreased PTH is achieved by decreasing the catabolism and increasing the synthesis of calcitriol. Currently, there are no diets available that are restricted in phosphate alone, so restriction of dietary phosphate is typically accomplished by restricting animal-source proteins.

In a study of cats with naturally occurring CRF, renal secondary hyperparathyroidism was successfully managed by dietary restriction of phosphorus; one-third of the cats also required treatment with phosphorus binders. Survival times in CRF cats eating the renal diet were over twice that of those eating maintenance diets: this effect was attributed to phosphorus control and control of PTH. Renal diets may provide sufficient dietary phosphate restriction during early stages of CRF, but often dietary phosphate binders are needed. Phosphorus-binding agents should be given with meals or within 2 hours of feeding to maximize their binding of dietary phosphorus. Commonly employed oral phosphorus binders include aluminum hydroxide, calcium carbonate, and calcium acetate.

Two nutritional supplements designed to limit intestinal phosphate absorption have been approved for use in cats in some countries. Epakitin (Vetoquinol, Buena, NJ) contains chitosan and calcium carbonate to provide intestinal phosphate binding for cats. One small study in CRF cats has shown that this product lowers serum phosphorus in those eating a normal diet after 35 days. Lanthanum carbonate is a potent phosphate binder that is an emerging favorite for use in human nephrology. Lanthanum carbonate has recently been approved as a nutritional supplement for cats in Europe and Japan (Renalzin, Bayer Animal Health, Pittsburgh, PA) and is designed to limit intestinal phosphate absorption. Several studies have shown the ability of this product to limit intestinal phosphate absorption from maintenance diets and from veterinary renal diets in both normal cats and those with reduced renal function.

Return of serum phosphorus to normal does not guarantee that PTH levels will return to normal, as phosphorus restriction works only in those that have enough active tubular machinery capable of calcitriol synthesis once the inhibitory effects of excess phosphorus are removed. Return of serum phosphorus to within the normal range is an initial goal, but achieving concentrations in the lower to midrange for normal serum phosphorus provides additional benefits in control of PTH.

Protein

Although widely advocated, the ability of dietary protein restriction to ameliorate clinical signs in dogs and cats with CRF remains unclear. Potential benefits would be obtained by decreasing the production of toxic metabolites of protein metabolism in patients with azotemia. Moderate protein restriction is indicated, but protein restriction as a single dietary change does not seem to provide protection against progression of renal disease in dogs and cats with advanced CRF.

When to start protein restriction in the course of CRF is unclear. It is not recommended early in the course of CRF prior to the accumulation of nitrogenous waste products. There is no evidence that dietary intervention provides any benefits to dogs or cats that are not yet azotemic. If there is evidence of progression of CRF (increasing proteinuria, progressively less concentrated urine), dietary intervention may be prescribed before the pet becomes overtly ill. Current guidelines suggest that dietary therapy for CRF should be instituted when serum urea nitrogen is less than 60–80 mg/dL and serum creatinine is less than 2.0–2.5 mg/dL.

The development of protein-calorie malnutrition is always a concern in dogs and cats with CRF, but even more so when patients are consuming low-protein diets. Cats have a higher protein requirement than do dogs. Enzymes in the cat's liver are unable to adapt to changes in dietary protein intake, and these enzymes function at a high rate of activity independent of the level of dietary protein. Thus, a large amount of protein is catabolized after every meal regardless of the amount of protein ingested. Cats also require higher levels of arginine and taurine. Cats synthesize only a small amount of taurine and cannot use glycine for bile acid conjugation if taurine is restricted. Thus, a source of taurine from animal sources is necessary in the diet to replace taurine loss. For these reasons, it is easier for cats to develop protein-calorie malnutrition as compared to dogs. Protein restriction should be considered when moderate to severe azotemia persists in the well-hydrated state. There must be a balance between reducing protein intake and the animal's willingness to eat. Maintenance of stable body weight and serum albumin concentration suggests adequate intake of calories and protein, whereas progressive declines in body weight and serum albumin concentration suggest malnutrition or progression of disease and are indications to increase the amount of protein fed.

Cats with CRF fed a protein-restricted, phosphorus-restricted veterinary diet survived a median of 633 days compared to 264 days for cats fed a conventional diet in one nonrandomized retrospective study. In a prospective randomized, blinded clinical trial, the feeding of a renal diet was superior to the feeding of an adult maintenance diet in minimizing uremic episodes and mortality rate in cats with spontaneous CRF. No renal-related deaths or uremic crises occurred in cats consuming the renal diet during the 24 months of this study compared to 22% deaths and 26% uremic episodes in CRF cats eating the maintenance diet. In a randomized, blinded prospective clinical study, dogs with mild to moderate renal failure fed a renal diet had a median survival time of 594 days and fewer uremic crises compared to a median survival time of 188 days in dogs fed the conventional diet. The observed results were compatible with a slower rate of progression of renal disease in the dogs fed the modified diet.

Energy

Adequate nonprotein calories to maintain body condition should be provided by carbohydrate and fat. Energy requirements for pets with CRF are similar to that of normal animals.

Lipid

Lipoprotein abnormalities have been poorly characterized in dogs and cats with CRF. Dogs and cats with CRF may show a mild increase in serum cholesterol concentration early in the course of disease, with a mild elevation of serum triglyceride concentration occurring later. Dogs with secondary hyperparathyroidism due to chronic renal failure exhibit a decrease in lipoprotein lipase activity, resulting in impaired removal of lipid from the circulation. Proteinuria may be associated with the urinary loss of heparin sulfate, an important cofactor for lipoprotein lipase. In humans with CRF, the progression of renal dysfunction has been shown to correlate with serum total cholesterol. Lipoprotein synthesis may also be altered in CRF.

Dietary fat may influence the progression of CRF by affecting serum cholesterol and triglyceride concentrations and changing platelet aggregation, immune responses, or blood pressure. Supplementation of diets with omega-3 polyunsaturated fatty acids (PUFAs) may have a renoprotective effect. The ideal ratio of omega-6 to omega-3 PUFA in the diet is not known. Fish oil can be supplemented at 1 g/10 lb body weight per day. Increasing the amount of omega-3 PUFA relative to omega-6 PUFA in the diet decreases production of the proinflammatory, platelet-aggregating, vasoconstrictive prostaglandin TXA_2 and increases production of vasodilatory prostaglandins (PGE, PGI), which have the potential to increase renal blood flow and glomerular filtration rate. These effects may slow the progression of CRF. Studies in dogs have demonstrated beneficial effects of omega-3 PUFA supplementation, with decreased cholesterol and triglyceride concentrations, reduction in proteinuria, preservation of glomerular filtration rate, and less severe renal damage. In a recent study of cats with CRF, the survival on one modified diet with a high level of omega-3 PUFA was the longest, suggesting benefit from the omega-3 PUFA supplementation.

Sodium Chloride

In dogs and cats with CRF and systemic hypertension, and in those with glomerular disease, sodium retention, and edema, sodium restriction is advisable. Many commercial pet foods provide more sodium than needed. It is probably wise to provide adequate dietary sodium, but to avoid excessive amounts.

Potassium

Excessive serum potassium is usually not a problem in CRF, as the kidneys can maintain normal serum potassium concentrations even when the glomerular filtration rate is about 5% of normal. Cats with CRF are prone to disorders of potassium homeostasis, resulting in a decrease in circulating potassium (hypokalemia). Potassium supplementation is indicated if hypokalemia is observed. Dietary potassium should be provided at adequate but not excessive levels.

Vitamins

Excess serum vitamin A concentrations are common in people with renal failure, and serum creatinine concentrations appear to correlate with vitamin A concentrations. Toxicity is uncommon though, because most of the vitamin A is bound to retinol-binding protein and is inactive. Little is known regarding vitamin A concentrations in dogs and cats with renal failure, thus no dietary recommendations have been made.

There is an increased risk for deficiency of B vitamins in renal failure, due to decreased intake and loss in vomit, diarrhea, and urine. Deficiency of some of the B vitamins may be linked to the anorexia seen in renal failure. Vitamins should be supplied in adequate quantities in the diet.

Dog Recipes for Renal Disease

Chicken and Rice   416
Ground Beef and Rice   417
Salmon and Potato   418
Chicken and Potato   419
Ground Beef and Potato   420
Ground Beef and Tapioca   421
Eggs and Rice   422
Eggs and Potato   423
Tofu and Rice   424

Cat Recipes for Renal Disease

Chicken and Rice   497
Ground Beef and Rice   498
Lamb and Rice   499
Tuna and Rice   500
Salmon and Couscous   501

Additional Reading

Allen TA, Polzin DJ, Adams LG. 2000. Renal disease. In *Small Animal Clinical Nutrition*, 4th edition. Hand MS, Thatcher CD, Remillard RL, Roudebush P (Eds). Mark Morris Institute, Topeka, KS, pp. 563–604.

Bauer JE, Markwell PJ, Rawlings JM, Senior DE. 1999. Effects of dietary fat and polyunsaturated fatty acids in dogs with naturally developing chronic renal failure. J Am Vet Med Assoc 215(11):1588–1591.

Brown SA, Finco DR, Barges JW, Brown CA, Barsanti JA. 1998. Interventional nutrition for renal disease. Clin Tech in Sm Anim Pract 13(4):217–223.

Buffington CA, Holloway C, Abood S. 2004. Clinical dietetics. In *Manual of Veterinary Dietetics*. Elsevier, St. Louis, pp. 49–142.

Case LP, Carey DP, Hirakawa DA, Daristotle L (Eds). 2000. Chronic renal failure. In *Canine and Feline Nutrition: A Resource for Companion Animal Professionals*, 2nd edition. Mosby, St. Louis, pp. 451–472.

Chew DJ, Buffington CAT, Schenck PA. 2004. Feeding the aging cat with chronic renal failure. Compendium on Continuing Education for the Practicing. Veterinarian 26(Suppl 2A):28–33.

DiBartola SP, Willard MD. 2006. Disorders of phosphorus: Hypophosphatemia and hyperphosphatemia. In *Fluid Therapy in Small Animal Practice*, 3rd edition. Dibartola S (Ed). Elsevier, St. Louis, pp. 195–209.

Elliott DA. 2006. Nutritional management of chronic renal disease in dogs and cats. Vet Clin North Am Small Anim Pract 36(6):1377–1384.

Elliott D, Lefebvre H. 2006. Chronic renal disease: The importance of nutrition. In *Encyclopedia of Canine Clinical Nutrition*. Pibot P, Biourge V, Elliott D (Eds). Aniwa SAS, Aimargues, France, pp. 252–282.

Elliott J, Elliott DA. 2008. Dietary therapy for feline chronic kidney disease. In *Encyclopedia of Feline Clinical Nutrition*. Pibot P, Biourge V, Elliott D (Eds). Aniwa SAS, Aimargues, France, pp. 249–283.

Jacob F, Polzin DJ, Osborne CA, Allen TA, Kirk CA, Neaton JD, et al. 2002. Clinical evaluation of dietary modification for treatment of spontaneous chronic renal failure in dogs. J Am Vet Med Assoc 220(8):1163–1170.

Laflamme DP. 2008. Pet food safety: Dietary protein. Top Companion Anim Med 23(3):154–157.

Pollen SM. 2001. Renal disease in small animals: A review of conditions and potential nutrient and botanical interventions. Altern Med Rev 6(Suppl):S46–S61.

Ross SJ, Osborne CA, Kirk CA, Lowry SR, Koehler LA, et al. 2006. Clinical evaluation of dietary modification for treatment of spontaneous chronic kidney disease in cats. J Am Vet Med Assoc 229(6):949–957.

Schenck PA, Chew DJ, Nagode LA, Rosol TJ. 2006. Disorders of calcium: Hypercalcemia and hypocalcemia. In *Fluid Therapy in Small Animal Practice*, 3rd edition. Dibartola S (Ed). Elsevier, St. Louis, pp. 122–194.

CHAPTER 15
Diet and Urinary Tract Stones

P.A. Schenck

D.J. Chew

Urinary tract stones (uroliths) are a relatively common problem in dogs and cats. The most common uroliths in dogs are struvite, oxalate, purine (urate and xanthine), cystine, and silicates. The most common uroliths in cats are struvite and oxalate.

A urolith is an organized concretion found in the urinary tract. When the solubility product of a solute is exceeded, crystals form, aggregate, and grow. Crystals must reside in the urinary tract for a sufficient period of time to allow a urolith to form. Diet, water intake, urine volume, urine concentration, urine pH, metabolic abnormalities, environment, and genetics all contribute to stone formation. Most uroliths have one major component. Crystals can be present in urine (crystalluria) when uroliths are not, and crystals may be absent in urine even though uroliths are present. A few crystals present in concentrated urine can be normal; however, large numbers of crystals in fresh urine sediment are a risk factor for recurrence of stone formation in those animals that have previously formed a urolith.

Some uroliths are large and remain in the bladder. Some uroliths are small enough to pass into the urethra and cause obstruction. Signs of uroliths include straining to urinate, frequent urination, urinary incontinence, and blood in the urine (hematuria). Uroliths can be present in the bladder for long periods of time before any clinical signs are present.

Quantitative stone analysis is essential for accurate identification of the uroliths present. Small stones may be aspirated from the bladder

195

through a urinary catheter; surgical removal of stones from the bladder (cystotomy) may be necessary if the uroliths are large. Radiographs or ultrasound of the urinary tract should be performed to ensure that all urinary stones have been removed after surgery or removal through a catheter.

General Treatment of Urolithiasis

The frequency of urolithiasis in dogs or cats is not high enough to justify dietary modification before a urolith forms, and treatment of crystalluria is unnecessary in dogs that have never formed a urolith. Initial therapy of urolithiasis is to either remove or dissolve the urolith, followed by therapy to decrease the risk of recurrence. Specific treatment recommendations are based on the type of urolith present.

Any animal that has formed a urolith is at increased risk for recurrence. Water is the most important nutrient in preventing recurrence. Increasing water intake to dilute urine and increase the frequency of urination is an important part of treatment. Urine specific gravity should be kept near 1.020 in dogs, and less than 1.030 in cats. A specific diet should be chosen that provides less precursor minerals for excretion and results in a favorable urinary pH to keep crystals in solution.

Medical dissolution protocols are available for struvite, urates, and cystine uroliths. There are no protocols available for dissolution of calcium oxalate uroliths; thus, these must be removed either by catheterization or surgery. Successful dissolution should be confirmed by radiographs or ultrasound. Periodic evaluation of the urine should be performed to make sure that there is no urinary infection and to assess the urine specific gravity. There should be few crystals present; if large numbers of crystals are present, then there needs to be a change in therapy.

Struvite Urolithiasis in Dogs

Struvite (magnesium ammonium phosphate hexahydrate) is the most common urolith type and accounts for about 50% of uroliths in dogs. Struvite stones can be single or multiple and can be very large. They are usually dense enough to be seen on radiographs.

Most struvite uroliths are associated with a urinary tract infection (UTI). Struvite urolithiasis is most common in female dogs between 2 and 9 years of age. The miniature schnauzer, Shih tzu, bichon frise, miniature poodle, Lhasa apso, and cocker spaniel are at increased risk.

Table 15.1. Dietary recommendations for struvite urinary stones in dogs.

Factor	Recommendation for Treatment	Recommendation for Future Prevention
Water	Encourage intake; keep USG < 1.020	Encourage intake; keep USG < 1.020
Protein	<8% DM	<25% DM
Phosphorus	<0.1% DM	<0.6% DM
Magnesium	<0.02% DM	0.04%–0.10% DM
Urine pH	Maintain in acidic range (pH 5.9–6.1)	Maintain in acidic range (pH 6.2–6.4)

USG, urine specific gravity; DM, dry matter.

Urinary tract infection usually precedes the development of struvite uroliths. Hydrolysis of urea by bacteria leads to increased generation of ammonia and carbon dioxide into the urine, which results in an increase in urinary pH. Increased availability of ammonium and phosphate ions results, which contributes to struvite formation. The solubility of struvite is markedly reduced in the alkaline urine. Failure to eliminate or prevent UTI is the main reason why struvite uroliths recur.

Diets designed for dissolution of struvite uroliths in dogs are severely protein-restricted, phosphate-restricted, and magnesium-restricted (Table 15.1). These diets also produce highly acidic urine. The severe protein restriction is designed to reduce urea generation; therefore, less urinary urea is available as a substrate for urease-producing bacteria in the urine. Mineral restriction reduces the urinary minerals available to form struvite uroliths.

Caution should be exercised when feeding these diets. Since these diets are very restricted in protein, they may decrease serum proteins, which affects fluid balance, and should not be used in dogs with heart failure, renal failure, or hypertension. Also, since these diets are typically high in fat, they should be used with caution in patients at risk for pancreatitis. Breeds at risk for pancreatitis (miniature schnauzers, bichon frisoco, Yorkshire terriers, Chihuahuas, Jack Russell terriers, Japanese spaniels, Labrador retrievers, Maltese, and Shetland sheepdogs) should be evaluated for pancreatitis before and during dietary therapy. Because of the protein and mineral restriction, these diets should only be fed when necessary, and they should not be fed long term.

Once the struvite urolith has dissolved, prevention of recurrence is aimed at eliminating UTI. Any underlying conditions predisposing to

UTI (excessive perivulvar skin folds, incontinence, hyperadrenocorticism, etc.) should be treated.

Calcium Oxalate Urolithiasis in Dogs

Calcium oxalate monohydrate and dihydrate stones account for about 30% of uroliths in dogs, and the incidence has increased in recent years. Calcium oxalate uroliths may be single or multiple and are visible on radiographs. The dehydrate form is often spicular, with sharp, jagged edges, and the monohydrate form is usually small, smooth, and round. Breeds at increased risk for calcium oxalate uroliths are miniature schnauzers, standard schnauzers, Lhasa apso, Yorkshire terrier, bichon frises, shih tzu, and miniature poodles. Breeds at decreased risk for development of calcium oxalate uroliths include German shepherds, golden retrievers, and cocker spaniels. Affected dogs are typically male and between 8 and 12 years of age, with an average age of 8–9 years. Overweight dogs are at increased risk, and dogs with hyperadrenocorticism are also at increased risk, possibly secondary to decreased renal tubular calcium reabsorption. An increase in serum calcium (hypercalcemia) has been detected in about 4% of dogs with calcium oxalate uroliths. Urinary tract infection is not typical in dogs with calcium oxalate uroliths. Calcium oxalate uroliths are relatively slow growing, and the recurrence rate is from 25% to 48%.

Supersaturation with calcium and oxalate in urine is required for calcium oxalate uroliths to form. Acidic urine is common in dogs with calcium oxalate uroliths and reflects systemic acid-base balance. The chronic feeding of an acidifying diet may cause leaching of calcium from bones as a buffering response, and this excess calcium is filtered by the kidneys, resulting in excess calcium excreted in urine (hypercalciuria). Hypercalciuria is a risk factor for calcium urolith formation.

Calcium oxalate uroliths need to be removed surgically or via catheterization. Dogs with concurrent hypercalcemia should be evaluated for the presence of primary hyperparathyroidism. To prevent the recurrence of calcium oxalate uroliths, a protein-restricted diet that produces an alkaline urine is typically recommended (Table 15.2). The diet should not be supplemented with additional sodium since this increases calcium excretion and contributes to increased calcium in the urine. The diet should also not be phosphorus-restricted as this can cause an increase in calcitriol production, resulting in increased

Table 15.2. Dietary recommendations for prevention of calcium oxalate urinary stones in dogs.

Factor	Recommendation for Future Prevention
Water	Encourage intake; keep USG < 1.020
Protein	10%–18% DM; avoid excess protein
Sodium	<0.3% DM; avoid excess sodium
Magnesium	0.04%–0.15% DM; avoid deficiency or excess
Oxalate	Avoid foods high in oxalates

USG, urine specific gravity; DM, dry matter.

calcium in the urine. Whether dietary calcium should be restricted is debated. High-calcium diets can result in decreased absorption of dietary calcium and oxalate. In addition, low calcium intake could cause an upregulation of calcitriol production, resulting in an increase in urinary calcium. Foods high in oxalates should be avoided (Table 15.3), and vitamin C should not be given as a supplement, as vitamin C can be converted to oxalates. The desired pH of the urine is about 7.0 and should be measured using a pH meter, not urinary dip strips. If diet does not sufficiently raise the urine pH, potassium citrate is added to the treatment regimen.

Urate Urolithiasis

Purine stones (urates and xanthin) account for about 8% of urinary uroliths in dogs. In dogs, urate uroliths are usually composed of the monobasic ammonium salt of uric acid (ammonium acid urate). Urate uroliths are small, brittle, spherical stones with concentric laminations. They are usually multiple in number and light yellow, brown, or green in color. They are most often found in the bladder and urethra. They usually form in urine that is neutral to acidic. Urate uroliths are not often seen on radiographs, and special procedures such as contrast radiography or ultrasound are usually required.

Urate uroliths are most common in Dalmatians and English bulldogs; other breeds affected include miniature schnauzers, Yorkshire terriers, and shih tzus. Males are more commonly affected because the small uroliths become lodged in the urethra, leading to signs of urinary tract obstruction. Urate stones usually occur in dogs between 1 and 4 years of age, and the risk of urate urolith formation greatly decreases after 5 years of age. The recurrence rate for urate uroliths is high (33%–50%).

Table 15.3. Oxalate contents of dietary ingredients.

	Ingredients Low in Oxalates	Ingredients High in Oxalates
Meats and eggs	Beef, fish, shellfish, lamb, pork, poultry, eggs	Sardines
Vegetables	Cabbage, cauliflower, mushrooms, green peas, radishes, white potatoes	Asparagus, broccoli, carrots, celery, corn, cucumber, eggplant, green beans, green peppers, lettuce, spinach, summer squash, sweet potatoes, tofu, tomatoes
Milk and dairy products	Cheese, milk, yogurt	—
Fruits	Avocado, banana, Bing cherries, grapefruit, green grapes, mangos, cantaloupe, casaba, honeydew, watermelon, plums	Apples, apricots, cherries, berries, oranges, peaches, pears, pineapple, tangerines
Breads, grains, nuts	White bread, macaroni, noodles, rice, spaghetti	Corn bread, fruit cake, grits, peanuts, pecans, soybeans, wheat germ

Urate uroliths are often found in dogs with portosystemic shunts, possibly due to reduced conversion of ammonia to urea and uric acid to allantoin. A defect in uric acid metabolism in the Dalmatian is a predisposing factor for urate urolithiasis. Uric acid is derived from the metabolic degradation of purines. In dogs other than Dalmatians, uric acid is converted to allantoin in the liver by the enzyme uricase. Dalmatian dogs have higher plasma uric acid concentrations and excrete much more uric acid in their urine than do other dogs. Impaired transport of uric acid into liver cells may reduce the rate of hepatic oxidation in Dalmatians. The proximal tubules of Dalmatians appear to reabsorb less and secrete more urate than do the kidneys of non-Dalmatian dogs. Many Dalmatian puppies have abundant urate crystalluria, although most will not develop urate urolithiasis. There is no

Table 15.4. Dietary recommendations for urate or cystine urinary stones in dogs.

Factor	Recommendation for Treatment and Future Prevention
Water	Encourage intake; keep USG <1.020
Protein	10%–18% DM; avoid excess protein
Urine pH	Maintain in an alkaline range (pH 7.1–7.7)

USG, urine specific gravity; DM, dry matter.

suitable method to predict which Dalmatians with urate crystalluria will develop clinical signs of urolithiasis and which will not.

A reduced intake of dietary purines and other purine precursors (diets low in organ-derived meats, especially) is recommended to reduce the risk for recurrence of urate urolithiasis (Table 15.4). The solubility of ammonium urate is greater in less-acid urine, thus diets that generate more alkaline urine are recommended. The protein content of these diets is low, and they should not be fed to growing dogs or pregnant or lactating bitches. These low-purine diets should also not be fed to English bulldogs due to the potential risk of the development of dilated cardiomyopathy. English bulldogs with urate stones may have defective renal reabsorption of cystine and carnitine, and the carnitine deficiency may contribute to dilated cardiomyopathy.

Allopurinol can be used as a treatment to help dissolve or prevent the recurrence of urate stones. Allopurinol is a competitive inhibitor of the enzyme xanthine oxidase, which converts hypoxanthine to xanthin and xanthine to uric acid in purine metabolism. Thus, allopurinol reduces the amount of uric acid generated. Dogs receiving allopurinol should be fed low-purine diets because feeding a diet high in purine with allopurinol increases the risk for development of xanthine stones. UTI is a common complication of urate urolithiasis, and can occur in a third of affected dogs.

Cystine Urolithiasis

Cystine stones account for about 1% of all urinary stones in dogs. Cystine uroliths have been reported in English bulldogs, Newfoundlands, dachshunds, Irish terriers, basset hounds, and bullmastiffs. Male dogs are typically affected, but both male and female Newfoundlands can be affected. Cystine stones usually develop in dogs about 4–6 years of age.

Cystine excretion in the urine (cystinuria) is an inherited disorder of renal tubular transport, and the presence of cystine in the urine is a predisposing factor for cystine uroliths. Cystine stones are small, spherical, and light yellow, brown, or green in color. Cystine crystals have a characteristic hexagonal shape. Multiple uroliths are usually present, and the recurrence rate may be as high as 75%. UTI is usually a complication.

Drugs used to treat cystine stones include D-penicillamine, or 2-mercaptopropionylglycine (2-MPG). A small number of dogs treated with 2-MPG may develop aggression as a side effect. A low-protein diet may result in lower urine specific gravity and increased urine pH (Table 15.4) and may help to prevent recurrence.

Silicate Urolithiasis

Silicate stones account for about 1% of all urinary stones in dogs. Silicate stones are gray-white or brownish and usually multiple in number. They frequently have a jack-like appearance, and should be surgically removed. The role of diet in silicate urolithiasis has not been determined, but diets high in corn gluten or soybean are suspected to contribute. There is no obvious relationship between silica urolithiasis and urine pH. Diets high in plant proteins (soybean) may predispose to recurrence and should be avoided.

Urolithiasis in Cats

The term *feline lower urinary tract disease* (FLUTD) encompasses a number of conditions. The incidence is unknown, but is estimated to be about 1%, based on the presence of clinical signs. Clinical signs of FLUTD include blood in the urine, urination outside of the litter box, straining to urinate, increased frequency of urination, or urinary blockage. Urolithiasis is a potential cause of FLUTD. The most common urinary stones in cats are struvite and calcium oxalate. Prior to the late 1980s, sterile struvite was the most common urolith found in cats. The proportion of struvite urolithiasis declined in subsequent years following changes in commercial cat food formulations. Unfortunately, the decline of struvite stones is associated with an increase in the number of calcium oxalate stones.

The frequency of urolithiasis does not appear to be greater in cats than in dogs, so no modification of the diet is necessary prior to formation of the first stone. Treatment of sporadic calcium oxalate or struvite crystalluria is not necessary in cats that have never formed a stone previously. However, all cats that have formed a stone are at increased risk for recurrence. Water is the most important nutrient to prevent recurrence of stone formation. Increased water intake will dilute the urine and increase the frequency of urination. Urine specific gravity should be approximately 1.030. Decreasing the concentration of potential stone-forming minerals in the urine and increasing the voiding frequency are primary therapies to reduce the risk of new stone formation.

Struvite Urolithiasis in Cats

Unlike dogs, most cats with struvite uroliths do not have UTI. Neutered cats are 3.5 times more likely to develop struvite uroliths as compared to sexually intact cats. Most cats develop struvite uroliths between 4 and 7 years of age, and breeds at risk include foreign shorthair, ragdoll, Chartreux, oriental shorthair, domestic shorthair, and Himalayan. The rex, Burmese, Abyssinian, Russian blue, Birman, Siamese, and mixed breed cats have a significantly lower risk of developing struvite uroliths.

Excess dietary protein should be avoided with struvite urolithiasis and should be restricted to 30%–45% DM (Table 15.5). Struvite stones can be dissolved over several weeks using a magnesium-restricted, acidifying, wet diet. Although magnesium-restricted acidifying diets are commonly employed to prevent recurrence of sterile struvite stones in cats, no data have demonstrated their effectiveness.

Calcium Oxalate Urolithiasis in Cats

Consumption of urine-acidifying diets and indoor housing are independent risk factors for calcium oxalate urolithiasis. Breeds at risk for calcium oxalate uroliths include ragdoll, British shorthair, foreign shorthair, Himalayan, Havana brown, Scottish fold, Persian, and exotic shorthair cats. The Birman, mixed breed, Abyssinian, and Siamese cats have significantly lower risks for developing calcium oxalate uroliths. Calcium oxalate stones usually form in cats between 7 and 10 years of age, and male cats and neutered cats are at much higher risk. About one-third of cats with calcium oxalate stones have idiopathic hypercalcemia as an association. Nephroliths from cat kidneys are most likely to be calcium oxalate.

Table 15.5. Dietary recommendations for struvite and oxalate stones in cats.

Factor	Struvite	Calcium Oxalate
Water	Encourage intake; keep USG <1.030	Encourage intake; keep USG <1.030
Protein	30%–45% DM	30%–50% DM
Calcium	—	0.5%–0.8% DM; 0.11%–0.20% ME
Phosphorus	0.5%–0.9% DM; 0.11%–0.24% ME	0.5%–0.7% DM; 0.10%–0.16% ME
Magnesium	Dissolution: 0.04%–0.06% DM; 0.009%–0.012% ME Prevention: 0.04%–0.10% DM; 0.009%–0.024% ME	0.04%–0.10% DM; 0.009%–0.024% ME
Sodium	Dissolution: 0.7%–0.9% DM; 0.15%–0.18% ME Prevention: 0.2%–0.6% DM; 0.06%–0.11% ME	0.10%–0.40% DM; 0.03%–0.10% ME
Urine pH	Dissolution: 5.9–6.1 Prevention: 6.2–6.4	6.6–6.8

USG, urine specific gravity; DM, dry matter; ME, metabolizable energy.

No medical regimen has been shown to successfully dissolve calcium oxalate uroliths, so surgery or catheterization is recommended. The frequency of recurrent calcium oxalate stone formation in cats is unknown. Although a decreased risk of recurrence of oxalate stones related to diet change has not been documented in cats, changing to a diet that is less acidifying and that has not been magnesium-restricted seems reasonable, as long as the resulting urine specific gravity is less than 1.030 (Table 15.5). Acidifying agents are contraindicated in cats with calcium oxalate urolithiasis. Foods high in oxalate content should not be used (Table 15.3).

Dog Recipes for Struvite Stone Prevention

Dog Recipes for Oxalate Stone Prevention

Chicken and Rice   428
Eggs and Rice   429

Dog Recipes for Cystine/Urate Stone Prevention

Chicken and Potato   430
Tofu and Rice   431

Cat Recipes for Struvite Stone Prevention

Venison and Rice   483
Pork and Barley   485
Chicken and Rice   505

Cat Recipes for Oxalate Stone Prevention

Chicken and Rice   502
Ground beef and Rice   503
Salmon and Rice   504

Additional Reading

Allen TA, Kruger JM. 2000. Feline lower urinary tract disease. In *Small Animal Clinical Nutrition*, 4th edition. Hand MS, Thatcher CD, Remillard RL, Roudebush P (Eds). Mark Morris Institute, Topeka, KS, pp. 689–724.

Bartges JW, Kirk CA. 2006. Nutrition and lower urinary tract disease in cats. Vet Clin Small Anim 36:1361–1376.

Bartges JW, Osborne CA, Lulich JP, Kruger JM, Sanderson SL, Koehler LA, et al. 1999. Canine urate urolithiasis. Etiopathogenesis, diagnosis, and management. Vet Clin North Am Small Anim Pract 29(1):161–191.

Case LP, Carey DP, Hirakawa DA, Daristotle L (Eds). 2000. Dietary management of urolithiasis in cats and dogs. In *Canine and Feline Nutrition: A Resource for Companion Animal Professionals*, 2nd edition. Mosby, St. Louis, pp. 409–428.

Gieg JA, Chew DJ, McLoughlin MA. 2006. Diseases of the urinary bladder. In *Manual of Small Animal Practice*, 3rd edition. Birchard SJ, Sherding RG (Eds). Elsevier, St. Louis, pp. 895–914.

Houston DM, Elliott DA. 2008. Nutritional management of feline lower urinary tract disorders. In *Encyclopedia of Feline Clinical Nutrition*. Pibot P, Biourge V, Elliott D (Eds). Aniwa SAS, Aimargues, France, pp. 285–321.

Houston DM, Moore AE, Favrin MG, Hoff B. 2004. Canine urolithiasis: A look at over 16000 urolith submissions to the Canadian veterinary urolith centre from February 1998 to April 2003. Can Vet J 45(3):225–230.

Lekcharoensuk C, Osborne CA, Lulich JP, Pusoonthornthum R, Kirk CA, Ulrich LK, et al. 2002. Associations between dietary factors in canned food and formation of calcium oxalate uroliths in dogs. Am J Vet Res 63(2):163–169.

Lulich JP, Osborne CA, Lekcharoensuk C, Allen TA, Nakagawa Y. 1999. Canine calcium oxalate urolithiasis. Vet Clin North Am Small Anim Pract 29(1):123–139.

Lulich JP, Osborne CA, Lekcharoensuk C, Kirk CA, Bartges JW. 2004. Effects of diet on urine composition of cats with calcium oxalate urolithiasis. J Am Anim Hosp Assoc 40:185–191.

Lulich JP, Osborne CA, Sanderson SL. 2005. Effects of dietary supplementation with sodium chloride on urinary relative supersaturation with calcium oxalate in healthy dogs. Am J Vet Res 66(2):319–324.

Lulich JP, Osborne CA, Thumchai R, Lekcharoensuk C, Ulrich LK, Koeler LA, et al. 1999. Epidemiology of canine calcium oxalate uroliths. Identifying risk factors. Vet Clin North Am Small Anim Pract 29(1):133–122.

Osborne CA, Bartges JW, Lulich JP, Polzin DJ, Allen TA. 2000. Canine urolithiasis. In *Small Animal Clinical Nutrition*, 4th edition. Hand MS, Thatcher CD, Remillard RL, Roudebush P (Eds). Mark Morris Institute, Topeka, KS, pp. 603–688.

Osborne CA, Sanderson SL, Lulich JP, Bartges JW, Ulrich LK, Loehler LA, et al. 1999. Canine cystine urolithiasis. Cause, detection, treatment and prevention. Vet Clin North Am Small Anim Pract 29(1):193–211.

Stevenson A, Rutgers C. 2006. Nutritional management of canine urolithiasis. In *Encyclopedia of Canine Clinical Nutrition*. Pibot P, Biourge V, Elliott D (Eds). Aniwa SAS, Aimargues France, pp. 284–315.

Stevenson AE, Blackburn JM, Markwell PJ, Robertson WG. 2004. Nutrient intake and urine composition in calcium oxalate stone-forming dogs: Comparison with health dogs and impact of dietary modification. Vet Ther 5(3):218–231.

Stevenson AE, Hynds WK, Markwell PJ. 2003. Effect of dietary moisture and sodium content on urine composition and calcium oxalate relative supersaturation in healthy miniature schnauzers and Labrador retrievers. Res Vet Sci 74(2):145–151.

Zentek J, Schulz A. 2004. Urinary composition of cats is affected by the source of dietary protein. J Nutr 134:2162S–2165S.

CHAPTER 16
Diet and Skin Disease

The skin is the largest organ and serves as a barrier between the pet and the environment. Skin is important in protecting against water loss and comprises about 14% of adult body weight in dogs. The skin and hair are important because they regulate body temperature and provide insulation. The growth rate of hair varies by breed, season, length of hair, and region of the body. Hair follicles can be in many different stages of hair-growth cycle at any time. The growing period is termed *anagen*, the resting period is *telogen*, and the transitional period is *catagen*. Hair growth rate is usually fastest during the summer and slowest in the winter, as growth rate responds mostly to the amount of daylight.

Dogs with long hair use more protein to maintain hair growth than do dogs with short hair. Small dogs with long hair may use about 30% of the dietary protein just to maintain hair growth compared to a large breed dog with a short hair coat that may only need about 10% of dietary protein for hair growth.

Normal skin slowly replenishes itself, with only about 1.5% of skin cells replicating at any given time. Actively growing hair rapidly renews itself, with about 24% of cells replicating.

Hair contains about 65%–95% protein, and the water content is dependent on the humidity. Hair has a low mineral content, and analysis of the hair is not very useful for the determination of nutritional deficiencies.

Skin disorders are common in small animals, with about 25% of veterinary visits dealing with the diagnosis of skin and hair coat problems. The most common skin disorders of the dog and cat are

Table 16.1. Common skin disorders in dogs and cats.

Dogs	Cats
Allergy (flea bite hypersensitivity, atopy)	Abscesses
Cutaneous neoplasms	Parasites of the skin
Bacterial pyoderma	Allergy (flea bite hypersensitivity, atopy)
Seborrhea	Miliary dermatitis
Parasites of the skin	Eosinophilic granuloma complex
Adverse reactions to food (food hypersensitivity or intolerance)	Fungal infections
Immune-mediated dermatoses	Adverse reactions to food
Endocrine disorders	Psychogenic dermatoses
	Seborrhea
	Neoplasia
	Immune-mediated disorders

listed in Table 16.1. Other than adverse reactions to food, skin diseases due to nutritional deficiencies are uncommon. Most skin diseases due to nutritional deficiencies occur in young, growing animals or in females during reproduction or lactation, as these are the stages in which nutrient requirements are highest. Changes in the hair or skin suggesting nutritional problems may include a dry, brittle, dull coat, with hair that falls out easily; slow regrowth of hair from areas that have been clipped; scale accumulation on the skin; loss of hair in areas of friction; poor wound healing; or changes in normal hair color.

For diagnosis, a routine complete blood count (CBC), serum biochemistry profile, urinalysis, and thyroid profile should be performed to help identify the presence of any other underlying disease. In addition, skin scrapings for parasites, bacterial and fungal cultures, skin biopsy, and examination of the hair may be performed. With nutritional deficiencies, examination of hair and examination of the skin biopsy tissues are usually the most helpful diagnostic tools. Hair that is malformed suggests nutritional or metabolic diseases. Hair with a normal shaft that is clearly broken suggests external trauma (licking, scratching, or grooming).

Protein and Energy Deficiency

For hair growth to occur, adequate protein and energy intake are required. Hair growth requires sulfur-containing amino acids, and dietary protein sources should be of high quality and be highly digestible. This is most important during growth, reproduction, and lactation, when nutrient requirements are highest. During protein deficiency, hair may not form correctly, there may be depigmentation of hair, and there are changes in skin lipids. The protective barrier of the skin is altered, and this can lead to secondary bacterial infections or impaired wound healing. These pets typically have dry, brittle hair coats, with patchy hair loss. Hair can be lost during the growth phase (anagen) or during the resting phase (telogen). Hair in telogen is usually lost when a stressful event occurs (illness, surgery, etc.). Hair loss in anagen is sudden, and coincides typically with the use of a drug, infectious disease, or metabolic disease. Dogs with primary seborrhea or severe pyoderma may also have higher protein requirements. Dietary recommendations for dogs and cats with skin and hair disorders are listed in Table 16.2.

Migratory necrolytic erythema (hepatocutaneous syndrome) is a severe skin disorder due to an amino acid deficiency. Migratory necrolytic erythema is usually the result of chronic liver disease or a pancreatic glucagonoma. Migratory necrolytic erythema can occur in any breed and is usually seen in older animals. Lesions are seen around the mouth, around the eyes, on the feet (pads), and around the anus. The lesions are very painful, but with nutritional therapy they can improve. Intravenous infusions of amino acid solution are usually

Table 16.2. Dietary recommendations for dogs and cats with skin and hair disorders.

Nutrient	Dogs		Cats	
	Adult	Puppy	Adult	Kitten
Protein	25%–30% DM	30%–45% DM	30%–45% DM	35%–50% DM
Fat	10%–15% DM	15%–30% DM	15%–25% DM	20%–35% DM
Zinc (mg/kg)	100–200	100–200	50–150	50–150
Copper (mg/kg)	5–10	5–10	15–30	15–30
Essential fatty acids	>3.0% DM	>3.0% DM	>1.5% DM	>1.5% DM

DM, dry matter.

given daily. Egg yolks, essential fatty acids, and zinc can be given as supplements.

Fatty Acid Deficiency

A dietary supply of the essential fatty acids is very important for maintenance of a healthy skin and coat. The skin lacks certain enzymes that are required to convert linoleic acid or linolenic acid into longer-chain fatty acids, thus fatty acids must be supplied in the diet and transported to the skin. In dogs and cats with fatty acid deficiency, scaly skin, matted hair, loss of hair, dull coat, and lack of hair regrowth are often observed. Deficiency is rapidly reversed by supplementing with essential fatty acids.

Fatty acids supplementation may improve the skin and hair coat in those with seborrhea. Dogs with seborrhea can have low levels of linoleic acids in their skin even though the dietary source and serum concentrations appear adequate. Supplementation with linoleic acid may be beneficial in those with seborrhea. Dry skin and dull coat in general may also benefit from supplementation with polyunsaturated fatty acid (PUFA) found in vegetable oils.

Mineral Deficiencies

Copper is an important mineral and is a cofactor for many enzymes in the body. Clinical signs of copper deficiency include a dull, rough hair coat, thinning of hair, and loss of normal hair coloration. The loss of hair color usually starts on the face and gradually extends to the whole body. The hair color is washed out and becomes gray. Copper deficiency can occur due to a lack of dietary copper, but it is more commonly caused by an excess of dietary zinc. Excess zinc can inhibit the absorption of copper. Copper is highly available in poultry and in poultry, beef, and sheep liver.

Zinc is also an important cofactor in many enzymatic reactions. Zinc deficiency has been characterized in many animal species. Skin lesions associated with zinc deficiency include loss of hair, ulceration, inflammation of the skin, and the development of crusty lesions, especially of the footpads, areas over joints, and around the mouth and eyes, the lower extremities, tail, armpits and groin, and ear canals. Zinc deficiency may also decrease the absorption of essential fatty acids. Zinc deficiency can occur from feeding diets high in phytates (such as bran), which chelates zinc. It can also result from diets that contain excessive calcium or can occur in breeds that have an inability to absorb zinc.

Zinc malabsorption occurs primarily in Nordic breeds (Siberian husky, Alaskan malamutes), but it can also occur in other breeds such as Great Danes, bull terriers, German shepherd dogs, and Boston terriers. These breeds typically develop clinical signs in early adulthood. Treatment involves zinc supplementation, and there is usually clinical improvement in less than 1 month. Treatment is lifelong.

Lethal acrodermatitis is an inherited disorder of bull terriers and is associated with defects in zinc absorption and metabolism. Clinical signs of zinc deficiency are present from about 2 weeks of age, and bronchopneumonia, bone abnormalities, cataracts, and gastroenteritis also occur. The disease is fatal.

Vitamin Deficiencies

Vitamin A is important for skin cell growth, reproduction, and vision. Sources of dietary vitamin A include vitamin A palmitate (retinyl esters) found in animal tissues and β-carotene from vegetable sources. Cats, however, require vitamin A from animal sources, since cats cannot convert β-carotene to vitamin A. The term *retinoid* refers to the group of vitamin A compounds.

Skin has a specific receptor for retinoic acid, and deficiency results in scaling and skin atrophy. Deficiency is rare since most dogs and cats consume adequate vitamin A. Retinoids have been used to treat a number of skin disorders, including disorders of skin keratinization or sebaceous gland abnormalities. Vitamin A–responsive dermatosis has been recognized primarily in cocker spaniels but also in Labrador retrievers and miniature schnauzers. Clinical signs appear in adults and include refractory seborrhea with plaques, primarily on the ventral and lateral thorax and abdomen. A waxy discharge from the ears and a poor hair coat are usually present. Dogs with this dermatosis respond within 3 to 4 weeks after starting oral vitamin A supplementation. Vitamin A supplementation should only be initiated when necessary. Side effects can occur and include an increase in serum calcium (hypercalcemia), conjunctivitis, an increase in serum triglycerides, decreased tear production, and an increase in liver enzymes.

Vitamin E activity includes eight different tocopherols, with α-tocopherol being the most active. Vitamin E is important as an antioxidant, especially when a higher concentration of polyunsaturated fatty acids is fed. Vitamin E deficiency has only been reported in cats that are consuming large quantities of highly unsaturated fatty acids (such as in red meat tuna). Clinical signs include fever, loss of appetite, anemia, an increase in white blood cells, and firm subcutaneous nodules. Treatment involves providing adequate dietary vitamin E and providing a balanced diet.

Even though not caused by a vitamin E deficiency, a number of skin disorders have been treated with supplemental vitamin E. Inflammatory disorders that may respond to supplemental vitamin E include discoid or systemic lupus erythematosus, pemphigus erythematosus, panniculitis, acanthosis nigricans, dermatomyositis, and ear margin vasculitis. Vitamin E may help stabilize membranes and protect them against damage from free radicals.

Deficiencies of B vitamins such as biotin, riboflavin, niacin, and pyridoxine can result in loss of appetite, weight loss, diarrhea, loss of hair, and dry, flaky skin. Clinical signs occur more commonly in young, growing animals. B vitamins are important cofactors in fatty acid metabolism. A deficiency of B vitamins can occur in pets eating homemade diets that are not supplemented with vitamins.

Dog Recipes for Skin Conditions

■ **Adult Dogs**

Chicken and Rice   277
Chicken and Pasta   278
Chicken and Potato   279
Ground Beef and Rice   280
Ground Beef and Pasta   281
Ground Beef and Potato   282
Tofu, Lentils, and Rice   290
Tofu, Lentils, and Pasta   292
Tofu, Lentils, and Potato   294
Chicken and Pasta   300
Salmon and Couscous   350
Chicken and Quinoa   384
Tuna and Rice   386
Tofu and Pasta   393
Pork and Sweet Potato   394

■ Puppies

Cat Recipes for Skin Conditions

■ Adult Cats

■ Kittens

Additional Reading

Fritsche K. 2006. Fatty acids as modulators of the immune response. Annu Rev Nutr 26:45–73.

Prelaud P, Harvey R. 2006. Nutritional dermatoses and the contribution of dietetics in dermatology. In *Encyclopedia of Canine Clinical Nutrition*. Pibot P, Biourge V, Elliott D (Eds). Aniwa SAS, Aimargues, France, pp. 58–91.

Mueller RS, Dethioux F. 2008. Nutritional dermatoses and the contribution of dietetics in dermatology. In *Encyclopedia of Feline Clinical Nutrition*. Pibot P, Biourge V, Elliott D (Eds). Aniwa SAS, Aimargues, France, pp. 51–75.

Mueller RS, Fettman MJ, Richardson K, Hansen RA, Miller A, Magowitz J, et al. 2005. Plasma and skin concentrations of polyunsaturated fatty acids before and after supplementation with n-3 fatty acids in dogs with atopic dermatitis. Am J Vet Res 66(5):868–873.

Roudebush P, Sousa CA, Logas DE. 2000. Skin and hair disorders. In *Small Animal Clinical Nutrition*, 4th edition. Hand MS, Thatcher CD, Remillard RL, Roudebush P (Eds). Mark Morris Institute, Topeka, KS, pp. 455–474.

Saevik BK, Bergvall K, Holm BR, Saijonmaa-Koulumies LE, Hedhammar A, Larsen S, et al. 2004. A randomized, controlled study to evaluate the steroid sparing effect of essential fatty acid supplementation in the treatment of canine atopic dermatitis. Vet Dermatol 15(3):137–145.

Schoenherr WD, Roudebush P, Swecker WS. 2000. Use of fatty acids in inflammatory disease. In *Small Animal Clinical Nutrition*, 4th edition. Hand MS, Thatcher CD, Remillard RL, Roudebush P (Eds). Mark Morris Institute, Topeka, KS, pp. 907–922.

CHAPTER 17
Diet and Endocrine Disease

Thyroid Disorders

■ Hypothyroidism

Hypothyroidism is the most common endocrine disorder in dogs, but is uncommon in cats. Clinical signs of hypothyroidism include weight gain, obesity, lethargy, cold intolerance, lack of tear production, poor hair coat, hair loss, and mental dullness. Hypothyroidism can be due to congenital lack of thyroid hormone production (uncommon) or due to destruction of the thyroid glands (common). Diagnosis is made by identifying low serum thyroid hormone concentrations with an elevation of thyroid-stimulating hormone (TSH). Medical treatment involves replacement therapy with thyroxine. Dietary management is aimed at treating obesity if present. Since hypothyroidism is associated with lipid metabolism disorders, feeding a low-fat diet may be beneficial.

■ Hyperthyroidism

Hyperthyroidism is the most common endocrine disorder in the cat, but is rare in dogs. In the cat, hyperthyroidism is due to a benign tumor in the thyroid gland (thyroid adenoma); thyroid carcinomas (cancer) are rare in the cat. Most cats with hyperthyroidism are over 10 years of age. Clinical signs include weight loss, an increase in appetite, a palpable thyroid tumor, increased urination, increased thirst, increased heart rate, hyperactivity, and diarrhea. Diagnosis is made by identifying increased levels of circulating thyroid hormones. The initiating cause of hyperthyroidism is still unknown. In several epidemiological studies, cats fed canned foods were at increased risk of developing hyperthyroidism compared to those fed dry or semi-moist cat foods. Variation in iodine content in cat diets has been suggested as a potential cause of hyperthyroidism, but this has not been proven. Further studies are necessary to determine the cause of feline hyperthyroidism. Treatment involves either surgical removal or radioactive iodine destruction of the thyroid tumor, or blockage of thyroid hormone production with medical therapy. Most cats with hyperthyroidism are thin and in an energy-deficient state. Many cats with hyperthyroidism also have some degree of renal disease, and excess dietary protein should be avoided with renal disease. Diets for hyperthyroidism should be aimed at providing adequate calorie intake. The fat content may be increased to provide higher energy to the diet.

Hyperthyroidism is rare in dogs and is caused by a thyroid carcinoma. Most thyroid carcinomas are nonfunctional and do not cause hyperthyroidism. Hyperthyroidism only occurs in about 10%–20% of thyroid carcinomas. Clinical signs include a visible neck mass, coughing, difficulty in swallowing, change in voice, weight loss, and hyperactivity. Treatment of canine hyperthyroidism includes surgery and chemotherapy. If the dog is thin, a diet providing increased energy is appropriate.

Adrenal Gland Disorders

■ Hyperadrenocorticism

Hyperadrenocorticism (Cushing's disease) is caused by an excess in cortisol secretion. Clinical signs of hyperadrenocorticism include increased urination, increased thirst, increased appetite, weight gain, pot-bellied appearance, panting, muscle wasting, and loss of hair. Hypertension is common, and diabetes mellitus may also be present. Hyperadrenocorticism is much more common in dogs than in cats. Medical treatment is necessary to control the clinical signs of hyperadrenocorticism. Diets designed for adult maintenance are suitable, and diets lower in fat and higher in fiber may be beneficial for weight loss. Excessive salt should be avoided if hypertension is present.

■ Hypoadrenocorticism

Hypoadrenocorticism (Addison's disease) is caused by deficiency of mineralocorticoid (aldosterone) secretion and a deficiency of cortisol production. Hypoadrenocorticism usually affects younger dogs and is characterized by vague clinical signs such as vomiting, diarrhea, weight loss, inappetite, and lethargy. Some dogs may have an addisonian crisis, with collapse, shock, or death. Medical treatment is required to control hypoadrenocorticism. Diets designed for adult maintenance (or growth if still a puppy) are suitable, although excessive dietary potassium should be avoided.

Parathyroid Gland Disorders

■ Hypoparathyroidism

Hypoparathyroidism is caused by a deficiency of parathyroid hormone (PTH) secretion by the parathyroid glands. Hypoparathyroidism is not common, but is more common in dogs than in cats. A decrease in PTH production can be due to destruction of the parathyroid glands or can be due to surgery in the neck that disrupts blood supply to the parathyroid glands. The parathyroid glands secrete PTH, which is a key hormone involved in calcium metabolism. With a deficiency of PTH production, serum calcium concentration decreases. Clinical signs of low serum calcium (hypocalcemia) include twitching, facial rubbing, self-mutilation, and seizures. Medical treatment includes the administration of calcium supplements, calcitriol (the active form of vitamin D), and possibly magnesium supplementation. These treatments cannot be provided in the diet, as doses must be closely monitored. Diets designed for adult maintenance are generally suitable.

■ Primary Hyperparathyroidism

Primary hyperparathyroidism is caused by a parathyroid gland tumor that secretes excessive PTH. Excessive PTH results in an increased serum calcium concentration, which leads to an increase in urination, increased thirst, lethargy, and loss of appetite. Diagnosis is made by measuring circulating serum concentrations of calcium and PTH. Primary hyperparathyroidism is more common in dogs, and there are some breeds that are predisposed to it (keeshonds). Treatment involves removal of the parathyroid tumor. After surgery, the serum calcium concentration may be low until the parathyroid glands return to function, and supplemented calcium may be required for a short period after surgery. Diets for adult maintenance are suitable.

■ Nutritional Secondary Hyperparathyroidism

Nutritional secondary hyperparathyroidism is caused by diets containing excessive phosphorus or inadequate calcium or vitamin D content. Deficient diets are typically homemade diets made primarily with meat. The imbalance of dietary calcium and phosphorus causes a decrease in the serum calcium concentration, which stimulates PTH secretion. Excess PTH production causes bone resorption in an effort to maintain a normal serum calcium concentration. Clinical signs include bone pain, lameness, limb deformities, and fractures and are more common in young, growing animals. Nutritional secondary hyperparathyroidism can also occur in animals with severe gastrointestinal disease that causes decreased absorption of calcium or vitamin D. Treatment is to provide a balanced diet.

■ Renal Secondary Hyperparathyroidism

Renal secondary hyperparathyroidism occurs when renal failure is present. With the progressive destruction of kidney cells, there is decreased ability to synthesize the active form of vitamin D (which occurs in the kidney). The lack of the active form of vitamin D (calcitriol) results in a decrease in the serum calcium concentration, which stimulates PTH secretion. In renal disease, the excess PTH causes bone resorption, particularly in the bones of the skull, resulting in "rubber jaw." Calcitriol is given to alleviate the excess PTH; dietary management includes feeding a renal diet with restricted phosphorus content.

■ Vitamin D Toxicity

Vitamin D toxicity can occur from oversupplementation with vitamin D, cholecalciferol rodenticide ingestion, ingestion of plants, such as *Cestrum diurnum*, containing vitamin D metabolites. The excess ingested vitamin D results in an increase in serum calcium with suppression of PTH production. Serum phosphorus is also increased as a result; calcium and phosphorus can bind and precipitate in organs, causing severe damage, especially in the kidneys. Clinical signs include an acute onset of increased urination, increased thirst, anorexia, depression, vomiting, and diarrhea. Acute renal failure is common. Medical treatment is designed to decrease serum calcium and phosphorus and to treat renal disease. Treatment may need to be prolonged since vitamin D is a fat-soluble vitamin, and excess can remain in the body for months. Renal diets with restricted phosphorus may be appropriate.

■ Idiopathic Hypercalcemia in Cats

Idiopathic hypercalcemia (IHC) was first described in the 1990s. IHC can occur in young to old cats, and long-haired cats have a higher incidence of IHC, suggesting a genetic predisposition. Many cats with IHC have no clinical signs, or there may be a history of weight loss, chronic constipation, and calcium oxalate–containing urinary stones. Some may develop renal failure. IHC is characterized by an elevated serum calcium concentration with a suppression of PTH production. No treatment has worked consistently. In some cats, increasing the fiber in the diet has been helpful in lowering the serum calcium. Further studies are needed to evaluate the effectiveness of dietary therapy and to determine the cause of IHC.

Pancreatic Disorders

■ Insulinoma

Insulinoma is a malignant tumor of the pancreas that results in an excessive secretion of insulin. Insulinomas are uncommon in dogs and rare in cats, but when present usually occur in older dogs. Medium to larger breed dogs are predisposed to insulinoma. Clinical signs may be episodic and are more common after eating. Clinical signs include lethargy, weakness, loss of coordination, dementia, seizures, and coma. Diagnosis is based on finding a low serum concentration of glucose with an excessive concentration of insulin. Surgical treatment is the best option to remove the tumor, but metastasis is often present or the tumor cannot be completely removed. Simple sugars should be avoided in the diet since these carbohydrates cause an excess secretion of insulin. Complex carbohydrates from starch are preferred. The fiber in the diet should also be less than 5% of the dry matter (Table 17.1). Amino acids also stimulate the release of insulin. Excessive dietary protein should be avoided. Protein in diets for those with insulinomas

Table 17.1. Dietary recommendations for dogs and cats with insulinoma.

Factor	Dogs	Cats
Protein	15%–25% DM	28%–45% DM
Fat	20%–25% DM	25%–30% DM
Crude fiber	<5% DM	<5% DM

DM, dry matter.

should be 15%–25% DM for dogs and 28%–45% DM for cats. Higher-fat diets may be beneficial for those with insulinoma, but this needs to be investigated. Multiple small meals should be fed throughout the day to try to maintain a constant energy intake and to prevent a large release of insulin that can occur after a big meal.

■ Diabetes Mellitus

Diabetes mellitus is a pancreatic disorder characterized by an increase in blood glucose concentration. Dogs typically have insulin-dependent diabetes mellitus (type 1), in which there is a lack of insulin produced from the pancreas. Cats, on the other hand, usually have non-insulin-dependent diabetes mellitus (NIDDM; type 2) in which cells become unresponsive to the effects of insulin (insulin resistance) and blood glucose elevates, causing further insulin release. Thus in NIDDM, both blood glucose and insulin concentrations are initially increased. NIDDM is most common in humans as well. With time, the cells secreting insulin eventually "burn out" and stop secreting insulin. Thus, these patients may become permanently insulin-dependent.

In dogs, the average age at diagnosis is 7 to 9 years and is more common in females. Breeds that appear to be predisposed include keeshonds, miniature and toy poodles, dachshund, miniature schnauzer, beagle, puli, Cairn terrier, and miniature pinscher. In cats more than 50% of those affected are older than 10 years of age. The incidence in cats is approximately 0.5%, and obesity increases the risk threefold to fivefold. Male cats have an increased risk, and neutered cats are at twice the risk for developing diabetes.

Clinical signs do not typically develop until the blood glucose concentration is greater than 180–200 mg/dL in dogs and 200–280 mg/dL in cats. Clinical signs include increased thirst, increased urination, and increased appetite. Rapid weight loss is common in dogs, and about 40% of dogs have cataracts. In dogs with type 1 diabetes mellitus, about 50% of patients have concurrent diseases. Dehydration, muscle wasting, and an increased liver size may be present. Diagnosis is

Table 17.2. Dietary recommendations for dogs and cats with diabetes mellitus.

Factor	Dogs	Cats
Protein	15%–25% DM	28%–45% DM
Carbohydrate	50%–55% DM	10%–30% DM
Fat	<20% DM	<20% DM
Crude fiber	10%–15% DM	10%–15% DM

DM, dry matter.

usually based on finding a persistent elevation in blood glucose (hyperglycemia) and the presence of glucose in urine (glycosuria). Ketones may also be present in urine (ketonuria), which confirms the presence of diabetic ketoacidosis.

The goal of therapy is to eliminate clinical signs and to prevent the development of complications. Insulin therapy is the major treatment for diabetes mellitus. Dietary management is also very important in diabetes. Dietary carbohydrate is probably the most important factor to manage.

Dietary Management of the Dog with Diabetes Mellitus

In people with diabetes mellitus, daily insulin therapy is constantly adjusted based on repeated blood glucose measurement, but this is not the way that diabetes is managed in dogs. Fixed daily insulin dosages are typically used to manage diabetic dogs, thus diets should provide a constant amount of carbohydrate each day. Dietary carbohydrate should be present at 50%–55% DM (Table 17.2). Rice is a highly digestible carbohydrate source, but it may elicit a higher glucose response than some other carbohydrate sources. Sorghum or barley may be better carbohydrate sources in diets for dogs with diabetes mellitus. The amount of dietary fiber is controversial in diabetes mellitus, but it appears that dogs with type 1 diabetes mellitus do not require any more fiber than those without diabetes mellitus. Moderate amounts of dietary fiber (10%–15% DM) are beneficial for management of diabetes mellitus, but high-fiber diets are not necessary.

Alterations in fat metabolism occur in diabetes mellitus, and increases in serum cholesterol and triglyceride are common. Atherosclerosis is not a typical problem in dogs as compared to humans, due to differences in lipid metabolism, but atherosclerosis has been reported in dogs with diabetes mellitus. Dogs with diabetes mellitus are also at increased risk for the development of pancreatitis, so some restriction in dietary fat may be beneficial. Dietary fat should be less than 20% DM or provide less than 30% of the total energy in the diet. However, low-fat diets are not recommended because they can contribute to undesirable weight loss. The protein content of the diet does not need to be restricted unless concurrent renal failure is present. Dietary protein content is typically 15%–25% DM.

Dietary Management of the Cat with Diabetes Mellitus

One of the goals of dietary therapy in the diabetic cat is to maintain good body condition and control excess body weight. The optimal diet for diabetic cats should be high in protein, moderate in energy and fat, and low in carbohydrate. Dietary protein should provide greater than 45% of the total energy, or 28%–45% DM (Table 17.2). Carbohydrate sources should provide less than 20% of the total energy and should be complex carbohydrates rather than simple sugars. Rice is highly digestible but elicits a high glycemic response; thus, it is not an optimal source of carbohydrate. Moderate- to high-fiber content is beneficial to slow GI transit time and helps to control body weight. Fiber is usually present at 10%–15% DM. The fat content of the diet should be less than 20% DM. An increased concentration of fish oil in the diet may be beneficial by providing omega-3 fatty acids. Omega-3 fatty acids may improve insulin sensitivity by activation of certain cellular receptors. Cats with diabetes mellitus should be fed twice daily to coincide with insulin injections.

Lipid Metabolic Disorders

Both dogs and cats can be affected with disorders that cause changes in lipid metabolism. Lipid metabolism is complex and involves many enzymes and organs. Dietary cholesterol and triglycerides are absorbed in the small intestine with the help of bile. The absorbed cholesterol and triglycerides are transported to the liver, where they can be stored, secreted in bile, or packaged into lipoproteins. Lipoproteins are then released from the liver and can transport cholesterol and triglycerides to many other tissues. Dogs and cats both produce chylomicrons, very low-density lipoproteins (VLDLs), low-density lipoproteins (LDLs), and high-density lipoproteins (HDLs), as do humans, but there are major metabolic differences in lipoprotein metabolism between pets and humans. Humans are very prone to atherosclerosis, whereas dogs and cats are not typically affected. Thus, the concern of atherosclerosis in humans surrounding the consumption of high-fat diets is not a problem in most pets.

Lipid metabolic disorders are classified as either primary, where there is a defect in some metabolic process, or secondary, where the lipid alterations are being caused by another disease. Diseases that can cause changes in lipid metabolism include hypothyroidism, hyperadrenocorticism, diabetes mellitus, kidney disease, pancreatitis, and some types of liver disease.

Normally, there will be high levels of lipid present in serum after a meal, but this lipid should be cleared from the serum as it is being delivered to the liver. When this clearing process is slow, excessive amounts of lipid remain in the serum (hyperlipidemia) for long periods of time. Thus, the most common clinical sign suggesting the presence of a lipid metabolic disorder is hyperlipidemia after a 12-hour fast. Hypothyroidism is a common cause of fasting hyperlipidemia in dogs, and dogs with fasting hyperlidemia are 3.2 times more likely to have hypothyroidism as compared to dogs with hyperlipidemia. Usually, with treatment of the underlying disorder, the lipid metabolism problems will be corrected. If there is no secondary cause of hyperlipidemia, then a primary lipid defect is suspected. Primary lipid disorders include idiopathic hyperlipoproteinemia in the dog and idiopathic hyperchylomicronemia in the cat.

Idiopathic hyperlipoproteinemia has been observed in a number of dog breeds, including the miniature schnauzer, Shetland sheepdog, beagle, miniature poodle, cocker spaniel, English cocker spaniel, and mixed-breed dogs. Miniature schnauzers have the highest incidence. Clinical signs associated with idiopathic hyperlipoproteinemia include abdominal pain (possibly due to concurrent pancreatitis) and seizures, but many dogs have no clinical signs. One of the defects present in idiopathic hyperlipoproteinemia is a lack of lipoprotein lipase (LPL) activity; LPL is an important enzyme required for clearance of lipoprotein from the serum. Long-term effects of chronic hyperlipidemia are unknown, but atherosclerosis, pancreatitis, diabetes mellitus, or renal damage may be sequelae.

In cats, the most common primary lipid disorder is idiopathic hyperchylomicronemia, which is most likely a hereditary condition. Idiopathic hyperchylomicronemia usually affects young cats, and the most common clinical signs are lipid deposits in the skin and organs and presence of lipid in the eye. Kittens may be weak, lethargic, and fail to grow due to the excessive lipid. Blood will often have a "cream of tomato soup" appearance. There is a severe decrease in LPL activity in cats with hyperchylomicronemia, which greatly slows the clearance of ingested and absorbed cholesterol and triglyceride. Atherosclerosis

Table 17.3. Dietary recommendations for dogs and cats with lipid disorders.

Factor	Dogs	Cats
Protein	>18% DM, >6% ME	>30% DM, >8.5% ME
Fat	<8% DM, <2.5% ME	<10% DM, <3% ME

DM, dry matter; ME, metabolizable energy.

has not been reported in cats even though there is excessive circulating lipid.

For treatment of the idiopathic hyperlipidemias, the main therapy involves a switch to feeding a low-fat diet with moderate protein content (Table 17.3). Diets low in protein may cause an increase in serum cholesterol concentration and therefore are not recommended unless the presence of other conditions (such as renal disease) warrants their use. A low-fat diet should be chosen on the basis of the total energy provided by fat rather than the percentage of fat in the diet on a dry matter basis. After feeding the low-fat diet for 6–8 weeks, the presence of hyperlipidemia should be reevaluated. If hyperlipidemia is still present in dogs, then fish oil supplementation at a dose 1 g fish oil/10 lb body weight is added to the treatment regimen. At this level of fish oil supplementation, the dog may have a fishy odor. Fish oil supplements containing high levels of long-chain omega-3 fatty acids are effective at lowering serum triglyceride, cholesterol, and lipoprotein concentrations. Fish oils may also be important in the prevention of pancreatitis and diabetes mellitus. Little is known regarding the use of fish oil supplementation in cats, but if high levels of fish oil are given, then additional vitamin E should be added to the diet as an antioxidant.

Other Disorders

■ Acromegaly

Acromegaly occurs when the secretion of growth hormone is excessive. Growth hormone is secreted by the pituitary gland and causes a release of insulin-like growth factor 1 (IGF-1) from the liver. The diagnosis of acromegaly is determined by an increase in IGF-1 concentrations. Excess growth hormone secretion causes a proliferation of bone cartilage and an increase in organ size. Clinical signs include broadening of the skull, an increase in tongue size, increased spacing between the teeth, and increased size of the paws. An increase in the size of the liver and heart is also typical. Acromegaly is much more common in older cats, especially those with diabetes mellitus. Diets for cats with acromegaly should contain highly digestible protein, should be low in fat (<12% DM), low in simple sugars, and have a moderate fiber content (8%–17% DM). Diets designed for diabetes mellitus are suitable.

■ Diabetes Insipidus

Diabetes insipidus (DI) is characterized by increased urination (polyuria) and increased intake of water (polydipsia). DI is usually diagnosed after all other causes of increased urination and drinking have been ruled out. Water deprivation testing is usually required for diagnosis. Antidiuretic hormone (ADH; also known as vasopressin) is secreted by the brain and acts in the kidney to cause reabsorption of water. DI is due either to a lack of secretion of ADH or kidney insensitivity to ADH. Medical treatment varies depending on the cause of DI. Diets recommended for adult maintenance are suitable, but excessive salt intake should be avoided. An ample supply of water must be available at all times.

Dog Recipes for Diabetes Mellitus

Chicken and Barley   359
Ground Beef and Potato   360
Eggs and Pasta   361
Tofu and Pasta   362

Dog Recipes for Insulinoma

Chicken and Pasta   363
Ground Beef and Rice   364
Tofu and Rice   289
Tofu and Potato   293

Dog Recipes for Lipid Disorders

Chicken and Potato   365
Pork and Rice   366
Whitefish and Rice   367

Cat Recipes for Diabetes Mellitus

Cat Recipes for Idiopathic Hypercalcemia

Cat Recipes for Insulinoma

Cat Recipes for Lipid Disorders

Additional Reading

Bennett N, Greco DS, Peterson ME, Kirk C, Mathes M, Fettman MJ. 2005. Comparison of a low carbohydrate-low fiber diet and moderate carbohydrate-high fiber diet in the management of feline diabetes mellitus. J Fel Med Surg 8:73–84.

Case LP, Carey DP, Hirakawa DA, Daristotle L (Eds). 2000. Diabetes mellitus. In *Canine and Feline Nutrition: A Resource for Companion Animal Professionals*, 2nd edition. Mosby, St. Louis, pp. 397–408.

Castillo VA, Lalia JC, Junco M, Sartorio G, Marquez A, Rodriguez MS, et al. 2001. Changes in thyroid function in puppies fed a high iodine commercial diet. Vet Jour 161:80–84.

de Oliveira LD, Carciofi AC, Oliveira MC, Vasconcellos RS, Bazolli RS, Pereira GT, et al. 2008. Effects of six carbohydrate sources on diet digestibility and postprandial glucose and insulin response in cats. J Anim Sci 86(9):2237–2246.

Fleeman L, Rand J. 2006. Diabetes mellitus: Nutritional strategies. In *Encyclopedia of Canine Clinical Nutrition*. Pibot P, Biourge V, Elliott D (Eds). Aniwa SAS, Aimargues, France, pp. 192–221.

Graham PA, Maskell IE, Rawlings JM, Nash AS, Markwell PJ. 2002. Influence of a high fibre diet on glycaemic control and quality of life in dogs with diabetes mellitus. J Small Anim Pract 43:67–73.

Kirk CA. 2006. Feline diabetes mellitus: Low carbohydrates versus high fiber? Vet Clin Small Anim 36:1297–1306.

Lutz TA. 2008. Feline diabetes mellitus: Nutritional strategies. In *Encyclopedia of Feline Clinical Nutrition*. Pibot P, Biourge V, Elliott D (Eds). Aniwa SAS, Aimargues, France, pp. 181–221.

Rand JS, Fleeman LM, Farrow HA, Appleton DJ, Lederer R. 2004. Canine and feline diabetes mellitus: Nature or nurture? J Nutr 134: 2072S–2080S.

Schachter S, Nelson RW, Kirk CA. 2001. Oral chromium picolinate and control of glycemia in insulin-treated diabetic dogs. J Vet Intern Med 15:379–384.

Schenck PA. 2004. Effects of dietary components on the development of hyperthyroidism in cats. Compendium on Continuing Education for the Practicing Veterinarian 26(Suppl 2A):18–22.

Schenck PA. 2006. Canine hyperlipidemia: Causes and nutritional management. In *Encyclopedia of Canine Clinical Nutrition*. Pibot P, Biourge V, Elliott D (Eds). Aniwa SAS, Aimargues, France, pp. 222–250.

Schenck PA. 2007. Calcium homeostasis in thyroid disease in dogs and cats. Vet Clin NA Sm Anim Pract 37(4):693–708.

Schenck PA. 2007. Nutritional secondary hyperparathyroidism. In *Clinical Veterinary Advisor: Dogs and Cats*. Cote E (Ed). Elsevier, St. Louis, pp. 758–759.

Schenck PA. 2008. Diagnostic approach to the hyperlipidemic cat and dietary treatment. In *Encyclopedia of Feline Clinical Nutrition*. Pibot P, Biourge V, Elliott D (Eds). Aniwa SAS, Aimargues, France, pp. 224–246.

Schenck PA, Chew DJ. 2005. Idiopathic hypercalcemia in cats. Waltham Focus 15(3):20–24.

Schenck PA, Chew DJ. 2006. Diseases of the parathyroid gland and calcium metabolism. In *Manual of Small Animal Practice*, 3rd edition. Birchard SJ, Sherding, RG (Eds). Elsevier, St. Louis, pp. 343–356.

Schenck PA, Chew DJ, Behrend EN. 2005. Updates on hypercalcemic disorders. In *Consultations in Feline Internal Medicine*. August J (Ed). Elsevier, St. Louis, pp. 157–168.

Schenck PA, Chew DJ, Nagode LA, Rosol TJ. 2006. Disorders of calcium: Hypercalcemia and hypocalcemia. In *Fluid Therapy in Small Animal Practice*, 3rd edition. Dibartola S (Ed). Elsevier, St. Louis, pp. 122–194.

Thiess S, Becskei C, Tomsa K, Lutz TA, Wanner M. 2004. Effects of high carbohydrate and high fat diet on plasma metabolite levels and on IV glucose tolerance test in intact and neutered male cats. J Fel Med Surg 6:207–218.

Wynn S. 2001. Nutrients and botanicals in the treatment of diabetes in veterinary practice. Altern Med Rev 6(Suppl):S17–S23.

Zicker SC, Ford RB, Nelson RW, Kirk CA. 2000. Endocrine and lipid disorders. In *Small Animal Clinical Nutrition*, 4th edition. Hand MS, Thatcher CD, Remillard RL, Roudebush P (Eds). Mark Morris Institute, Topeka, KS, pp. 849–886.

CHAPTER 18
Diet and Heart Disease

Heart disease is common in older dogs and cats. There are many types of heart disease, and most have different breed predispositions. Dilated cardiomyopathy (DCM) was once very common in cats, but since the discovery that taurine deficiency was the cause, supplementation of cat diets with taurine is common and the incidence of DCM in cats has decreased. Hypertrophic cardiomyopathy is now the most common cause of heart disease in cats. Dilated cardiomyopathy has become more common in dogs, especially in large breeds. Hypertension in dogs and cats is more common now, most likely due to increased awareness and monitoring of blood pressure in dogs and cats. The most common heart disorders that require dietary management are congestive heart failure, hypertension, and heart diseases related to deficiency of a specific nutrient (taurine, carnitine).

Congestive heart failure (CHF) is a general term and not a specific disease. In general, heart failure is characterized by a heart that is unable to pump adequately and cannot deliver nutrients (especially oxygen) to tissues. Clinical signs of heart failure include weakness, exercise intolerance, fainting, coughing, abnormal breath sounds, and fluid retention. Renal disease is commonly present in association with heart disease.

Weight Management

Pets with CHF commonly have weight loss, which is termed cardiac cachexia. In dogs and cats with CHF, amino acids serve as the primary source of energy, and lean body mass is lost. Loss of muscle mass is commonly noted in the shoulders, back, and facial muscles. Cardiac cachexia is most common in dogs with DCM. Weight loss is caused by a decrease in food intake, increased energy requirements, or alterations in metabolism. Decreased appetite (anorexia) is common in CHF because in this condition the production of inflammatory mediators is increased, and these mediators can cause anorexia. Dietary therapy should provide adequate energy to prevent weight loss. Supplementation with omega-3 fatty acids, such as those present in fish oils, may be beneficial in decreasing the production of inflammatory mediators.

Some dogs with CHF may be obese. Obesity contributes to the clinical signs of CHF, and a weight reduction program should be initiated. Careful attention must be paid to the amount of treats given, as these can be a significant source of calories. Any treats given should be both low in calories and low in sodium.

Dietary Sodium

The restriction of dietary sodium has been debated in patients with CHF. Recent studies have suggested that severe sodium restriction may not be beneficial when the early stages of cardiac disease are present. If asymptomatic heart disease is present, there is a heart murmur or arrhythmia, but clinical signs of heart disease are not noted. In these patients, severe sodium restriction is not necessary, but diets, treats, and table foods high in sodium (greater than 100 mg/100 kcal) should be avoided. If there is enlargement of the heart ventricles, then the sodium content of the diet should be restricted to 50–80 mg/100 kcal. With mild to moderate CHF, clinical signs are present with mild exercise or at rest. Coughing, exercise intolerance, mild respiratory distress is usually noted. Sodium content should be restricted to 50–80 mg/100 kcal or should be restricted to less than 50 mg/100 kcal if increasing doses of diuretics are needed to control clinical signs. With advanced heart failure, clinical signs of heart failure are severe. Sodium content in the diet should be restricted to less than 50 mg/100 kcal, and sodium intake from treats or table foods must be restricted. On a dry matter basis, sodium should be restricted to 0.07%–0.25% DM in dogs and 0.3% DM in cats (Table 18.1). Chloride levels are usually 1.5 times the sodium intake. Recommended and nonrecommended ingredients for cardiac diets based on sodium content are listed in Table 18.2.

Table 18.1. Nutrient recommendations for dogs and cats with cardiac disease.

Factor	Condition	Recommendation
Sodium	Hypertension, congestive heart failure	Restrict sodium to 0.07%–0.25% DM in dogs and to 0.3% DM in cats
Potassium	Hypokalemia (associated with many diuretics)	Ensure adequate potassium in diet
Magnesium	Hypomagnesemia (associated with diuretic use)	Make sure diet contains adequate magnesium; could supplement with 20–40 mg magnesium/kg body weight daily
Phosphorus	Hyperphosphatemia (if renal failure is present)	Restrict phosphorus if necessary
Taurine	Dog: dilated cardiomyopathy	Supplement taurine 500 mg taurine twice daily
	Cat: dilated cardiomyopathy	Diet should contain adequate levels of taurine (in a wet food, 2000–3000 mg/kg DM diet)
Carnitine	Dog: dilated cardiomyopathy	Supplement carnitine 50–100 mg L-carnitine/kg body weight three times daily

Protein

In the past it was recommended that dietary protein be restricted in dogs and cats with CHF. This restriction is no longer recommended as it could contribute to cardiac cachexia and loss of lean body mass. Dietary protein should not be restricted unless chronic kidney disease is also present.

Taurine

Taurine deficiency is the most common cause of DCM in cats. Cats lose large amounts of taurine in bile acids, and the synthesis of taurine

Table 18.2. Ingredients for cardiac diets based on sodium content.

	Recommended Ingredients	Not Recommended
Starches	Potatoes, rice, macaroni	Bread, pretzels, potato chips, etc.
Fats	Vegetable shortening, unsalted margarine	Mayonnaise
Dairy products	None	Milk, cream cheese, cottage cheese, butter, cheese
Meats	Fresh beef, chicken (skinless), lamb, pork, turkey	Eggs, bacon, ham, frankfurters, canned tuna, sausage
Vegetables	Green beans, peas, green pepper, tomato, lettuce, corn, cucumber	Canned vegetables
Fruits	Most are low in sodium	
Other		Pizza, peanut butter, macaroni and cheese

can not overcome this continued loss. DCM is uncommon in cats since cat diets are routinely supplemented with taurine.

DCM has become more prevalent in dogs. Some breeds with DCM also appear to have an increased incidence of taurine deficiency (cocker spaniel, Newfoundland, golden retriever, Scottish terrier, border collie), thus plasma taurine should be measured in these breeds. Dogs with DCM that are consuming lamb and rice and high-fiber or very low-protein diets should also have plasma taurine measured. In dogs with low levels of taurine, 500–1000 mg taurine should be given twice daily.

Fat

Fat provides an important source of calories. Dogs with DCM have significantly lower circulating concentrations of long-chain omega-3 fatty acids, specifically eicosapentaenoic acid (EPA) and docosahexaenoic acid (DHA). EPA and DHA are found in fish oil. Fish oil therapy reduces the production of inflammatory mediators and improves the anorexia present in some patients with CHF. Fish oil has been supplemented at a dose of 1 capsule/10 lb body weight. Sources of omega-3 fatty acids other than fish oil, such as flaxseed oil, should not be used.

Potassium

Potassium is an important electrolyte for proper cardiac function. A decrease in potassium (hypokalemia) causes muscle weakness and decreases the effectiveness of some cardiac drugs. The use of some diuretics (furosemide) can predispose a patient with CHF to hypokalemia. The potassium content of the diet should be high enough to provide adequate potassium intake.

Magnesium

Magnesium is important in many enzymatic reactions, and serum magnesium concentration is often low in CHF. A decrease in serum magnesium can increase the risk of arrhythmias and can decrease the contraction of the heart. If deficient, magnesium can be supplemented at 20–40 mg/kg body weight/day. Excess magnesium should also be avoided.

L-Carnitine

Animals use lysine and methionine to synthesize L-carnitine. This compound is classified as a water-soluble vitamin or a nonessential amino acid. It is needed to transport free fatty acids into the mitochondria of cardiac muscle. Carnitine is esterified with fatty acids to facilitate their movement across cell membranes. Inside mitochondria, oxidation of fatty acids generates energy in the form of ATP. Carnitine remaining after fat oxidation forms esters with potentially toxic waste products and transports them from the mitochondria.

Carnitine is usually present in high concentration in cardiac muscle, and carnitine deficiency has been associated with heart disease in humans. Carnitine is abundant in red meat. Feeding nonmeat-based diets to dogs results in plasma carnitine levels that are 50% lower than in those consuming meat-based diets. It is unclear whether L-carnitine supplementation is beneficial in pets with heart disease. The recommended dose is 50–100 mg/kg body weight every 8 hours. Few side effects have been noted with carnitine supplementation, but L-carnitine is expensive, which may be a deterrent to treatment.

Coenzyme Q10

Coenzyme Q10 is required for energy production, and deficiency may play a role in heart disease. Coenzyme Q10 supplementation has been used in patients with DCM and may provide increased antioxidant protection. The recommended dose is 30–90 mg twice daily, depending on the body weight. Controlled studies are needed to evaluate the benefits of coenzyme Q10.

Dog Recipes for Heart Disease

■ **Adult Dogs**

Chicken and Rice   391
Ground Beef and Potato   392
Tofu and Pasta   393
Pork and Sweet Potato   394
Whitefish and Barley   395
Lamb and Pasta   396

■ **Puppies**

Chicken and Rice   397
Ground Beef and Potato   398

Cat Recipes for Heart Disease

Chicken and Rice   486
Ground Beef and Rice   487
Whitefish and Rice   488

Additional Reading

Backus RC, Ko KS, Fascetti AJ, Kittleson MD, Macdonald KA, Maggs DJ, et al. 2006. Low plasma taurine concentration in Newfoundland dogs is associated with low plasma methionine and cyst(e)ine concentrations and low taurine synthesis. J Nutr 136(10):2525–2533.

Chetboul V, Biourge V. 2008. Acquired cardiovascular diseases in cats: The influence of nutrition. In *Encyclopedia of Feline Clinical Nutrition*. Pibot P, Biourge V, Elliott D (Eds). Aniwa SAS, Aimargues, France, pp. 323–354.

Fascetti AJ, Reed JR, Rogers QR, Backus RC. 2003. Taurine deficiency in dogs with dilated cardiomyopathy: 12 cases. J Am Vet Med Assoc 223(11):1565.

Freeman LM. 1998. Interventional nutrition for cardiac disease. Clin Tech Small Anim Pract 13(4):232–237.

Freeman LM, Rush JE. 2006. Cardiovascular diseases: Nutritional modulation. In *Encyclopedia of Canine Clinical Nutrition*. Pibot P, Biourge V, Elliott D (Eds). Aniwa SAS, Aimargues, France, pp. 316–347.

Freeman LM, Rush JE, Markwell PJ. 2006. Effects of dietary modification in dogs with early chronic valvular disease. J Vet Intern Med 20:1116–1126.

Sanderson SL. 2006. Taurine and carnitine in canine cardiomyopathy. Vet Clin Small Anim 36:1325–1343.

Sanderson SL, Gross KL, Ogburn PN, Calvert C, Jacobs G, Lowry SR, et al. 2001. Effects of dietary fat and L-carnitine on plasma and whole blood taurine concentrations and cardiac function in healthy dogs fed protein-restricted diets. Am J Vet Res 62:1616–1623.

Torres CL, Blackus RC, Fascetti AJ, Rogers QR. 2003. Taurine status in normal dogs fed a commercial diet associated with taurine deficiency and dilated cardiomyopathy. J Anim Physiol Anim Nutr (Berl) 87(9–10):359–372.

Roudebush P, Keene BW, Mizelle HL. 2000. Cardiovascular disease. In *Small Animal Clinical Nutrition*, 4th edition. Hand MS, Thatcher CD, Remillard RL, Roudebush P (Eds). Mark Morris Institute, Topeka, KS, pp. 529–562.

CHAPTER 19
Diet and Pancreatic Disease

There are several diseases of the pancreas that can be managed in part with diet. Both dogs and cats can be affected with pancreatitis, the condition in which the pancreas is inflamed. Exocrine pancreatic insufficiency can also affect both dogs and cats, and these two conditions can benefit from dietary modification.

Exocrine Pancreatic Insufficiency

The pancreas plays a critical role in the digestion of nutrients by synthesizing and secreting enzymes that digest fat, carbohydrate, and proteins. The pancreas also secretes bicarbonate to maintain the pH of the intestinal tract in an optimal range for digestion and secretes a factor necessary for the absorption of vitamin B_{12}. When functional pancreatic mass is lost, there is a decrease in production of these digestive enzymes, which decreases the digestion and absorption of nutrients.

Chronic diarrhea is usually present in dogs with exocrine pancreatic insufficiency (EPI). Large amounts of feces are produced that are gray or yellow in color, and stools have the consistency of cow feces. Dogs typically are affected with flatulence and defecate more than three times per day. Weight loss may be mild to extreme, and these dogs have a poor body condition. Dogs with EPI often have a ravenous appetite, and coprophagia and pica are common. The hair coat is usually poor, and there may be muscle loss.

EPI is uncommon in cats. In cats with EPI, the clinical signs are typically weight loss and soft voluminous feces. Diarrhea is not as common in cats as it is in dogs.

The biochemistry profile is usually normal in dogs with EPI. Dogs with EPI do not typically have low plasma protein concentrations. Concentrations of vitamins B_{12}, A, and E are decreased in dogs with EPI, and folate concentrations are often increased. A decrease in serum trypsin-like immunoreactivity (TLI) is definitive for EPI. A feline-specific TLI (fTLI) is now available, and a decrease in fTLI is diagnostic for EPI in cats.

Atrophy of the pancreas is the common cause of EPI in dogs less than 5 years old; in older dogs the cause is usually chronic pancreatitis. In cats, chronic pancreatitis is the common cause of EPI and occurs in older cats. Atrophy of the pancreas has not been noted in cats. German shepherd dogs, collies, and English setters are at increased risk for atrophy of the pancreas and development of EPI. Miniature schnauzers are predisposed to chronic pancreatitis and have a higher incidence of developing EPI. In cats there is no breed predisposition to EPI.

For treatment of EPI, enzyme preparations must be added to the food to help the dog or cat digest the nutrients. Powdered enzyme preparations must be fresh and stored properly to be effective. The goal is to use the lowest dose of enzymes that is effective due to the cost of these preparations. Powdered enzymes should be mixed with the food immediately prior to feeding; preincubating the food with the enzyme preparation is not necessary. As an alternative to powdered enzyme preparations, raw fresh pancreas can be fed. Cow pancreas is safest, but there is always the risk of bacterial infection causing GI upset from raw meat. Fresh pancreas can be stored frozen for several months. The pancreas tissue cannot be cooked, as this will destroy the digestive enzymes present in the tissue. In addition to enzyme preparations, vitamin B_{12} should be supplemented, since the enzyme supplements do not improve the absorption of vitamin B_{12}. An injection of vitamin B_{12} once per month is adequate to prevent deficiency.

Diets designed for pets with EPI need to be highly digestible. Typical protein sources include egg, cottage cheese, and muscle meats, and carbohydrate sources usually include rice or barley. The fiber content of these diets should be low (less than 2% DM). The fat content of the diet does not need to be restricted. Diets with up to 19% DM fat or diets providing 43% calories from fat have been well tolerated by dogs with EPI (Table 19.1). Several small meals should be fed each day rather than feeding one large meal.

Table 19.1. Dietary recommendations for dogs and cats with EPI.

Nutrient	Dietary Recommendation
Fiber	<2% DM
Fat	≤19% DM; ≤43% energy

EPI, exocrine pancreatic insufficiency; DM, dry matter.

Pancreatitis

Pancreatic inflammation is relatively common, and it can be life-threatening. Acute pancreatitis can be difficult to diagnose. In dogs, the typical clinical signs are vomiting, anorexia, and abdominal pain. Other signs include depression, fever, diarrhea, abdominal distention, dehydration, shock, respiratory distress, and cardiac arrhythmias. In cats, the most common clinical signs include lethargy, anorexia, and dehydration, which are nonspecific signs. Vomiting and abdominal pain are uncommon clinical signs in the cat. Chronic pancreatitis is more difficult to recognize since it is characterized by subclinical inflammation and clinical signs can be mild and nonspecific. Anorexia and weight loss may be the only clinical signs associated with chronic pancreatitis. Chronic pancreatitis may lead to the development of diabetes mellitus or EPI.

The cause of pancreatitis is poorly understood. In dogs, dietary indiscretion, obesity, or the consumption of a high-fat meal may be related to the development of pancreatitis. Dogs over 5 years of age are at higher risk for pancreatitis, and miniature schnauzers, Yorkshire terriers, silky terriers, and miniature poodles are more commonly affected. In cats, dietary indiscretion, obesity, or the consumption of high-fat meals do not appear to predispose them to pancreatitis. The risk of chronic pancreatitis increases with age in the cat, but there is no breed or sex predisposition.

Previously, increases in serum amylase and lipase activities have been used to diagnose pancreatitis, but these enzymes can be elevated in animals without pancreatitis. Assays for pancreatic-specific enzymes have been developed. In dogs with acute pancreatitis, TLI, trypsinogen activation peptide (TAP), and pancreatic lipase immunoreactivity (PLI) have been elevated. Elevations in PLI may be the most specific for pancreatitis, but TLI, TAP, and PLI may also be elevated in renal disease. Serum amylase and lipase can not be used to diagnose pancreatitis in cats. Feline-specific TLI is not very useful for diagnosing pancreatitis in cats, but feline-specific PLI appears to be more sensitive.

Abdominal ultrasound is useful in the diagnosis of pancreatitis, especially in cats with chronic pancreatitis. Normally, the pancreas is not visible on ultrasound, but if inflammation is present, the pancreas can be seen.

Pancreatitis occurs when digestive enzymes are activated in the pancreas. Chronic inflammation may lead to the development of diabetes mellitus or EPI in dogs. The activation of pancreatic enzymes causes the release of tumor necrosis factor (TNF-α), interleukin-1 (IL-1), and platelet-activating factor (PAF), which result in increased inflammation of the pancreas. Thus, the cycle of inflammation is somewhat self-perpetuating.

Treatment for pancreatitis involves both medical and dietary management. Intravenous fluids and antibiotics are essential in the treatment of acute pancreatitis. Initially, no food is given orally to dogs because food in the duodenum stimulates the release of more pancreatic enzymes, which can worsen the inflammation. However, there is debate as to the use of parenteral (intravenous) versus enteral nutrition. Enteral nutrition can be provided via the placement of a jejunostomy tube through which a liquid diet is placed directly into the jejunum. Patients receiving a combination of both enteral and parenteral nutrition appear to have an increased survival rate as compared to those receiving parenteral nutrition alone.

In dogs, oral feeding can be reinitiated when vomiting stops. Cats rarely exhibit vomiting, but typically do not want to eat early in the course of acute pancreatitis. Cats should not be forced to eat orally, as this can cause food aversion, and it is difficult to force-feed an adequate number of calories.

Oral diets for dogs and cats recovering from pancreatitis should be highly digestible. Some amino acids can excessively stimulate pancreatic enzyme release, so excess dietary protein should be avoided. Dietary protein levels in dogs should be between 15% and 30% DM and in cats should be between 30% and 45% DM (Table 19.2). The fat content of the diet is important and varies depending on other factors. Dogs that are obese or who have hypertriglyceridemia should be fed a low-fat diet (less than 10% DM). If these conditions are not present, then a moderate fat diet (10%–15% fat DM) can be fed. Cats recovering from pancreatitis should receive a moderate-fat diet.

Table 19.2. Dietary recommendations for dogs and cats with pancreatitis.

Nutrient	Dogs	Cats
Protein	15%–30% DM	30%–45% DM
Fat	<10% if obese or hypertriglyceridemic; otherwise 10%–15% DM	10%–15% DM

DM, dry matter.

The use of dietary antioxidants in pancreatitis may be beneficial, but there is currently little evidence to support their use in dogs or cats. Supplementation with omega-3 fatty acids from fish oil can modify inflammation in pancreatitis in humans, but their effect is unknown in the dog and cat. Probiotics may be helpful in treating pancreatitis, since probiotics appear to improve the intestinal barrier and suppress inflammation. Vitamin B_{12} supplementation may be beneficial since serum vitamin B_{12} is often low in pancreatitis patients. Injectable vitamin B_{12} can be given weekly to treat deficiency.

Dog Recipes for Exocrine Pancreatic Insufficiency

Chicken and Rice   409
Cottage Cheese and Rice   410
Chicken and Rice   412
Eggs and Rice   413
Cottage Cheese and Rice   414
Whitefish and Rice   298
Cottage Cheese and Rice   371
Rabbit and Rice   372
Pork and Rice   374
Chicken and Rice   375
Ground Beef and Rice   376
Egg and Rice   377
Chicken and Rice   383
Tuna and Rice   386

Dog Recipes for Pancreatitis

■ Low-Fat Diets

Chicken and Rice   409
Cottage Cheese and Rice   410
Pork and Potato   411

■ Moderate-Fat Diets

Chicken and Rice   412
Eggs and Rice   413
Cottage Cheese and Rice   414
Pork and Potato   415
Chicken and Rice   277

Cat Recipes for Exocrine Pancreatic Insufficiency

Cat Recipes for Pancreatitis

Additional Reading

Biourge VC, Fontaine J. 2004. Exocrine pancreatic insufficiency and adverse reaction to food in dogs: A positive response to a high-fat, soy isolate hydrolysate-based diet. J Nutr 134:2166S–2168S.

Davenport DJ, Remillard RL, Simpson KW, Pidgeon GL. 2000. Gastrointestinal and exocrine pancreatic disease. In *Small Animal Clinical Nutrition*, 4th edition. Hand MS, Thatcher CD, Remillard RL, Roudebush P (Eds). Mark Morris Institute, Topeka, KS, pp. 725–810.

Kerl ME, Johnson PA. 2004. Nutritional plan: Matching diet to disease. Clin Tech Small Anim Pract 19(1):9–21.

Nicholson A, Watson AD, Mercer JR. 1989. Fat malassimilation in three cats. Aust Vet J 66(4):110–113.

Rutgers HC, Biourge V. 2008. Nutritional management of hepatobiliary and pancreatic diseases. In *Encyclopedia of Feline Clinical Nutrition*. Pibot P, Biourge V, Elliott D (Eds). Aniwa SAS, Aimargues, France, pp. 139–179.

Simpson KW. 2002. Feline pancreatitis. J Feline Med Surg 4(3):183–184.

Simpson KW. 2006. The role of nutrition in the pathogenesis and the management of exocrine pancreatic disorders. In *Encyclopedia of Canine Clinical Nutrition*. Pibot P, Biourge V, Elliott D, (Eds). Aniwa SAS, Aimargues, France, pp. 162–191.

Westermarck E, Wiberg ME. 2006. Effects of diet on clinical signs of exocrine pancreatic insufficiency in dogs. J Am Vet Med Assoc 228(2):225–229.

Wynn SG. 2009. Probiotics in veterinary practice. J Am Vet Med Assoc 234(5):606–613.

Zoran DL. 2006. Pancreatitis in cats: Diagnosis and management of a challenging disease. J Am Anim Hosp Assoc 42(1):1–9.

CHAPTER 20
Diet and Hepatic Disease

The liver is a major metabolic organ and carries out over 1500 biochemical functions. The liver is important in drug metabolism; in removal of toxic substances; in the synthesis of albumin, clotting factors, bile salts, and lipoproteins; and in the digestion and metabolism of nutrients. Protein metabolic functions of the liver include the synthesis of albumin, acute-phase proteins, coagulation factors, the regulation of amino acid metabolism, and detoxification of ammonia and the synthesis of urea. The liver is important in carbohydrate metabolism for glycogen metabolism and storage, glucose homeostasis, and the synthesis of glucose. Lipid metabolic functions include the synthesis of triglycerides, phospholipids, cholesterol, lipoproteins, and bile acids. The liver is also important for clearance and storage of lipid, lipid oxidation, ketone production, and excretion of cholesterol. Vitamin C is synthesized by the liver, and vitamin D is hydroxylated by the liver. Vitamins B and K are also activated by and stored in the liver. The liver is important for the degradation of polypeptides and steroid hormones, and stores vitamins, lipids, glycogen, copper, iron, and zinc. The liver plays a role in digestion by synthesizing bile acids and participating in the enterohepatic circulation, absorbing the fat-soluble vitamins (A, D, E, and K), and digesting and absorbing lipids.

The liver is a large organ with tremendous reserve and regenerative capabilities. This is important to maintain adequate function since the liver is so critical to metabolism. However, this also means that by the time clinical signs of liver disease are evident, liver damage is often advanced. Early clinical signs of liver disease are vague and nonspecific and often go unnoticed. Early signs include loss of appetite, weight loss, lethargy, vomiting, diarrhea, increased thirst, and increased urination. Once advanced liver disease is present, pets may be jaundiced, have fluid accumulation in the abdomen (ascites), have hepatic encephalopathy, and blood coagulation problems. If there is major bile duct obstruction, feces may be pale or gray in color. Jaundice is not a common sign of liver disease and may be due to severe hemolysis or compression of the bile duct by pancreatitis or neoplasia. Ascites is common in dogs, but uncommon in cats, and is typically caused by portal hypertension. With chronic liver disease, the liver is usually decreased in size. The liver may be enlarged in cases of neoplasia and with feline hepatic lipidosis.

Laboratory Testing

Serum biochemistry is useful when looking for evidence of hepatic disease. Many serum enzymes can be elevated in liver disease, including alkaline phosphatase (ALP), alanine aminotransferase (ALT), aspartate aminotransferase (AST), and gamma-glutamyltransferase (GGT). Other parameters such as bilirubin, albumin, globulin, urea nitrogen, glucose, and cholesterol may be altered in liver disease. Serum bile acids also increase in liver disease. Unfortunately, there are no specific tests for the different liver disorders. Abdominal radiographs can provide an estimate of liver size and shape, but abdominal ultrasound gives more specific information about the liver, bile ducts, and blood vessels. Liver biopsy is often necessary to identify the underlying cause of liver disease. Liver copper levels can also be determined from a biopsy sample.

Causes of Liver Disease

Liver diseases can be the result of inflammatory, noninflammatory, or biliary causes. Infectious inflammatory liver disease can be caused by bacteria (leptospirosis, toxoplasmosis, cholangiohepatitis), or viruses (infectious canine hepatitis, feline infectious peritonitis). Noninfectious inflammatory causes include chronic hepatitis, cirrhosis and fibrosis, lymphocytic cholangitis, or toxins and drugs. Noninflammatory liver disease can be caused by vacuolar hepatopathy (storage disorders, steroid therapy, diabetes mellitus, chronic illness, hepatocutaneous syndrome), portosystemic shunts, or neoplasia. Bile duct disease can be caused by obstruction, secondary to liver disease, or inflammation.

Risk Factors

Any breed can be affected by liver disease; however, some breeds are predisposed to particular disorders. Bedlington terriers are at increased risk for genetic copper-associated hepatic disease; West Highland white terriers, Skye terriers, and Doberman pinschers are at increased risk for chronic hepatitis; cocker spaniels, standard poodles, Labrador retrievers, and Scottish terriers are prone to idiopathic cirrhosis; and German shepherd dogs are at increased risk for idiopathic hepatic fibrosis. Copper accumulation in association with liver disease is common in Doberman pinschers, Dalmatians, West Highland white terriers, Skye terriers, and cocker spaniels. Portosystemic shunts occur more frequently in purebred dogs, especially miniature schnauzers, Irish wolfhounds, and Yorkshire terriers. Inflammatory liver disease is more common in female dogs, and male dogs are more prone to congenital liver disease.

Obese cats that become anorexic for any reason are at risk for developing hepatic lipidosis. Cholangiohepatitis is more common in cats that have pancreatitis, bile duct obstruction, or inflammatory bowel disease.

Treatment with certain medications may predispose to liver disease. The anticonvulsant drug phenobarbital is associated with chronic hepatitis, and acute hepatic toxicity is associated with potentiated sulfonamides, carprofen, and mebendazole. Glucocorticoid therapy or endogenous excess glucocorticoids (as in hyperadrenocorticism) can cause steroid hepatopathy.

Nutrient Alterations in Liver Disease

■ Protein Alterations

The liver is responsible for the synthesis of the majority of the circulating proteins; albumin makes up about 60% of the total plasma proteins. Albumin has many roles, helps maintain plasma oncotic pressure, and serves as a binding and carrier protein for hormones, steroids, amino acids, vitamins, fatty acids, calcium, and other drugs. Other important proteins synthesized by the liver include the clotting factors. With severe liver disease, there is a decrease in synthesized albumin (hypoalbuminemia), which can lead to edema and ascites.

The liver is also important in degradation of excess dietary proteins, and amino acids not needed for protein synthesis are deaminated and oxidized by the liver. The aromatic amino acids (tyrosine, phenylalanine, and tryptophan) are normally removed from the portal circulation and metabolized by the liver; with liver disease, these amino acids accumulate in the circulation. The concentrations of most other amino acids are decreased because of increased use by muscle and fat tissue. Alterations in amino acid concentrations may play a role in the development of hepatic encephalopathy.

Nitrogen metabolism is also altered in liver disease, with an increase in circulating ammonia. Hyperammonemia may be due to amino acid deamination, impaired production of urea, and inadequate return of ammonia to the liver as a result of portosystemic shunts.

■ Carbohydrate Alterations

The liver plays a major role in carbohydrate metabolism. Liver is the storage organ for glycogen, which can be readily mobilized when glucose is needed. There is adequate liver glycogen to normally meet the needs for glucose for about 24 to 36 hours, but with cirrhosis, glycogen is depleted in 10 to 12 hours. With liver disease, there is increased protein breakdown to provide amino acids for glucose production, which occurs in the liver. Blood glucose concentrations can be maintained with as little as one-fourth of the functional liver tissue, but a decrease in circulating glucose (hypoglycemia) can occur with cirrhosis, hepatic failure, or hepatic neoplasia. An excess of circulating glucose (hyperglycemia) can occur in cats with hepatic lipidosis. With liver cirrhosis, there may be an increase in circulating glucagon, resulting in a necrotizing skin disease (hepatocutaneous syndrome).

■ Lipid Alterations

The liver is very important in lipid metabolism. Fatty acids are synthesized in the liver and can be stored as triglycerides. When liver glycogen becomes depleted, fatty acids are released from fat tissue and are oxidized by the liver. Ketone bodies are produced and can be an important energy source. Carnitine is a cofactor necessary for transport of fatty acids from the cytoplasm into mitochondria, and the liver is important in carnitine metabolism. With liver disease, there may be decreased synthesis of carnitine or increased carnitine turnover. Carnitine supplementation may be beneficial in the prevention of hepatic lipidosis in cats.

Lipoprotein metabolism is altered with liver failure since the liver plays a major role in cholesterol synthesis, storage, and secretion. Bile salt production may be decreased, and with cholestasis, hypercholesterolemia and hypertriglyceridemia may be present. A decrease in serum cholesterol (hypocholesterolemia) has been observed in patients with portosystemic shunts or liver necrosis. Lipoprotein patterns in dogs and cats with liver disease have not been well studied.

■ Vitamins and Minerals

Fat-soluble vitamins (A, D, E, and K) are stored in the liver. Vitamin E deficiency is common in chronic liver disease and results in an increase in oxidative damage to the liver. Vitamin K deficiency is also common with liver disease and causes an increase in coagulation times. B vitamins may be deficient in chronic liver disease, especially vitamin B_{12}. Vitamin C synthesis is also affected by liver disease.

Iron, zinc, and copper are stored in the liver. Copper accumulation can cause hepatic damage. Copper can accumulate either as a result of a primary defect in copper metabolism or secondary to decreased copper excretion. Zinc deficiency is common in liver disease, and manganese concentrations may be decreased with cirrhosis.

Liver Disorders

■ Hepatic Encephalopathy

Hepatic encephalopathy is a metabolic disorder that affects the nervous system and develops secondary to advanced liver disease. It usually occurs as a result of portosystemic shunts (PSS). Clinical signs of hepatic encephalopathy include loss of appetite, vomiting, diarrhea, disorientation, blindness, and seizures. Signs may be intermittent and associated with the ingestion of a meal high in protein.

The cause of hepatic encephalopathy is not known, but may be due to excess ammonia, amino acids, or altered neurotransmitters. An increase in circulating ammonia is common in both dogs and cats with PSS. Amino acid alterations are present in hepatic encephalopathy. Excess dietary methionine should be avoided in animals with PSS since this can result in signs of hepatic encephalopathy. Arginine deficiency can also lead to signs of hepatic encephalopathy. Animal-source proteins are high in arginine, but vegetable-based diets for pets with liver disease should be supplemented with arginine. Dietary protein levels are typically reduced for patients with hepatic encephalopathy. Frequent small meals should be fed, and soy proteins may help decrease the risk of this disease.

■ Portosystemic Vascular Shunts

In the normal dog, blood draining the intestines (portal venous blood) enters the liver before entering the systemic circulation. In dogs affected with a congenital portosystemic shunt (PSS), the portal venous blood bypasses the liver and directly empties into the systemic circulation. A PSS may arise from any part of the portal venous system and typically empties into the caudal vena cava. Why these shunts occur remains unknown. Congenital PSS has not been shown to be hereditary, although more than one puppy in a litter may be affected. Many dogs with congenital PSS are also cryptorchid. Acquired PSS typically occur in response to portal hypertension with fibrosis and cirrhosis, but it may be due to urea cycle deficiencies in Irish wolfhounds. PSSs are uncommon in cats, but Persians and Himalayans may be predisposed.

Portal venous blood drains the intestines and contains toxins, nutrients, intestinal and pancreatic hormones, and bacteria. When this blood bypasses the liver, the liver does not develop normally and remains small in size. Toxic substances are subsequently not metabolized in the liver and reach the systemic circulation, leading to clinical signs. PSS is most commonly diagnosed in dogs less than 1 year of age. Central nervous system (CNS) signs are most common and are termed *hepatic encephalopathy*, since the CNS signs are related to the liver dysfunction. CNS signs range from depression and lethargy to seizures. Signs are typically intermittent and progressive and may be related to food or medication ingestion. Dogs with PSS are often thin and small for their age and breed. Some dogs with PSS have signs of urinary tract disease. Crystals, most commonly ammonium biurate, may occur in the urine. Ammonia absorbed from the gut is normally converted to urea by the liver. In PSS, this conversion does not occur, leading to increased ammonia in the blood and increased ammonia excretion in the kidney. The increased concentration of ammonia in the kidney leads to the formation of ammonium biurate crystals.

Diagnosis is tentatively based on history and clinical signs. Special tests that may be performed in addition to a serum biochemistry profile are determination of serum bile acids or ammonia levels, abdominal radiographs or ultrasound, and liver biopsy. PSS is usually managed medically until surgery can be performed. Providing adequate energy intake is important, and most dogs or cats with PSS require the same caloric intake as a normal healthy adult dog or cat. Adequate energy is necessary to allow for protein synthesis and to prevent ammonia production. Carbohydrate and fat are important sources of calories for patients with PSS. Dietary protein concentra-

Table 20.1. Dietary recommendations for dogs and cats with liver disease.

Factor	Dogs	Cats
Protein	15%–30% DM[a]	30%–45% DM[a]
Fat	15%–30% DM	20%–40% DM
Carbohydrate	45%–55% DM	30%–40% DM
Fiber	3%–8% DM	3%–8% DM
Sodium	0.1%–0.25% DM	0.20%–0.35% DM
Potassium	0.8%–1.0% DM	0.8%–1.0% DM
Chloride	0.25%–0.40% DM	0.30%–0.45% DM
Arginine	1.2%–2.0% DM	1.5%–2.0% DM
Taurine	—	2500–5000 ppm

DM, dry matter.
[a]Protein should be reduced if hepatic encephalopathy is present.

tions are usually between 15% and 30% DM for dogs and 30% and 45% DM for cats (Table 20.1). If hepatic encephalopathy is present, dietary protein should be decreased. Vegetable and dairy sources of protein may provide better control of signs of encephalopathy. Oral antibiotics are typically used to decrease intestinal bacteria that may also produce ammonia. A few animals have been managed medically for up to 4 years, but these animals have not functioned normally. Most dogs managed medically (without surgery) show a progressive worsening of clinical signs associated with the progression of liver failure, leading to death or euthanasia.

The goal of surgery is to occlude the shunt, allowing portal blood to go through the liver. Mortality during surgery may be as high as 21%. A good prognosis is expected in dogs surviving the surgical procedure. The liver increases in size, and liver function tests approach normal. Clinical signs disappear if the PSS is totally ligated, but mild signs may persist if the shunt can be only partially corrected. Dogs diagnosed with PSS at an earlier age seem to do better after surgery than older dogs. The best prognosis is for young dogs in which the PSS can be totally ligated.

■ Acute Liver Disease

Acute liver disease is usually caused by toxins, infections, trauma, or heat stroke. Clinical signs include vomiting, diarrhea, bleeding, hepatic encephalopathy, or clotting disorders. In the acute phase, nutrition is usually provided via nasogastric tube feeding. Frequent small meals are offered once food is accepted. Dietary protein should not be restricted unless hepatic encephalopathy is present. Antioxidants such as vitamin E and S-adenosylmethionine (SAMe) may be given. SAMe has both antioxidant and anti-inflammatory properties.

■ Chronic Hepatitis and Cirrhosis in Dogs

Chronic hepatitis is a general term used to describe necrosis and inflammation of the liver. There are many causes of hepatitis, including drugs and toxins. It is important to provide a palatable diet that should be fed in small portions multiple times per day. Dietary protein levels should be adequate for an adult dog, unless hepatic encephalopathy is present. Soy protein may help to reduce the risk of hepatic encephalopathy. Diets should also contain adequate zinc concentrations.

■ Copper-Associated Hepatotoxicosis

Bedlington terriers can be affected by an inherited recessive disorder characterized by accumulation of copper in the liver due to decreased excretion of copper in bile. Approximately 25% of Bedlington terriers are affected, and 50% are carriers. DNA testing is available to identify affected and carrier animals. By the time affected dogs are 2 to 4 years of age, toxic levels of copper accumulate in their livers. Copper causes oxidative injury in hepatocytes, with damage to the mitochondria. Hepatitis occurs when liver copper concentration exceeds 2000 ppm. Necrosis of the liver occurs when liver copper exceeds 3000 ppm. Cirrhosis develops after massive liver necrosis if the dog survives.

A number of other breeds exhibit an increase in liver copper in chronic hepatitis and cirrhosis, but it is unclear whether excess copper occurs prior to liver disease or is a result of decreased copper excretion from chronic cholestasis. In breeds such as West Highland white terriers, Skye terriers, Kerry blue terriers, Doberman pinschers, and cocker spaniels, liver copper concentrations are lower than in Bedlington terriers, and concentrations do not increase with age. Hepatic copper accumulation is rare in cats, but has been described in Siamese.

Dietary protein requirements for dogs with copper toxicosis are similar to other adult dogs. If hepatic encephalopathy is present, dietary protein should be restricted.

Excess dietary copper should be avoided, and foods containing high levels of copper should not be fed (Table 20.2). Some fiber sources and zinc can block copper absorption. Supplemental zinc induces

Table 20.2. Copper content in dietary ingredients.

Foods High in Copper	Foods Low in Copper
Legumes	Cheese
Liver	Cottage cheese
Muscle meats	Rice
Shellfish	Tofu

production of metallothionein by the intestine, which binds very efficiently to copper, blocking it from being absorbed. Zinc is given as a supplement and not in the diet. Penicillamine is another compound that is often used as a treatment to chelate copper and block the absorption. Vitamin E supplementation has also been recommended as a treatment in copper toxicosis.

■ Feline Hepatic Lipidosis

Hepatic lipidosis occurs in cats and is characterized by extreme accumulation of fat within the liver. This accumulation of fat causes liver dysfunction and blockage of the bile ducts, resulting in cholestasis. Hepatic lipidosis is common in obese cats that suddenly undergo rapid weight loss. Middle-aged to older cats are most commonly affected, and any breed can develop feline hepatic lipidosis (FHL).

Cats are carnivores and require high amounts of dietary protein and fatty acids. Cats tend to accumulate fat in their liver cells (hepatocytes), and in FHL this accumulation exceeds the mobilization of fat for oxidation and utilization. Fat accumulates in hepatocytes due to rapid mobilization of peripheral fat. There is decreased production of lipoproteins by the liver in FHL, so fat remains in the liver. Decreased levels of antioxidants such as vitamin E and glutathione lead to increased oxidative damage, causing further liver damage.

Clinical signs of FHL include loss of appetite, rapid weight loss, excess salivation, and vomiting. Many cats have jaundice and a loss of muscle mass. The liver is enlarged, and there is an increase in serum liver enzyme concentrations. Hepatic encephalopathy may occur. Diagnosis requires either a fine needle aspirate of liver cells, or a liver biopsy.

Aggressive therapy is necessary since the mortality rate is high with FHL. Nutritional support is important, and most cats require feeding via a nasogastric tube for a short period of time because these cats are usually anorexic. Cats should never be force-fed orally as they develop food aversions very easily. Providing adequate calories is important, especially in protein. Cats with FHL should be fed a diet containing 30%–45% DM protein (Table 20-1). If hepatic encephalopathy is present, then the protein concentration should be decreased.

A decrease in serum potassium (hypokalemia) is common in FHL due to decreased intake of potassium and the loss of potassium with vomiting. L-Carnitine supplementation may be beneficial in FHL (250mg/cat/day). B vitamins and vitamin E should be provided in adequate amounts.

■ Cholangiohepatitis/Cholangitis in Cats

Cholangitis is inflammation of the bile duct system, and cholangio-hepatitis is inflammation of both the liver and bile duct system that occurs primarily in cats. Mainly dogs are affected by inflammation of the liver (hepatitis), but in cats, inflammation typically involves the bile ducts. Persian cats are predisposed to this condition. Suppurative cholangitis occurs usually due to a bacterial infection ascending into the bile ducts from the intestines and frequently is a result of pancreatitis or inflammatory bowel disease (IBD). Clinical signs are acute and include fever, vomiting, loss of appetite, and jaundice. Obstruction of bile ducts can result from cholangitis. Early treatment usually involves feeding via a nasogastric tube and antibiotic therapy. Later in the course of treatment, oral feeding with a typical liver diet is instituted.

Cholangitis with inflammation due to lymphocytes is usually due to an immune-mediated process. The disease is chronic and slowly progressive and characterized by weight loss, anorexia, jaundice, and enlarged liver, and ascites. Cats with cholangiohepatitis or cholangitis are treated nutritionally similar to cats with hepatic lipidosis.

■ Hepatic Amyloidosis

Hepatic amyloid accumulation may affect young adult Siamese and Oriental shorthair cats. Clinical signs are vague, but rupture of the liver can occur. There is no treatment.

■ Portal Hypertension

Portal hypertension is an increase in the blood pressure in the portal venous system as a result of chronic fibrosis and cirrhosis of the liver. The blood pressure gradually increases to continue to provide perfusion to the diseased liver. As the portal blood pressure increases, portosystemic shunts can develop. Shunting can lead to hepatic encephalopathy. As the liver becomes more diseased, the flow of lymph is impaired, and ascites is the result. Energy and protein requirements in portal hypertension are similar to those in other liver disorders. If ascites is present, sodium should be restricted to 0.1%–0.25% DM in dogs and 0.20%–0.35% DM in cats.

General Nutritional Considerations

Dietary fat does not need to be restricted in most cases of liver disease unless there is significant bile duct obstruction or concurrent fat malabsorption. In liver disease, dietary fat of 15%–30% DM for dogs and 20%–40% DM for cats appears to be tolerated. Medium-chain triglycerides (MCT) may have some advantages as a fat source since they are easily absorbed and hydrolyzed; however, MCT oil is expensive and not very palatable. Omega-3 fatty acid supplementation may also be beneficial in liver disease.

An increase in dietary fiber reduces the amount of nitrogenous waste that is absorbed. Increased fiber can also bind bile acids and bacteria. Dietary fiber for dogs and cats with liver disease is typically between 3% to 8% DM.

A decrease in serum potassium is common due to vomiting and decreased intake. Dietary potassium should be provided in adequate amounts. Iron and zinc deficiency often occur with liver disease, and adequate amounts should be provided in the diet. Excess dietary iron should be avoided. Water-soluble vitamins (especially B vitamins) are often deficient in liver disease due to loss in vomit and urine. Vitamin K is synthesized in the liver and may be low in those with liver disease. Vitamin K deficiency can lead to clotting problems and bleeding. All vitamins should be provided in adequate amounts in the diet.

Dog Recipes for Liver Disease

Dog Recipes for Hepatic Encephalopathy

Chicken and Rice   406
Tofu and Rice   407

Dog Copper-Restricted Recipes

Tofu and Rice   408

Cat Recipes for Liver Disease

Tofu and Chicken   489
Tofu and Ground Beef   490
Tofu and Cottage Cheese   491
Tofu and Tuna   492

Cat Recipes for Hepatic Encephalopathy

Tofu and Lentils   493

Additional Reading

Bauer JE, Schenck PA. 1989. Nutritional management of hepatic disease. Vet Clin N Amer Sm Anim 19(3):513–526.

Case LP, Carey DP, Hirakawa DA, Daristotle L (Eds). 2000. Feline hepatic lipidosis. In *Canine and Feline Nutrition: A Resource for Companion Animal Professionals*, 2nd edition. Mosby, St. Louis, pp. 473–476.

Ibrahim WH, Bailey N, Sunvold FD, Bruckner GG. 2003. Effects of carnitine and taurine on fatty acid metabolism and lipid accumulation in the liver of cats during weight gain and weight loss. Am J Vet Res 64(10):1265–1277.

Roudebush P, Davenport DJ, Dimski DS. 2000. Hepatobiliary disease. In *Small Animal Clinical Nutrition*, 4th edition. Hand MS, Thatcher CD, Remillard RL, Roudebush P (Eds). Mark Morris Institute, Topeka, KS, pp. 811–848.

Rutgers HC, Biourge V. 2006. Nutrition of dogs with liver disease. In *Encyclopedia of Canine Clinical Nutrition*. Pibot P, Biourge V, Elliott D (Eds). Aniwa SAS, Aimargues, France, pp. 134–161.

Rutgers HC, Biourge V. 2008. Nutritional management of hepatobiliary and pancreatic diseases. In *Encyclopedia of Feline Clinical Nutrition*. Pibot P, Biourge V, Elliott D (Eds). Aniwa SAS, Aimargues, France, pp. 139–179.

CHAPTER 21
Diet and Cancer

With the improvements in pet health care, many dogs and cats are living to advanced ages. Cancer has become a relatively common disease in older pets. There are many different types of cancer with different biological properties that can affect pets. Both treatment regimens and current nutritional status have an impact on nutritional recommendations, thus there is no one diet that is perfect for all cancer patients.

Cancer Cachexia

Cancer cachexia is a specific term used to describe the involuntary weight loss that occurs with malignancy. The weight loss associated with cancer can be severe: fatigue, anemia, and a depletion of both lean body mass and fat mass occur. Weight loss is clinically significant as it can affect the quality of life and the prognosis for survival. Patients with poor nutritional status are less likely to respond to therapy and may be more prone to toxic effects of chemotherapy.

The cachexia that occurs with cancer can be primary and secondary. Secondary cachexia occurs as a result of the location of the tumor (interference with intake or ability to digest nutrients) or as a side effect of cancer treatment. Chemotherapy can alter the sense of smell and taste in humans and can most likely have the same effect in pets. Chemotherapy can also directly cause nausea, vomiting, and anorexia. Both radiation therapy and chemotherapy can destroy the gastrointestinal tract cell lining, decreasing food intake and leading to maldigestion and malabsorption of nutrients.

Primary cancer cachexia is a poorly understood syndrome and cannot be entirely reversed, even with apparently adequate nutritional intake. Cancer affects the metabolism of the patient, which leads to an inefficient utilization of energy. As a result, fat stores become depleted and lean body mass decreases. Metabolism of fat, protein, and carbohydrate is altered. In the early stages of cancer, there may be no obvious clinical signs, but metabolic changes are already taking place. During this stage, the animal may appear normal, may be starting to slow down, or aging a little more rapidly. At this point, increases in insulin and lactate are present, and there are alterations in the circulating concentrations of amino acids. In the second phase of cancer, patients start to exhibit loss of appetite, lethargy, and weight loss. During the third phase of cancer, there is further loss of appetite, lethargy, and more profound weight loss. The increases in insulin and lactate are more pronounced, and there are further alterations in amino acids. There is marked debilitation, with weakness and decreased body carbohydrate and fat stores, and evidence of a negative nitrogen balance (decreased circulating albumin). Vomiting and diarrhea may also occur. The fourth phase of cancer is either recovery or remission. Metabolic changes may persist, however, even though the patient has apparently recovered.

Carbohydrate Metabolism

Carbohydrate metabolism is significantly altered in cancer. Tumors preferentially utilize glucose for energy, which results in an excess of lactate formation. To convert the excess lactate to a usable form of energy, the animal must expend energy. Thus, extra calories are burned, which leads to a net loss of energy. Carbohydrate-rich foods should be avoided in pets with cancer, as these foods tend to increase the amount of lactate produced. Carbohydrates should comprise less than 25% of the dry matter of the diet or less than 20% of the metabolizable energy of the diet (Table 21.1).

Protein Metabolism

Patients with cancer typically have a decreased body muscle mass, decreased protein synthesis, and altered nitrogen balance. Tumors will use amino acids for growth, and this becomes significant because the amino acid utilization is greater than amino acid (protein) intake. With

Table 21.1. Dietary recommendations for cancer diets.

Nutrient	Dietary Recommendation
Protein	Dogs: 30%–45% DM; 25%–40% of total kcal
	Cats: 40%–50% DM; 35%–45% of total kcal
Carbohydrate	<25% DM; <20% of total kcal
Fat	25%–40% DM; 50%–65% of total kcal
Fatty acids	>5% DM of omega-3 fatty acids; omega-6/omega-3 ratio <3.0
Arginine	>2% DM

a negative protein balance, gastrointestinal and immune functions decrease and wound healing is impaired. Dogs with a variety of cancers can show a decrease in circulating concentrations of threonine, glutamine, glycine, valine, cystine, and arginine, and an increase in isoleucine and phenylalanine. Once these amino acid changes take place, they do not reverse, even after the tumor is removed, which suggests that cancer induces long-term metabolic changes.

Supplementation with branched-chain amino acids (BCAA) may be beneficial to cancer patients. Branched chain amino acids include isoleucine, leucine, and valine. BCAA may help suppress tumor growth. BCAA may also help prevent lean body wasting and may increase lean body mass. Leucine, especially, increases protein synthesis in skeletal muscle. There are no studies evaluating the use of BCAA in dogs or cats, but supplementation in rodents has been safe at a level of 5% of the diet. A safe dose for dogs and cats may be 100–200 mg/kg/day, but further studies are needed.

Methionine and asparagine are required by some tumors for growth. Replacement of methionine with homocysteine appears to be beneficial, increasing the sensitivity to chemotherapy. Glycine may decrease the toxicity of some chemotherapeutic regimens. Arginine and glutamine may have particular benefit. In some studies, the addition of arginine decreased tumor growth and the rate of metastases. In dogs with lymphoma, the circulating concentration of arginine showed a positive correlation with survival time. Glutamine is an important source of energy for intestinal cells and can improve GI function. Supplementation with glutamine may be beneficial in cancers with intestinal injury. Glutamine may have suppressive effects on tumor growth, and it also stimulates the immune system.

In cancer, it is important to avoid a deficiency of protein, and dietary protein should be provided in excess of healthy adult requirements. For dogs, protein should be provided at 30%–45% of the dry matter of the diet, or 25%–40% of the metabolizable energy of the diet. For cats, protein should be provided at 40%–50% of the dry matter of the diet, or 35%–45% of the metabolizable energy of the diet. Arginine should be provided in the diet at a level greater than 2% on a dry matter basis.

Lipid Metabolism

The majority of weight loss in cancer is due to the loss of body fat. Not only is less energy consumed with cancer, but cancer can also result in an increase in fat breakdown, with a decrease in fat production in the body. Once lipid metabolic changes take place, they do not reverse, even with treatment or during remission, suggesting that cancer induces long-term changes in fat metabolism. Diets for pets with cancer should supply a large proportion of energy from fat. Fat should supply 25%–40% of dry matter or 50%–60% of the metabolizable energy of the diet.

There has been a considerable amount of research focusing on the effect of omega-3 fatty acids on cancer. The omega-3 fatty acids are less inflammatory than are omega-6 fatty acids and thus may be beneficial in the treatment of some cancers. Omega-3 fatty acids, especially the longest chain omega-3 fatty acids (eicosapentaenoic acid [EPA] and docosahexaenoic acid [DHA]), appear to have the potential to inhibit the growth of some tumors. In some species, dietary supplementation with EPA and DHA can prevent cancer cachexia and can limit metastasis of some tumors. A possible mechanism of EPA and DHA in limiting tumor growth and metastasis is that these fatty acids alter the membrane properties as they are incorporated into tumor tissue. The omega-3 fatty acids make membranes more fluid and alters their permeability, which makes tumor cells more susceptible to chemotherapy and the patient's own immune system. Thus, tumor cells can be destroyed more readily by therapy. There is also evidence that omega-3 fatty acid supplementation may help prevent the recurrence of cancer after remission.

Therapeutic trials with omega-3 fatty acid supplementation in humans have shown significant benefit in cancer, with improvement in nitrogen balance, better wound healing, and a reduction in the incidence of complications from therapy. In dogs with lymphoma, supplementation with EPA, DHA, and arginine resulted in a decrease in circulating lactate. This same supplementation regimen for dogs with nasal tumors resulted in a decrease in lactate and an improvement in the quality of life. Diets for cancer should be designed with increased levels of omega-3 fatty acids (greater than 5% DM), and the omega-6-to-omega-3 fatty acid ratio should be less than 3.

Vitamins

There are a number of studies that have focused on the effects of different vitamins on tumor growth and metastasis. Vitamin A has the potential to regulate cancer cells, and some cancers can be treated with vitamin A derivatives. Vitamin A may make cancer cells more susceptible to treatment. However, since vitamin A is a fat-soluble vitamin, it can potentially be toxic if supplemented at high levels.

Vitamin C (ascorbic acid) may be helpful in prevention of cancer of the stomach and esophagus. In some species, vitamin C can prevent drug resistance of some cancers to chemotherapy. This association has not been directly shown in dogs or cats, however.

Vitamin E may be helpful in the prevention of mammary and colon cancer in some species. Vitamin E is a potent antioxidant and can help prevent oxidative damage that leads to cell death. Vitamin E may prevent tumor proliferation and augments the immune system. β-Carotene is an important antioxidant and has been extensively studied in humans. β-Carotene may be beneficial in some cancers, but other studies have shown an increased risk of cancer with increased levels of β-carotene. Thus, more work is needed in pets before a recommendation for β-carotene can be made.

Minerals

Many studies have focused on selenium and its impact on cancer. In humans, low selenium concentrations have been observed in association with gastrointestinal cancer, and in rodents, selenium supplementation inhibits mammary, stomach, and colon cancers.

Increased iron concentrations have been associated with lung, colon, bladder, and esophageal cancer in humans. In rodents, low serum concentrations of iron are associated with slower tumor growth. Low levels of zinc have been correlated with esophageal, pancreatic, and bronchial cancer in humans; however, zinc deficiency is associated with increased cancer in some laboratory animal species.

Selenium supplementation at 2–4 mg/kg body weight/day may be helpful in pets with neoplasia.

Other Ingredients and Supplements

Phytochemicals are the source of nearly all phenolics found in animals. Phenolics essential for animals, such as tyrosine, come either directly from plants or are modified from essential plant precursors. Phenolic phytochemicals are grouped into flavonoids (such as anthocyanins, genistein, and daidzein), tannins, lignins, and simple phenols such as the benzoic and cinnamic acids. These chemicals protect plants and have beneficial effects in animals. They protect animal cells by chelating, or quenching free radicals, which provides antioxidant activity. Phytochemicals are found in fruits, vegetables, grains, and legumes. Phytochemicals are beneficial only from dietary levels in naturally occurring foods; excess phytochemicals can be toxic.

Soybean products are rich in flavonoids. Other beans are also rich in phytochemicals. In addition, naturally blue, purple, red, orange, and yellow foods are abundant in flavonoids. Isolated factors from soybeans have been shown to suppress cancer growth in animal models of cancer, including colon and liver cancer. Soy isolates can also protect against the intestinal damage caused by some cancer-therapy agents.

Garlic consumption has been associated with a reduced risk of cancer in some human studies. In rodent models, dietary garlic extracts have antitumor properties and have a direct effect on human mammary and melanoma cancer. There are no studies that have shown a benefit of dietary garlic in the prevention or treatment of cancer in humans or pets.

Green and black teas may also have anticancer properties. The active agents in these teas act as antioxidants and can inhibit cancer-causing agents. Black tea is soothing and reduces oral discomfort associated with radiation therapy. Other ingredients in tea, such as tannins, can act as an oral astringent and have some anesthetic properties when the mouth is rinsed with tea two or three times per day.

Energy Requirements in Cancer Patients

The energy requirement for dogs and cats with cancer can vary from patient to patient, thus each animal must be evaluated individually.

In general, studies suggest that the daily energy requirement in dogs and cats with uncomplicated cancer is similar to that of normal healthy pets. Radiation, chemotherapy, or surgery can affect nutritional status, depending on the location of the cancer. Cancer therapies do not appear to increase the energy requirement, but they do interfere with ingestion or absorption of nutrients, which can lead to nutritional deficiencies and a loss of weight. Increasing food intake is an important step in the nutritional treatment of cancer patients.

Enhancing Intake of Food

The first step to increase the intake of food is to provide a quiet and nonstressful environment for eating. Meals should be given on a regular schedule, and the person feeding the pet should be calm and nonstressful.

The next step to increase the intake of food is to increase the palatability of the diet. Most homemade diets are highly palatable and should be readily consumed. The increased moisture of homemade diets helps to increase their intake. Also, the variety of ingredients and aromas present in homemade diets enhance their palatability. Slight warming of the diet (to no higher than body temperature) can increase the aroma.

Extra fat can be added to the diet to increase palatability. Additional fat also increases the energy density of the diet so that less diet needs to be consumed to meet daily energy requirements. Adding extra fat to diets should be avoided in patients with alterations in GI motility or in those prone to pancreatitis.

Some increase in dietary protein may also increase palatability. An increase in protein should be avoided in those with liver disease or renal failure.

For dogs, the addition of a sweet or salty ingredient on the top of the food may increase palatability. Artificial sweeteners should not be used since they provide no calories. Xylitol, especially, should not be fed because it can cause a large decrease in the glucose concentration and can lead to a hypoglycemic crisis. Corn syrup can be used in dogs to increase sweetness, but should not be used in cats as it can cause fructosuria. In general, cats do not respond to sweet tastes since they lack sweet receptors. For dogs, only a small amount of sugar or corn syrup should be added, and the supplement should provide less than 10% of the total daily calories. Additional salt sprinkled on the top of the food may increase palatability in the dog, but cats do not respond to extra salt. Salt should not be added to diets for dogs with hypertension, heart disease, or renal disease.

Despite all the attempts to increase food intake, some patients just will not consume enough food on their own to meet their daily energy needs. These patients will require assisted feeding via either a feeding tube or parenteral nutrition. Assisted feeding should be initiated early in the process to prevent severe wasting and nutritional deficiencies.

Dog Recipes for Cancer

Cat Recipes for Cancer

Additional Reading

Baracos VE. 2006. Cancer-associated cachexia and underlying biological mechanisms. Annu Rev Nutr 26:435–461.

Case LP, Carey DP, Hirakawa DA, Daristotle L (Eds). 2000. Nutritional care of cancer patients. In *Canine and Feline Nutrition: A Resource for Companion Animal Professionals*, 2nd edition. Mosby, St. Louis, pp. 505–514.

Colomer R, Moreno-Nogueira JM, Garcia-Luna PP, Garcia-Peris P, Garcia-de-Lorenzo A, Zarazaga A, et al. 2007. n-3 Fatty acids, cancer and cachexia: A systematic review of the literature. Brit J Nutr 97:823–831.

Delaney SJ. 2006. Management of anorexia in dogs and cats. Vet Clin Small Anim 36:1243–1249.

Mauldin GE. 2007. Nutritional management of the cancer patient. In *Small Animal Clinical Oncology*, 4th edition. Withrow SJ, Vail DM (Eds). Elsevier, St. Louis, pp. 3074–326.

Michel KE, Sorenmo KU. 2008. Nutritional status of cats with cancer: Nutritional evaluation and recommendations. In *Encyclopedia of Feline Clinical Nutrition*. Pibot P, Biourge V, Elliott D (Eds). Aniwa SAS, Aimargues, France, pp. 386–402.

Morley JE, Thomas DR, Wilson MG. 2006. Cachexia: Pathophysiology and clinical relevance. Am J Clin Nutr 83:735–743.

Ogilvie GK, Marks SL. 2000. Cancer. In *Small Animal Clinical Nutrition*, 4th edition. Hand MS, Thatcher CD, Remillard RL, Roudebush P (Eds). Mark Morris Institute, Topeka, KS, pp. 887–905.

Ogilvie GK, Fettman MJ, Mallinckrodt CH, Walton JA, Hansen RA, Davenport DJ, et al. 2000. Effect of fish oil, arginine, and doxorubicin chemotherapy on remission and survival time for dogs with lymphoma: A double-blind, randomized placebo-controlled study. Cancer 88(8):1916–1928.

Ogilvie GK. 1998. Interventional nutrition for the cancer patient. Clin Tech Small Anim Pract 13(4):224–231.

Perez Alenza D, Rutteman GR, Pena L, Beynen AC, Cuesta P. 1998. Relation between habitual diet and canine mammary tumors in a case-control study. J Vet Intern Med 1998 12(3):132–139.

Perez Alenza MD, Pena L, del Castillo N, Nieto AI. 2000. Factors influencing the incidence and prognosis of canine mammary tumours. J Small Anim Pract 41(10):476.

Raghavan M, Knapp DW, Bonney PL, Dawson MH, Glickman LT. 2005. Evaluation of the effect of dietary vegetable consumption on reducing risk of transitional cell carcinoma of the urinary bladder in Scottish terriers. J Am Vet Med Assoc 227(1):94–100.

Wakshlag JJ, Kallfelz FA. 2006. Nutritional status of dogs with cancer: Dietetic evaluation and recommendations. In *Encyclopedia of Canine Clinical Nutrition*. Pibot P, Biourge V, Elliott D (Eds). Aniwa SAS, Aimargues, France, pp. 408–425.

SECTION II
Home-Prepared Diets

Tools Needed

1. You will need a good scale to weigh your pet. An accurate body weight is necessary to determine the kilocalories per day your pet needs.
2. A good food scale that can accurately weigh in grams and ounces is important. This piece of equipment is vital for accurate preparation of diets.
3. A good set of measuring spoons and measuring cups is necessary.
4. A pill crusher is needed to crush the vitamin and mineral tablets. A pill splitter is also useful for cutting some tablets in half.
5. A calculator is helpful to perform the calculations needed to determine how much diet to feed your pet.

Choosing a Diet

1. Determine the life stage or special conditions that may be present to choose an appropriate diet. Most diets are complete and balanced; however, some special diets are not, and this is noted in the recipe. Diets that are not complete and balanced should only be fed under the direct supervision of your veterinarian.
2. Obtain an accurate body weight of your dog or cat.
3. Determine how many calories per day are needed using the tables in Chapter 4.

4. Determine how many grams of the chosen recipe should be fed per day. Divide the kilocalories per day needed by the kilocalories per gram of the diet.
5. Prepare the recipe and feed the correct amount to provide adequate kilocalories.

Let's use an 18-lb adult female spayed dog as an example. This dog is in good body condition, has no special conditions, and does not need to lose weight.

1. We will choose the Eggs and Rice diet (p. 284) formulated for adult dogs.
2. The body weight of the dog is 18 lb.
3. Using Table 4.2, Daily Energy Requirements for Neutered Adult Dogs, an 18-lb dog requires approximately 542 kilocalories per day.
4. According to the Eggs and Rice adult diet, this recipe as prepared makes approximately 693 g of diet and provides a total of 1066 kcal. Thus, this is a 1066 kcal/693 g diet, or a 1.54 kcal/g diet.

If this dog needs 542 kcal/day, then how many grams of this diet should be fed per day? Divide the kilocalories per day needed by the kilocalories per gram of diet to get the answer.

$$\frac{542\ \text{kcal/day}}{1.54\ \text{kcal/g diet}} = 352\ \text{g prepared diet/day to supply adequate kcal}$$

As another example, let's use a 55-lb intact male dog. This dog is in good body condition, has no special conditions, and does not need to lose weight.

1. Choose the Chicken and Rice diet (p. 277) formulated for adult dogs.
2. The body weight of the dog is 55 lb.
3. Using Table 4.1, Daily Energy Requirements for Intact Adult Dogs, a 55-lb intact male dog requires 1409 kcal/day.
4. According to the Chicken and Rice adult diet, this recipe as prepared makes approximately 459 g of diet and provides a total of 726 kcal. Thus, this is 726 kcal/459 g diet, or 1.58 kcal/g diet.

Divide the kilocalories per day needed by the kilocalories per gram of diet.

$$\frac{1409\ \text{kcal/day}}{1.58\ \text{kcal/g diet}} = 892\ \text{g prepared diet/day to supply adequate kcal}$$

5. One batch of this recipe makes only 459 g of diet. This dog needs more than this amount, so double the recipe. Multiply all ingredients by 2 to make a double batch, that is, 4 cups cooked rice, 8 ounces cooked chicken breast, etc.

Preparing Diets

1. Follow the recipes as written and do NOT omit or substitute ingredients. These diets have been carefully formulated to meet the nutritional needs of dogs or cats. This is especially important for the vitamin/mineral supplements included in the recipes.
2. Ingredients should be cooked as stated in the recipe prior to preparation. Recipes were formulated using the nutritional value provided by cooked ingredients.
3. Chop ingredients into small pieces so that ingredients can be well mixed. Any vitamins or minerals provided in tablet form should be crushed before adding them to the diet.
4. Only prepare as much diet as you will feed your pet in a day. Store unused portions either in the refrigerator (for no longer than 1 day) or in the freezer. These diets do not contain any preservatives, and bacteria can easily grow in these diets if left at room temperature.
5. Diets should be fed at room temperature. If ingredients are cold, palatability is decreased and the pet may not consume adequate diet. Diets can be slightly warmed to increase palatability if needed, but diets should NOT be heated until hot as this can destroy some of the vitamins present.
6. Small amounts of vegetables (less than 1/2 cup) can be added to most diets. Vegetables will increase the fiber content and decrease the caloric density of the diet. If vegetables are added, make sure that the pet consumes all of the diet necessary to provide adequate caloric and nutrient intake.

Dog Diet Recipes

Diets for Healthy Dogs

Adults

Gestation

Senior

Weight Loss

Diets for Dogs with Special Conditions

Allergy

Cancer

Endocrine

Diabetes Mellitus

Insulinoma

Lipid Disorders

Gastrointestinal

Megaesophagus

Esophagitis

Diet: Chicken and Rice

Species: Dog
Life Stage: Adult
Special Conditions: Pancreatitis (diet provides moderate fat); esophagitis; skin conditions

Ingredient	Quantity	Measure
Chicken breast, roasted, without skin	4	ounces
Rice, white, long-grain, cooked	2	cup
Canola oil	1	tbsp
Salt substitute (potassium chloride)	½	tsp
Bone meal powder	2	tsp
Salt, iodized (sodium chloride)	¾	tsp
Multivitamin & mineral tablet, kids complete	1	each
Zinc, 100 mg tablet	½	tablet

Prepared weight (approximately) = 459 g
Total kcal as prepared = 726 kcal
kcal/g prepared diet = 1.58 kcal/g diet

Nutrient	DM%[a]	As-Fed (g/100 g diet)	ME% (g/100 kcal)	% of total kcal
Protein	26	9.5	6.0	24
Fat	11	4.1	2.6	26
Carbohydrate	53	19.6	12.4	50
Fiber	1	0.3	0.2	—

[a]DM%, dry matter percent. If all the water was removed from this diet, this is the percentage of nutrient that would be present.

Diet: Chicken and Pasta

Species: Dog
Life Stage: Adult
Special Conditions: Esophagitis, gastric motility disorders; skin conditions

Ingredient	Quantity	Measure
Chicken breast, without skin, roasted	4	ounces
Pasta, enriched, cooked	3	cup
Canola oil	1½	tbsp
Sardines, with bone, in tomato sauce	2	each
Salt substitute (potassium chloride)	¾	tsp
Bone meal powder	2	tsp
Salt, iodized (sodium chloride)	1½	tsp
Multivitamin & mineral tablet, kids complete	1	each
Zinc, 100 mg tablet	½	tablet

Prepared weight (approximately) = 651 g
Total kcal as prepared = 1182 kcal
kcal/g prepared diet = 1.81 kcal/g diet

Nutrient	DM%[a]	As-Fed (g/100 g diet)	ME% (g/100 kcal)	% of total kcal
Protein	28	11.6	6.4	25
Fat	14	5.7	3.1	30
Carbohydrate	49	20.2	11.1	44
Fiber	3	1.2	0.6	—

[a]DM%, dry matter percent. If all the water was removed from this diet, this is the percentage of nutrient that would be present.

Diet: Chicken and Potato

Species: Dog
Life Stage: Adult
Special Conditions: Pancreatitis (diet provides moderate fat); esopha-
gitis; skin conditions

Ingredient	Quantity	Measure
Chicken breast, roasted, without skin	4	ounces
Potatoes, cooked in skin, diced	3	cup
Canola oil	1	tbsp
Salt substitute (potassium chloride)	½	tsp
Bone meal powder	2	tsp
Salt, iodized (sodium chloride)	¾	tsp
Multivitamin & mineral tablet, kids complete	1	each
Zinc, 100 mg tablet	½	tablet

Prepared weight (approximately) = 611 g
Total kcal as prepared = 722 kcal
kcal/g prepared diet = 1.18 kcal/g diet

Nutrient	DM%[a]	As-Fed (g/100 g diet)	ME% (g/100 kcal)	% of total kcal
Protein	25	7.2	6.1	24
Fat	10	3.0	2.6	24
Carbohydrate	54	15.6	13.2	52
Fiber	5	1.4	1.2	—

[a]DM%, dry matter percent. If all the water was removed from this diet, this is the
percentage of nutrient that would be present.

Diet: Ground Beef and Rice

Species: Dog
Life Stage: Adult
Special Conditions: Esophagitis, gastric motility disorders; skin conditions

Ingredient	Quantity	Measure
Ground beef, 10% fat, pan-browned	5	ounces
Rice, white, long-grain, cooked	2	cup
Canola oil	2	tsp
Salt substitute (potassium chloride)	½	tsp
Bone meal powder	2	tsp
Salt, iodized (sodium chloride)	¾	tsp
Multivitamin & mineral tablet, kids complete	1	each
Zinc, 100 mg tablet	½	tablet

Prepared weight (approximately) = 482 g
Total kcal as prepared = 824 kcal
kcal/g prepared diet = 1.71 kcal/g diet

Nutrient	DM%[a]	As-Fed (g/100 g diet)	ME% (g/100 kcal)	% of total kcal
Protein	27	10.1	5.9	24
Fat	15	5.7	3.3	32
Carbohydrate	49	18.7	10.9	44
Fiber	5	2.1	0.2	—

[a]DM%, dry matter percent. If all the water was removed from this diet, this is the percentage of nutrient that would be present.

Diet: Ground Beef and Pasta

Species: Dog
Life Stage: Adult
Special Conditions: Esophagitis, gastric motility disorders; pancreatitis (diet provides moderate fat), skin conditions

Ingredient	Quantity	Measure
Ground beef, 10% fat, pan-browned	5	ounces
Pasta, enriched, cooked	3	cup
Canola oil	2	tsp
Salt substitute (Potassium chloride)	½	tsp
Bone meal powder	2	tsp
Salt, iodized (sodium chloride)	1¼	tsp
Multivitamin & mineral tablet, kids complete	1	each
Zinc, 100 mg tablet	½	tablet

Prepared weight (approximately) = 589 g
Total kcal as prepared = 1076 kcal
kcal/g prepared diet = 1.83 kcal/g diet

Nutrient	DM%[a]	As-Fed (g/100 g diet)	ME% (g/100 kcal)	% of total kcal
Protein	26	11.0	6.0	24
Fat	12	5.1	2.8	27
Carbohydrate	53	22.2	12.1	49
Fiber	3	1.3	0.7	

[a]DM%, dry matter percent. If all the water was removed from this diet, this is the percentage of nutrient that would be present.

Diet: Ground Beef and Potato

Species: Dog
Life Stage: Adult
Special Conditions: Pancreatitis (diet provides moderate fat); esopha-
gitis, gastric motility disorders; skin conditions

Ingredient	Quantity	Measure
Ground beef, 10% fat, pan-browned	5	ounces
Potatoes, cooked in skin, diced	3	cup
Canola oil	2	tsp
Salt substitute (potassium chloride)	½	tsp
Bone meal powder	2	tsp
Salt, iodized (sodium chloride)	¾	tsp
Multivitamin & mineral tablet, kids complete	1	each
Zinc, 100 mg tablet	½	tablet

Prepared weight (approximately) = 634 g
Total kcal as prepared = 820 kcal
kcal/g prepared diet = 1.29 kcal/g diet

Nutrient	DM%[a]	As-Fed (g/100 g diet)	ME% (g/100 kcal)	% of total kcal
Protein	26	7.7	6.0	23
Fat	14	4.2	3.3	31
Carbohydrate	50	15.0	11.6	46
Fiber	4	2.0	1.0	—

[a]DM% = dry matter percent. If all the water was removed from this diet, this is the percentage of nutrient that would be present.

Diet: Ground Beef and Quinoa

Species: Dog
Life Stage: Adult
Special Conditions:

Ingredient	Quantity	Measure
Ground beef, 10% fat, pan-browned	5	ounces
Quinoa, cooked	1½	cup
Canola oil	2	tsp
Salt substitute (potassium chloride)	½	tsp
Bone meal powder	2	tsp
Salt, iodized (sodium chloride)	¾	tsp
Multivitamin & mineral tablet, kids complete	1	Each
Zinc, 100 mg tablet	½	tablet

Prepared weight (approximately) = 444 g
Total kcal as prepared = 746 kcal
kcal/g prepared diet = 1.70 kcal/g diet

Nutrient	DM%[a]	As-Fed (g/100 g diet)	ME% (g/100 kcal)	% of total kcal
Protein	32	11.8	7.0	28
Fat	20	7.2	4.3	41
Carbohydrate	37	13.6	8.1	32
Fiber	4.8	1.8	1.0	—

[a]DM%, dry matter percent. If all the water was removed from this diet, this is the percentage of nutrient that would be present.

Diet: Eggs and Rice

Species: Dog
Life Stage: Adult
Special Conditions:

Ingredient	Quantity	Measure
Eggs, whole, large, hard-boiled	4	each
Rice, white, long-grain, cooked	2	cup
Canola oil	2	tsp
Sardines, with bone, in tomato sauce	4	each
Salt substitute (potassium chloride)	½	tsp
Bone meal powder	2	tsp
Salt, iodized (sodium chloride)	¾	tsp
Multivitamin & mineral tablet, kids complete	1	each
Zinc, 100 mg tablet	½	tablet

Prepared weight (approximately) = 693 g
Total kcal as prepared = 1066 kcal
kcal/g prepared diet = 1.54 kcal/g diet

Nutrient	DM%[a]	As-Fed (g/100 g diet)	ME% (g/100 kcal)	% of total kcal
Protein	29	9.4	6.0	24
Fat	21	6.8	4.3	42
Carbohydrate	41	13.5	8.6	34
Fiber	1	0.2	0.1	—

[a]DM%, dry matter percent. If all the water was removed from this diet, this is the percentage of nutrient that would be present.

Diet: Eggs and Pasta

Species: Dog
Life Stage: Adult
Special Conditions:

Ingredient	Quantity	Measure
Eggs, whole, large, hard-boiled	4	each
Pasta, enriched, cooked	2	cup
Canola oil	1	tsp
Salt substitute (potassium chloride)	½	tsp
Bone meal powder	2	tsp
Salt, iodized (sodium chloride)	¾	tsp
Multivitamin & mineral tablet, kids complete	1	each
Zinc, 100 mg tablet	½	tablet

Prepared weight (approximately) = 500 g
Total kcal as prepared = 774 kcal
kcal/g prepared diet = 1.55 kcal/g diet

Nutrient	DM%[a]	As-Fed (g/100 g diet)	ME% (g/100 kcal)	% of total kcal
Protein	23	8.3	5.2	21
Fat	16	5.7	3.6	34
Carbohydrate	51	17.9	11.2	45
Fiber	3	1.0	0.6	—

[a]DM%, dry matter percent. If all the water was removed from this diet, this is the percentage of nutrient that would be present.

Diet: Eggs and Potato

Species: Dog
Life Stage: Adult
Special Conditions:

Ingredient	Quantity	Measure
Eggs, whole, large, hard-boiled	4	each
Potatoes, cooked in skin, diced	3	cup
Canola oil	2	tsp
Sardines, with bone, in tomato sauce	4	each
Salt substitute (potassium chloride)	½	tsp
Bone meal powder	2	tsp
Salt, iodized (sodium chloride)	¾	tsp
Multivitamin & mineral tablet, kids complete	1	each
Zinc, 100 mg tablet	½	tablet

Prepared weight (approximately) = 845 g
Total kcal as prepared = 1063 kcal
kcal/g prepared diet = 1.26 kcal/g diet

Nutrient	DM%[a]	As-Fed (g/100 g diet)	ME% (g/100 kcal)	% of total kcal
Protein	28	7.8	6.0	24
Fat	20	5.6	4.3	41
Carbohydrate	42	11.7	9.1	35
Fiber	4	1.0	0.8	—

[a]DM%, dry matter percent. If all the water was removed from this diet, this is the percentage of nutrient that would be present.

Diet: Cottage Cheese and Pasta

Species: Dog
Life Stage: Adult
Special Conditions:

Ingredient	Quantity	Measure
Cottage cheese, 2% fat	1	cup
Pasta, enriched, cooked	2½	cup
Canola oil	2	tbsp
Sardines, with bone, in tomato sauce	1	each
Salt substitute (potassium chloride)	¾	tsp
Bone meal powder	2	tsp
Salt, iodized (sodium chloride)	1	tsp
Multivitamin & mineral tablet, kids complete	1	each
Zinc, 100 mg tablet	½	tablet

Prepared weight (approximately) = 660 g
Total kcal as prepared = 1070 kcal
kcal/g prepared diet = 1.62 kcal/g diet

Nutrient	DM%[a]	As-Fed (g/100 g diet)	ME% (g/100 kcal)	% of total kcal
Protein	23	8.3	5.1	20
Fat	17	6.2	3.8	36
Carbohydrate	50	17.8	11.0	44
Fiber	3	1.0	0.6	—

[a]DM%, dry matter percent. If all the water was removed from this diet, this is the percentage of nutrient that would be present.

Diet: Liver, Red Beans, and Rice

Species: Dog
Life Stage: Adult
Special Conditions:

Ingredient	Quantity	Measure
Liver, beef, braised	4	ounces
Rice, white, long-grain, cooked	2½	cup
Beans, red kidney, canned, drained	1	cup
Canola oil	4	tsp
Salt substitute (potassium chloride)	¾	tsp
Bone meal powder	2	tsp
Salt, iodized (sodium chloride)	1¼	tsp
Multivitamin & mineral tablet, kids complete	1	each
Zinc, 100 mg tablet	½	tablet

Prepared weight (approximately) = 803 g
Total kcal as prepared = 1201 kcal
kcal/g prepared diet = 1.50 kcal/g diet

Nutrient	DM%[a]	As-Fed (g/100 g diet)	ME% (g/100 kcal)	% of total kcal
Protein	21	7.8	5.2	21
Fat	9	3.4	2.2	22
Carbohydrate	60	21.6	14.4	57
Fiber	8.4	3.0	2.0	—

[a]DM%, dry matter percent. If all the water was removed from this diet, this is the percentage of nutrient that would be present.

Diet: Tofu and Rice

Species: Dog
Life Stage: Adult
Special Conditions: Insulinoma

Ingredient	Quantity	Measure
Tofu, extra firm	12	ounces
Rice, white, long-grain, cooked	1½	cup
Canola oil	1	tbsp
Salt substitute (potassium chloride)	½	tsp
Bone meal powder	2	tsp
Salt, iodized (sodium chloride)	¾	tsp
Multivitamin & mineral tablet, kids complete	1	each
Zinc, 100 mg tablet	½	tablet
Vitamin B_{12} liquid, 1000 mcg B_{12} per mL	0.25	mL

Prepared weight (approximately) = 606 g
Total kcal as prepared = 746 kcal
kcal/g prepared diet = 1.23 kcal/g diet

Nutrient	DM%[a]	As-Fed (g/100 g diet)	ME% (g/100 kcal)	% of total kcal
Protein	24	6.6	5.4	20
Fat	21	5.7	4.6	42
Carbohydrate	44	12.3	10.0	38
Fiber	1.4	0.4	0.3	—

[a]DM%, dry matter percent. If all the water was removed from this diet, this is the percentage of nutrient that would be present.

Diet: Tofu, Lentils, and Rice

Species: Dog
Life Stage: Adult
Special Conditions: Skin conditions

Ingredient	Quantity	Measure
Tofu, extra firm	12	ounces
Rice, white, long-grain, cooked	1½	cup
Beans, lentils, cooked	1	cup
Canola oil	1	tbsp
Salt substitute (potassium chloride)	½	tsp
Bone meal powder	2	tsp
Salt, iodized (sodium chloride)	1	tsp
Multivitamin & mineral tablet, kids complete	1	each
Zinc, 100 mg tablet	½	tablet
Vitamin B_{12} liquid, 1000 mcg B_{12} per mL	0.25	mL

Prepared weight (approximately) = 806 g
Total kcal as prepared = 975 kcal
kcal/g prepared diet = 1.21 kcal/g diet

Nutrient	DM%[a]	As-Fed (g/100 g diet)	ME% (g/100 kcal)	% of total kcal
Protein	25	7.2	5.9	23
Fat	15	4.4	3.6	33
Carbohydrate	50	14.2	11.7	44
Fiber	7.8	2.2	1.8	—

[a]DM%, dry matter percent. If all the water was removed from this diet, this is the percentage of nutrient that would be present.

Diet: Tofu and Pasta

Species: Dog
Life Stage: Adult
Special Conditions:

Ingredient	Quantity	Measure
Tofu, extra firm	12	ounces
Pasta, enriched, cooked	2	cup
Canola oil	1	tbsp
Salt substitute (potassium chloride)	½	tsp
Bone meal powder	2	tsp
Salt, iodized (sodium chloride)	1	tsp
Multivitamin & mineral tablet, kids complete	1	each
Zinc, 100 mg tablet	½	tablet
Vitamin B_{12} liquid, 1000 mcg B_{12} per mL	0.25	mL

Prepared weight (approximately) = 651 g
Total kcal as prepared = 880 kcal
kcal/g prepared diet = 1.35 kcal/g diet

Nutrient	DM%[a]	As-Fed (g/100 g diet)	ME% (g/100 kcal)	% of total kcal
Protein	25	7.7	5.7	21
Fat	18	5.6	4.1	38
Carbohydrate	47	14.5	10.7	41
Fiber	3.2	1.0	0.7	—

[a]DM%, dry matter percent. If all the water was removed from this diet, this is the percentage of nutrient that would be present.

Diet: Tofu, Lentils, and Pasta

Species: Dog
Life Stage: Adult
Special Conditions: Skin conditions

Ingredient	Quantity	Measure
Tofu, extra firm	12	ounces
Pasta, enriched, cooked	2	cup
Beans, lentils, cooked	1	cup
Canola oil	1	tbsp
Salt substitute (potassium chloride)	½	tsp
Bone meal powder	2	tsp
Salt, iodized (sodium chloride)	1¼	tsp
Multivitamin & mineral tablet, kids complete	1	each
Zinc, 100 mg tablet	½	tablet
Vitamin B_{12} liquid, 1000 mcg B_{12} per mL	0.25	mL

Prepared weight (approximately) = 851 g
Total kcal as prepared = 1110 kcal
kcal/g prepared diet = 1.30 kcal/g diet

Nutrient	DM%[a]	As-Fed (g/100 g diet)	ME% (g/100 kcal)	% of total kcal
Protein	26	8.0	6.1	23
Fat	14	4.4	3.4	31
Carbohydrate	51	15.8	12.1	46
Fiber	8.4	2.6	2.0	—

[a]DM%, dry matter percent. If all the water was removed from this diet, this is the percentage of nutrient that would be present.

Diet: Tofu and Potato

Species: Dog
Life Stage: Adult
Special Conditions: Insulinoma

Ingredient	Quantity	Measure
Tofu, extra firm	12	ounces
Potatoes, cooked in skin, diced	2	cup
Canola oil	1	tbsp
Salt substitute (potassium chloride)	½	tsp
Bone meal powder	2	tsp
Salt, iodized (sodium chloride)	¾	tsp
Multivitamin & mineral tablet, kids complete	1	each
Zinc, 100 mg tablet	½	tablet
Vitamin B_{12} liquid, 1000 mcg B_{12} per mL	0.25	mL

Prepared weight (approximately) = 682 g
Total kcal as prepared = 709 kcal
kcal/g prepared diet = 1.04 kcal/g diet

Nutrient	DM%[a]	As-Fed (g/100 g diet)	ME% (g/100 kcal)	% of total kcal
Protein	24	5.8	5.5	20
Fat	21	5.0	4.8	43
Carbohydrate	43	10.4	10.0	37
Fiber	4.2	1.0	1.0	—

[a]DM%, dry matter percent. If all the water was removed from this diet, this is the percentage of nutrient that would be present.

Diet: Tofu, Lentils, and Potato

Species: Dog
Life Stage: Adult
Special Conditions: Skin Conditions

Ingredient	Quantity	Measure
Tofu, extra firm	12	ounces
Potatoes, cooked in skin, diced	2	cup
Beans, lentils, cooked	1	cup
Canola oil	1	tbsp
Salt substitute (potassium chloride)	½	tsp
Bone meal powder	2	tsp
Salt, iodized (sodium chloride)	1	tsp
Multivitamin & mineral tablet, kids complete	1	each
Zinc, 100 mg tablet	½	tablet
Vitamin B_{12} liquid, 1000 mcg B_{12} per mL	0.25	mL

Prepared weight (approximately) = 881 g
Total kcal as prepared = 939 kcal
kcal/g prepared diet = 1.07 kcal/g diet

Nutrient	DM%[a]	As-Fed (g/100 g diet)	ME% (g/100 kcal)	% of total kcal
Protein	25	6.5	6.1	23
Fat	15	4.0	3.7	33
Carbohydrate	49	12.5	11.8	44
Fiber	10.0	2.6	2.4	—

[a]DM%, dry matter percent. If all the water was removed from this diet, this is the percentage of nutrient that would be present.

Diet: Tofu, Black Beans, and Quinoa

Species: Dog
Life Stage: Adult
Special Conditions:

Ingredient	Quantity	Measure
Tofu, extra firm	12	ounces
Quinoa, cooked	1½	cup
Black beans, cooked	1½	cup
Canola oil	4	tsp
Salt substitute (potassium chloride)	½	tsp
Bone meal powder	2	tsp
Salt, iodized (sodium chloride)	1¼	tsp
Multivitamin & mineral tablet, kids complete	1	each
Zinc, 100 mg tablet	½	tablet
Vitamin B_{12} liquid, 1000 mcg B_{12} per mL	0.25	mL

Prepared weight (approximately) = 913 g
Total kcal as prepared = 1152 kcal
kcal/g prepared diet = 1.26 kcal/g diet

Nutrient	DM%[a]	As-Fed (g/100 g diet)	ME% (g/100 kcal)	% of total kcal
Protein	26	7.5	6.0	22
Fat	17	5.0	3.9	36
Carbohydrate	48	14.0	11.1	42
Fiber	11.8	3.5	2.7	—

[a]DM%, dry matter percent. If all the water was removed from this diet, this is the percentage of nutrient that would be present.

Diet: Chicken and Pasta

Species: Dog
Life Stage: Adult
Special Conditions: Gestation

Ingredient	Quantity	Measure
Chicken breast, without skin, roasted	4	ounces
Pasta, enriched, cooked	2½	cup
Canola oil	4	tsp
Sardines, with bone, in tomato sauce	2	each
Salt substitute (potassium chloride)	½	tsp
Bone meal powder	2½	tsp
Salt, iodized (sodium chloride)	1¼	tsp
Multivitamin & mineral tablet, kids complete	1	each
Zinc, 100 mg tablet	½	tablet

Prepared weight (approximately) = 578 g
Total kcal as prepared = 1051 kcal
kcal/g prepared diet = 1.82 kcal/g diet

Nutrient	DM%[a]	As-Fed (g/100 g diet)	ME% (g/100 kcal)	% of total kcal
Protein	30	12.3	6.8	27
Fat	14	5.9	3.2	31
Carbohydrate	46	19.0	10.4	42
Fiber	2.7	1.1	0.6	—

[a]DM%, dry matter percent. If all the water was removed from this diet, this is the percentage of nutrient that would be present.

Diet: Ground Beef and Rice

Species: Dog
Life Stage: Adult
Special Conditions: Gestation

Ingredient	Quantity	Measure
Ground beef, 10% fat, pan-browned	6	ounces
Rice, white, long-grain, cooked	1½	cup
Canola oil	1	tbsp
Salt substitute (potassium chloride)	½	tsp
Bone meal powder	2½	tsp
Salt, iodized (sodium chloride)	1	tsp
Multivitamin & mineral tablet, kids complete	1	each
Zinc, 100 mg tablet	½	tablet

Prepared weight (approximately) = 439 g
Total kcal as prepared = 827 kcal
kcal/g prepared diet = 1.88 kcal/g diet

Nutrient	DM%[a]	As-Fed (g/100 g diet)	ME% (g/100 kcal)	% of total kcal
Protein	31	12.5	6.6	26
Fat	20	8.0	4.2	41
Carbohydrate	38	15.4	8.2	33
Fiber	0.5	0.2	0.1	—

[a]DM%, dry matter percent. If all the water was removed from this diet, this is the percentage of nutrient that would be present.

Diet: Whitefish and Rice

Species: Dog
Life Stage: Adult
Special Conditions: Gestation, exocrine pancreatic insufficiency

Ingredient	Quantity	Measure
Whitefish, fillet, baked or broiled	6	ounces
Rice, white, long-grain, cooked	1½	cup
Canola oil	1	tbsp
Salt substitute (potassium chloride)	¼	tsp
Bone meal powder	2	tsp
Salt, iodized (sodium chloride)	¾	tsp
Multivitamin & mineral tablet, kids complete	1	each
Zinc, 100 mg tablet	½	tablet

Prepared weight (approximately) = 435 g
Total kcal as prepared = 728 kcal
kcal/g prepared diet = 1.67 kcal/g diet

Nutrient	DM%[a]	As-Fed (g/100 g diet)	ME% (g/100 kcal)	% of total kcal
Protein	30	11.0	6.6	26
Fat	17	6.3	3.8	36
Carbohydrate	42	15.6	9.3	37
Fiber	0.6	0.2	0.1	—

[a]DM%, dry matter percent. If all the water was removed from this diet, this is the percentage of nutrient that would be present.

Diet: Tofu and Rice

Species: Dog
Life Stage: Adult
Special Conditions: Gestation

Ingredient	Quantity	Measure
Tofu, extra firm	16	ounces
Rice, white, long-grain, cooked	1¼	cup
Canola oil	1	tbsp
Salt substitute (potassium chloride)	½	tsp
Bone meal powder	1¾	tsp
Salt, iodized (sodium chloride)	¾	tsp
Vitamin B_{12} liquid, 1000 mcg B_{12} per mL	0.25	mL
Multivitamin & mineral tablet, kids complete	1	each
Zinc, 100 mg tablet	½	tablet

Prepared weight (approximately) = 680 g
Total kcal as prepared = 797 kcal
kcal/g prepared diet = 1.17 kcal/g diet

Nutrient	DM%[a]	As-Fed (g/100 g diet)	ME% (g/100 kcal)	% of total kcal
Protein	28	7.4	6.3	23
Fat	23	6.0	5.1	46
Carbohydrate	37	9.7	8.2	31
Fiber	1.5	0.4	0.3	—

[a]DM%, dry matter percent. If all the water was removed from this diet, this is the percentage of nutrient that would be present.

Diet: Chicken and Pasta

Species: Dog
Life Stage: Adult
Special Conditions: Lactation, skin conditions

Ingredient	Quantity	Measure
Chicken breast, without skin, roasted	9	ounces
Pasta, enriched, cooked	2½	cup
Canola oil	4	tbsp
Salt substitute (potassium chloride)	¾	tsp
Bone meal powder	5	tsp
Salt, iodized (sodium chloride)	1¼	tsp
Multivitamin & mineral tablet, kids complete	2	each
Zinc, 100 mg tablet	½	tablet
Kelp, 150 mcg iodine per tablet	1	tablet

Prepared weight (approximately) = 697 g
Total kcal as prepared = 1477 kcal
kcal/g prepared diet = 2.12 kcal/g diet

Nutrient	DM%[a]	As-Fed (g/100 g diet)	ME% (g/100 kcal)	% of total kcal
Protein	32	14.3	6.7	26
Fat	22	9.8	4.6	44
Carbohydrate	36	15.8	7.5	29
Fiber	2.0	0.9	0.4	—

[a]DM%, dry matter percent. If all the water was removed from this diet, this is the percentage of nutrient that would be present.

Diet: Ground Beef and Rice

Species: Dog
Life Stage: Adult
Special Conditions: Lactation, megaesophagus, obstructive swallowing disorders

Ingredient	Quantity	Measure
Ground beef, 10% fat, pan-browned	10	ounces
Rice, white, long-grain, cooked	1½	cup
Canola oil	2	tbsp
Salt substitute (potassium chloride)	¾	tsp
Bone meal powder	4	tsp
Salt, iodized (sodium chloride)	1	tsp
Kelp, 150 mcg iodine per tablet	1	tablet
Multivitamin & mineral tablet, kids complete	1	each
Zinc, 100 mg tablet	½	tablet

Prepared weight (approximately) = 578 g
Total kcal as prepared = 1212 kcal
kcal/g prepared diet = 2.10 kcal/g diet

Nutrient	DM%[a]	As-Fed (g/100 g diet)	ME% (g/100 kcal)	% of total kcal
Protein	35	15.0	7.2	28
Fat	25	10.9	5.2	50
Carbohydrate	27	11 7	5 6	??
Fiber	0.4	0.2	0.1	—

[a]DM%, dry matter percent. If all the water was removed from this diet, this is the percentage of nutrient that would be present.

Diet: Whitefish and Rice

Species: Dog
Lifestage: Adult
Special Conditions: Lactation

Ingredient	Quantity	Measure
Whitefish, fillet, baked or broiled	10	ounces
Rice, white, long-grain, cooked	1½	cup
Canola oil	2	tbsp
Salt substitute (potassium chloride)	½	tsp
Bone meal powder	2¾	tsp
Salt, iodized (sodium chloride)	¾	tsp
Kelp, 150 mcg iodine per tablet	1	tablet
Multivitamin & mineral tablet, kids complete	1	each
Zinc, 100 mg tablet	½	tablet

Prepared weight (approximately) = 571 g
Total kcal as prepared = 1047 kcal
kcal/g prepared diet = 1.83 kcal/g diet

Nutrient	DM%[a]	As-Fed (g/100 g diet)	ME% (g/100 kcal)	% of total kcal
Protein	34	13.3	7.2	29
Fat	22	8.8	4.8	46
Carbohydrate	30	11.9	6.5	26
Fiber	0.4	0.2	0.1	—

[a]DM%, dry matter percent. If all the water was removed from this diet, this is the percentage of nutrient that would be present.

Diet: Tofu and Rice

Species: Dog
Life Stage: Adult
Special Conditions: Lactation, megaesophagus, obstructive swallowing disorders

Ingredient	Quantity	Measure
Tofu, extra firm	20	ounces
Rice, white, long-grain, cooked	1¼	cup
Canola oil	4	tsp
Salt substitute (potassium chloride)	¾	tsp
Bone meal powder	2½	tsp
Salt, iodized (sodium chloride)	¾	tsp
Vitamin B_{12} liquid, 1000 mcg B_{12} per mL	0.25	mL
Kelp, 150 mcg iodine per tablet	1	tablet
Multivitamin & mineral tablet, kids complete	1	each
Zinc, 100 mg tablet	½	tablet

Prepared weight (approximately) = 806 g
Total kcal as prepared = 942 kcal
kcal/g prepared diet = 1.17 kcal/g diet

Nutrient	DM%[a]	As-Fed (g/100 g diet)	ME% (g/100 kcal)	% of total kcal
Protein	29	7.6	6.5	24
Fat	25	6.5	5.5	50
Carbohydrate	32	8.4	7.2	27
Fiber	1.5	0.4	0.3	—

[a]DM%, dry matter percent. If all the water was removed from this diet, this is the percentage of nutrient that would be present.

Diet: Pork and Potato

Species: Dog
Life Stage: Adult
Special Conditions: Performance (sprinting)

Ingredient	Quantity	Measure
Pork loin, broiled	5	ounces
Potatoes, cooked in skin, diced	3	cup
Canola oil	1	tsp
Salt substitute (potassium chloride)	½	tsp
Bone meal powder	3	tsp
Salt, iodized (sodium chloride)	¾	tsp
Multivitamin & mineral tablet, kids complete	1	each
Zinc 100 mg tablet	½	tablet

Prepared weight (approximately) = 633 g
Total kcal as prepared = 732 kcal
kcal/g prepared diet = 1.16 kcal/g diet

Nutrient	DM%[a]	As-Fed (g/100 g diet)	ME% (g/100 kcal)	% of total kcal
Protein	25	7.3	6.4	25
Fat	10	2.9	2.5	24
Carbohydrate	52	15.0	13.0	51
Fiber	4.5	1.3	1.2	—
Calcium	1.7	0.50	0.4	
Magnesium	0.14	0.04	0.03	

[a]DM, dry matter percent. If all the water was removed from this diet, this is the percentage of nutrient that would be present.

Diet: Chicken and Pasta

Species: Dog
Life Stage: Adult
Special Conditions: Performance (sprinting)

Ingredient	Quantity	Measure
Chicken breast, without skin, roasted	3	ounces
Pasta, enriched, cooked	4	cup
Canola oil	2½	tsp
Sardines, with bone, in tomato sauce	2	each
Salt substitute (potassium chloride)	¾	tsp
Bone meal powder	3½	tsp
Salt, iodized (sodium chloride)	1½	tsp
Multivitamin & mineral tablet, kids complete	1	each
Zinc 100 mg tablet	½	tablet

Prepared weight (approximately) = 758 g
Total kcal as prepared = 1274 kcal
kcal/g prepared diet = 1.68 kcal/g diet

Nutrient	DM%[a]	As-Fed (g/100 g diet)	ME% (g/100 kcal)	% of total kcal
Protein	25	9.8	5.9	24
Fat	9	3.7	2.2	21
Carbohydrate	57	23.0	13.7	55
Fiber	3.3	1.3	0.8	—
Calcium	1.3	0.51	0.30	
Magnesium	0.1	0.04	0.02	

[a]DM%, dry matter percent. If all the water was removed from this diet, this is the percentage of nutrient that would be present.

Diet: Ground Beef and Potato

Species: Dog
Life Stage: Adult
Special Conditions: Performance (moderate work)

Ingredient	Quantity	Measure
Ground beef, 10% fat, pan-browned	6	ounces
Potatoes, cooked in skin, diced	3	cup
Canola oil	1	tbsp
Salt substitute (potassium chloride)	½	tsp
Bone meal powder	2½	tsp
Salt, iodized (sodium chloride)	1	tsp
Multivitamin & mineral tablet, kids complete	1	each
Zinc 100 mg tablet	½	tablet

Prepared weight (approximately) = 670 g
Total kcal as prepared = 926 kcal
kcal/g prepared diet = 1.38 kcal/g diet

Nutrient	DM%[a]	As-Fed (g/100 g diet)	ME% (g/100 kcal)	% of total kcal
Protein	27	8.5	6.2	24
Fat	17	5.2	3.8	36
Carbohydrate	45	14.2	10.3	40
Fiber	4	1.3	0.9	—
Calcium	1.3	0.4	0.29	
Magnesium	0.11	0.04	0.03	

[a]DM%, dry matter percent. If all the water was removed from this diet, this is the percentage of nutrient that would be present.

Diet: Chicken and Barley

Species: Dog
Life Stage: Adult
Special Conditions: Performance (moderate work)

Ingredient	Quantity	Measure
Chicken breast, without skin, roasted	6	ounces
Barley, pearled, cooked	2	cup
Canola oil	3	tbsp
Salt substitute (potassium chloride)	½	tsp
Bone meal powder	2½	tsp
Salt, iodized (sodium chloride)	¾	tsp
Multivitamin & mineral tablet, kids complete	1	each
Zinc 100 mg tablet	½	tablet

Prepared weight (approximately) = 543 g
Total kcal as prepared = 1042 kcal
kcal/g prepared diet = 1.92 kcal/g diet

Nutrient	DM%[a]	As-Fed (g/100 g diet)	ME% (g/100 kcal)	% of total kcal
Protein	27	11.0	5.7	22
Fat	23	9.1	4.7	45
Carbohydrate	42	16.5	8.6	33
Fiber	5.5	2.2	1.2	—
Calcium	1.2	0.49	0.26	
Magnesium	0.10	0.04	0.02	

[a]DM%, dry matter percent. If all the water was removed from this diet, this is the percentage of nutrient that would be present.

Diet: Salmon and Pasta

Species: Dog
Life Stage: Adult
Special Conditions: Performance (strenuous work)

Ingredient	Quantity	Measure
Salmon, Atlantic, fillet, baked/broiled	12	ounces
Pasta, cooked	3	cup
Canola oil	6	tbsp
Salt substitute (potassium chloride)	¾	tsp
Bone meal powder	4½	tsp
Salt, iodized (sodium chloride)	1½	tsp
Multivitamin & mineral tablet, kids complete	2	each
Zinc 100 mg tablet	½	tablet

Prepared weight (approximately) = 885 g
Total kcal as prepared = 2034 kcal
kcal/g prepared diet = 2.30 kcal/g diet

Nutrient	DM%[a]	As-Fed (g/100 g diet)	ME% (g/100 kcal)	% of total kcal
Protein	26	12.5	5.5	21
Fat	27	13.1	5.7	54
Carbohydrate	31	14.9	6.5	25
Fiber	1.8	0.9	0.4	—
Calcium	1.1	0.54	0.24	
Magnesium	0.09	0.04	0.02	

[a]DM%, dry matter percent. If all the water was removed from this diet, this is the percentage of nutrient that would be present.

Diet: Ground Beef and Rice

Species: Dog
Life Stage: Adult
Special Conditions: Performance (strenuous work)

Ingredient	Quantity	Measure
Ground beef, 10% fat, pan-browned	14	ounces
Rice, white, long-grain, cooked	3	cup
Canola oil	6	tbsp
Salt substitute (potassium chloride)	1	tsp
Bone meal powder	4½	tsp
Salt, iodized (sodium chloride)	1½	tsp
Multivitamin & mineral tablet, kids complete	2	each
Zinc 100 mg tablet	½	tablet
Kelp 150 mcg iodine per tablet	2	tablet

Prepared weight (approximately) = 997 g
Total kcal as prepared = 2280 kcal
kcal/g prepared diet = 2.29 kcal/g diet

Nutrient	DM%[a]	As-Fed (g/100 g diet)	ME% (g/100 kcal)	% of total kcal
Protein	29	12.6	5.5	22
Fat	30	13.4	5.8	55
Carbohydrate	31	13.6	6.0	23
Fiber	0.4	0.19	0.1	—
Calcium	1.1	0.49	0.21	
Magnesium	0.08	0.04	0.03	

[a]DM%, dry matter percent. If all the water was removed from this diet, this is the percentage of nutrient that would be present.

Diet: Ground Beef and Rice

Species: Dog
Life Stage: Adult
Special Conditions: Performance (endurance)

Ingredient	Quantity	Measure
Ground beef, 25% fat, pan-browned	24	ounces
Rice, white, long-grain, cooked	1	cup
Canola oil	¾	cup
Salt substitute (potassium chloride)	1½	tsp
Bone meal powder	7	tsp
Salt, iodized (sodium chloride)	1½	tsp
Multivitamin & mineral tablet, kids complete	3	each
Zinc 100 mg tablet	½	tablet
Kelp, 150 mcg iodine per tablet	6	tablets

Prepared weight (approximately) = 1080 g
Total kcal as prepared = 3588 kcal
kcal/g prepared diet = 3.32 kcal/g diet

Nutrient	DM%[a]	As-Fed (g/100 g diet)	ME% (g/100 kcal)	% of total kcal
Protein	30	17.0	5.1	19
Fat	49	27.1	8.1	76
Carbohydrate	8	4.4	1.3	5
Fiber	0.1	0.06	0.02	—
Calcium	1.3	0.70	0.21	
Magnesium	0.08	0.04	0.01	

[a]DM%, dry matter percent. If all the water was removed from this diet, this is the percentage of nutrient that would be present.

Diet: Chicken and Rice

Species: Dog
Life Stage: Puppy, adult
Special Conditions: Skin conditions

Ingredient	Quantity	Measure
Chicken breast, without skin, roasted	4	ounces
Rice, white, long-grain, cooked	2	cup
Sardines, with bone, in tomato sauce	2	each
Canola oil	4	tsp
Salt substitute (potassium chloride)	½	tsp
Bone meal powder	2¾	tsp
Salt, iodized (sodium chloride)	1	tsp
Multivitamin & mineral tablet, kids complete	1	each
Zinc, 100 mg tablet	½	tablet

Prepared weight (approximately) = 543 g
Total kcal as prepared = 908 kcal
kcal/g prepared diet = 1.67 kcal/g diet

Nutrient	DM%[a]	As-Fed (g/100 g diet)	ME% (g/100 kcal)	% of total kcal
Protein	29	11.0	6.6	26
Fat	16	5.8	3.5	34
Carbohydrate	45	16.7	10.0	40
Fiber	0.7	0.3	0.2	

[a]DM%, dry matter percent. If all the water was removed from this diet, this is the percentage of nutrient that would be present.

Diet: Chicken and Rice

Species: Dog
Life Stage: Puppy, adult
Special Conditions:

Ingredient	Quantity	Measure
Chicken breast, roasted, without skin	8	ounces
Rice, white, long-grain, cooked	2	cup
Canola oil	3	tbsp
Broccoli, cooked, chopped	1	cup
Salt substitute (potassium chloride)	½	tsp
Bone meal powder	4	tsp
Salt, iodized (sodium chloride)	1½	tsp
Multivitamin & mineral tablet, kids complete	1	each
Zinc, 100 mg tablet	½	tablet

Prepared weight (approximately) = 767 g
Total kcal as prepared = 1215 kcal
kcal/g prepared diet = 1.58 kcal/g diet

Nutrient	DM%[a]	As-Fed (g/100g diet)	ME% (g/100kcal)	% of total kcal
Protein	31	10.8	6.8	27
Fat	20	6.7	4.2	40
Carbohydrate	38	13.2	8.3	33
Fiber	2.4	0.8	0.5	—

[a]DM%, dry matter percent. If all the water was removed from this diet, this is the percentage of nutrient that would be present.

Diet: Chicken and Pasta

Species: Dog
Life Stage: Puppy, adult
Special Conditions: Skin conditions

Ingredient	Quantity	Measure
Chicken breast, without skin, roasted	4	ounces
Pasta, enriched, cooked	2	cup
Sardines, with bone, in tomato sauce	2	each
Canola oil	4	tsp
Salt substitute (potassium chloride)	½	tsp
Bone meal powder	1	tbsp
Salt, iodized (sodium chloride)	1	tsp
Multivitamin & mineral tablet, kids complete	1	each
Zinc, 100 mg tablet	½	tablet

Prepared weight (approximately) = 508 g
Total kcal as prepared = 940 kcal
kcal/g prepared diet = 1.85 kcal/g diet

Nutrient	DM%[a]	As-Fed (g/100 g diet)	ME% (g/100 kcal)	% of total kcal
Protein	32	13.2	7.2	28
Fat	16	6.6	3.5	34
Carbohydrate	42	17.3	9.4	37
Fiber	2.4	1.0	0.5	

[a]DM%, dry matter percent. If all the water was removed from this diet, this is the percentage of nutrient that would be present.

Diet: Chicken and Potato

Species: Dog
Life Stage: Puppy, adult
Special Conditions: Skin conditions

Ingredient	Quantity	Measure
Chicken breast, without skin, roasted	4	ounces
Potatoes, cooked in skin, diced	2	cup
Sardines, with bone, in tomato sauce	2	each
Canola oil	4	tsp
Salt substitute (potassium chloride)	½	tsp
Bone meal powder	2½	tsp
Salt, iodized (sodium chloride)	¾	tsp
Multivitamin & mineral tablet, kids complete	1	each
Zinc, 100 mg tablet	½	tablet

Prepared weight (approximately) = 537 g
Total kcal as prepared = 769 kcal
kcal/g prepared diet = 1.43 kcal/g diet

Nutrient	DM%[a]	As-Fed (g/100 g diet)	ME% (g/100 kcal)	% of total kcal
Protein	33	10.6	7.4	29
Fat	18	5.8	4.0	38
Carbohydrate	37	12.0	8.4	33
Fiber	3.3	1.1	0.7	—

[a]DM%, dry matter percent. If all the water was removed from this diet, this is the percentage of nutrient that would be present.

Diet: Chicken and Quinoa

Species: Dog
Life Stage: Puppy, adult
Special Conditions:

Ingredient	Quantity	Measure
Chicken breast, roasted, without skin	4	ounces
Quinoa, cooked	1½	cup
Canola oil	1	tbsp
Salt substitute (potassium chloride)	½	tsp
Bone meal powder	2	tsp
Salt, iodized (sodium chloride)	¾	tsp
Multivitamin & mineral tablet, kids complete	1	each
Zinc, 100 mg tablet	½	tablet

Prepared weight (approximately) = 420 g
Total kcal as prepared = 648 kcal
kcal/g prepared diet = 1.54 kcal/g diet

Nutrient	DM%[a]	As-Fed (g/100 g diet)	ME% (g/100 kcal)	% of total kcal
Protein	32	11.3	7.3	29
Fat	16	5.6	3.6	34
Carbohydrate	41	14.3	9.3	37
Fiber	5	1.9	1.2	—

[a]DM%, dry matter percent. If all the water was removed from this diet, this is the percentage of nutrient that would be present.

Diet: Ground Beef and Rice

Species: Dog
Life Stage: Puppy, adult
Special Conditions: Skin conditions

Ingredient	Quantity	Measure
Ground beef, 10% fat, pan-browned	12	ounces
Rice, white, long-grain, cooked	1½	cup
Canola oil	1	tbsp
Salt substitute (potassium chloride)	½	tsp
Bone meal powder	4	tsp
Salt, iodized (sodium chloride)	1½	tsp
Multivitamin & mineral tablet, kids complete	1	each
Zinc, 100 mg tablet	½	tablet

Prepared weight (approximately) = 617 g
Total kcal as prepared = 1219 kcal
kcal/g prepared diet = 1.97 kcal/g diet

Nutrient	DM%[a]	As-Fed (g/100 g diet)	ME% (g/100 kcal)	% of total kcal
Protein	41	16.7	8.5	34
Fat	22	9.0	4.6	44
Carbohydrate	27	11.0	5.6	22
Fiber	0.4	0.2	0.1	—

[a]DM%, dry matter percent. If all the water was removed from this diet, this is the percentage of nutrient that would be present.

Diet: Ground Beef and Pasta

Species: Dog
Life Stage: Puppy, adult
Special Conditions: Skin Conditions

Ingredient	Quantity	Measure
Ground beef, 10% fat, pan-browned	12	ounces
Pasta, enriched, cooked	2	cup
Canola oil	1	tbsp
Salt substitute (potassium chloride)	½	tsp
Bone meal powder	4	tsp
Salt, iodized (sodium chloride)	1¾	tsp
Multivitamin & mineral tablet, kids complete	1	each
Zinc, 100 mg tablet	½	tablet

Prepared weight (approximately) = 662 g
Total kcal as prepared = 1353 kcal
kcal/g prepared diet = 2.04 kcal/g diet

Nutrient	DM%[a]	As-Fed (g/100 g diet)	ME% (g/100 kcal)	% of total kcal
Protein	39	17.1	8.4	33
Fat	20	8.7	4.3	41
Carbohydrate	30	13.2	6.5	26
Fiber	1.7	0.8	0.4	—

[a]DM%, dry matter percent. If all the water was removed from this diet, this is the percentage of nutrient that would be present.

Diet: Ground Beef and Pasta

Species: Dog
Life Stage: Puppy, adult
Special Conditions:

Ingredient	Quantity	Measure
Ground beef, 10% fat, pan-browned	8	ounces
Pasta, enriched, cooked	2	cup
Peas, frozen, cooked	1	cup
Canola oil	1	tbsp
Salt substitute (potassium chloride)	½	tsp
Bone meal powder	4	tsp
Salt, iodized (sodium chloride)	1¾	tsp
Multivitamin & mineral tablet, kids complete	1	each
Zinc, 100 mg tablet	½	tablet

Prepared weight (approximately) = 708 g
Total kcal as prepared = 1216 kcal
kcal/g prepared diet = 1.71 kcal/g diet

Nutrient	DM%[a]	As-Fed (g/100 g diet)	ME% (g/100 kcal)	% of total kcal
Protein	32	12.6	7.3	29
Fat	16	6.3	3.6	35
Carbohydrate	40	15.6	9.1	36
Fiber	5.0	2.0	1.1	—

[a]DM%, dry matter percent. If all the water was removed from this diet, this is the percentage of nutrient that would be present.

Diet: Ground Beef and Potato

Species: Dog
Life Stage: Puppy, adult
Special Conditions: Skin conditions

Ingredient	Quantity	Measure
Ground beef, 10% fat, pan-browned	12	ounces
Potatoes, cooked in skin, diced	2	cup
Canola oil	1	tbsp
Salt substitute (potassium chloride)	½	tsp
Bone meal powder	4	tsp
Salt, iodized (sodium chloride)	1½	tsp
Multivitamin & mineral tablet, kids complete	1	each
Zinc, 100 mg tablet	½	tablet

Prepared weight (approximately) = 692 g
Total kcal as prepared = 1182 kcal
kcal/g prepared diet = 1.71 kcal/g diet

Nutrient	DM%[a]	As-Fed (g/100 g diet)	ME% (g/100 kcal)	% of total kcal
Protein	41	14.8	8.7	34
Fat	22	8.0	4.7	45
Carbohydrate	25	9.2	5.4	21
Fiber	2.5	0.9	0.5	—

[a]DM%, dry matter percent. If all the water was removed from this diet, this is the percentage of nutrient that would be present.

Diet: Lamb and Rice

Species: Dog
Life Stage: Puppy, adult
Special Conditions: Skin conditions

Ingredient	Quantity	Measure
Lamb, cooked	6	ounces
Rice, white, long-grain, cooked	1½	cup
Canola oil	1	tsp
Sardines, canned, in tomato sauce	2	each
Salt substitute (potassium chloride)	½	tsp
Bone meal powder	1	tbsp
Salt, iodized (sodium chloride)	1¼	tsp
Multivitamin & mineral tablet, kids complete	1	each
Zinc, 100 mg tablet	½	tablet

Prepared weight (approximately) = 509 g
Total kcal as prepared = 956 kcal
kcal/g prepared diet = 1.88 kcal/g diet

Nutrient	DM%[a]	As-Fed (g/100 g diet)	ME% (g/100 kcal)	% of total kcal
Protein	33	12.9	6.9	27
Fat	22	8.6	4.6	44
Carbohydrate	34	13.4	7.2	28
Fiber	0.5	0.2	0.1	—

[a]DM%, dry matter percent. If all the water was removed from this diet, this is the percentage of nutrient that would be present.

Diet: Eggs and Rice

Species: Dog
Life Stage: Puppy, adult
Special Conditions: Skin conditions

Ingredient	Quantity	Measure
Eggs, hard-boiled	5	each
Rice, white, long-grain, cooked	1½	cup
Sardines, with bone, in tomato sauce	4	each
Canola oil	2	tsp
Salt substitute (potassium chloride)	½	tsp
Bone meal powder	2½	tsp
Salt, iodized (sodium chloride)	¾	tsp
Multivitamin & mineral tablet, kids complete	1	each
Zinc, 100 mg tablet	½	tablet

Prepared weight (approximately) = 665 g
Total kcal as prepared = 1065 kcal
kcal/g prepared diet = 1.60 kcal/g diet

Nutrient	DM%[a]	As-Fed (g/100 g diet)	ME% (g/100 kcal)	% of total kcal
Protein	32	10.4	6.5	26
Fat	24	7.9	4.9	47
Carbohydrate	33	10.8	6.7	27
Fiber	0.5	0.2	0.1	—

[a]DM, dry matter percent. If all the water was removed from this diet, this is the percentage of nutrient that would be present.

Diet: Eggs and Pasta

Species: Dog
Life Stage: Puppy, adult
Special Conditions: Skin conditions

Ingredient	Quantity	Measure
Eggs, hard-boiled	5	each
Pasta, enriched, cooked	1½	cup
Sardines, with bone, in tomato sauce	4	each
Canola oil	2	tsp
Salt substitute (potassium chloride)	½	tsp
Bone meal powder	2½	tsp
Salt, iodized (sodium chloride)	¾	tsp
Multivitamin & mineral tablet, kids complete	1	each
Zinc, 100 mg tablet	½	tablet

Prepared weight (approximately) = 638 g
Total kcal as prepared = 1089 kcal
kcal/g prepared diet = 1.71 kcal/g diet

Nutrient	DM%[a]	As-Fed (g/100 g diet)	ME% (g/100 kcal)	% of total kcal
Protein	34	11.8	6.9	27
Fat	24	8.4	4.9	47
Carbohydrate	32	10.9	6.4	25
Fiber	1.8	0.6	0.4	—

[a]DM%, dry matter percent. If all the water was removed from this diet, this is the percentage of nutrient that would be present.

Diet: Eggs and Potato

Species: Dog
Life Stage: Puppy, adult
Special Conditions: Skin conditions

Ingredient	Quantity	Measure
Eggs, hard-boiled	5	each
Potatoes, cooked in skin, diced	2	cup
Sardines, with bone, in tomato sauce	4	each
Canola oil	2	tsp
Salt substitute (potassium chloride)	½	tsp
Bone meal powder	2½	tsp
Salt, iodized (sodium chloride)	¾	tsp
Multivitamin & mineral tablet, kids complete	1	each
Zinc, 100 mg tablet	½	tablet

Prepared weight (approximately) = 740 g
Total kcal as prepared = 1028 kcal
kcal/g prepared diet = 1.39 kcal/g diet

Nutrient	DM%[a]	As-Fed (g/100 g diet)	ME% (g/100 kcal)	% of total kcal
Protein	33	9.3	6.7	26
Fat	25	7.0	5.1	48
Carbohydrate	32	9.2	6.6	26
Fiber	2.7	0.8	0.6	—

[a]DM%, dry matter percent. If all the water was removed from this diet, this is the percentage of nutrient that would be present.

Diet: Tofu and Rice

Species: Dog
Life Stage: Puppy, adult
Special Conditions: Allergy

Ingredient	Quantity	Measure
Tofu, extra firm	16	ounces
Rice, white, long-grain, cooked	1¼	cup
Canola oil	1	tbsp
Salt substitute (potassium chloride)	½	tsp
Bone meal powder	2¼	tsp
Salt, iodized (sodium chloride)	¾	tsp
Multivitamin & mineral tablet, kids complete	1	each
Zinc, 100 mg tablet	½	tablet
Vitamin B_{12} liquid, 1000 mcg B_{12} per mL	0.25	mL

Prepared weight (approximately) = 681 g
Total kcal as prepared = 797 kcal
kcal/g prepared diet = 1.17 kcal/g diet

Nutrient	DM%[a]	As-Fed (g/100 g diet)	ME% (g/100 kcal)	% of total kcal
Protein	28	7.4	6.3	23
Fat	23	6.0	5.1	46
Carbohydrate	37	9.7	8.2	31
Fiber	1.5	0.4	0.3	—

[a]DM%, dry matter percent. If all the water was removed from this diet, this is the percentage of nutrient that would be present.

Diet: Tofu, Black Beans, and Rice

Species: Dog
Life Stage: Puppy, adult
Special Conditions: Allergy

Ingredient	Quantity	Measure
Tofu, extra firm	16	ounces
Rice, white, long-grain, cooked	1	cup
Black beans, cooked	1½	cup
Canola oil	4	tsp
Salt substitute (potassium chloride)	½	tsp
Bone meal powder	1	tbsp
Salt, iodized (sodium chloride)	1¼	tsp
Multivitamin & mineral tablet, kids complete	1	each
Zinc, 100 mg tablet	½	tablet
Vitamin B_{12} liquid, 1000 mcg B_{12} per mL	0.25	mL

Prepared weight (approximately) = 910 g
Total kcal as prepared = 1128 kcal
kcal/g prepared diet = 1.24 kcal/g diet

Nutrient	DM%[a]	As-Fed (g/100 g diet)	ME% (g/100 kcal)	% of total kcal
Protein	27	7.9	6.4	24
Fat	18	5.2	4.2	38
Carbohydrate	44	12.7	10.3	38
Fiber	9.5	2.7	2.2	—

[a]DM%, dry matter percent. If all the water was removed from this diet, this is the percentage of nutrient that would be present.

Diet: Chicken and Rice

Species: Dog
Life Stage: Puppy (large breed), adult
Special Conditions: Designed for large-breed puppies

Ingredient	Quantity	Measure
Chicken breast, without skin, roasted	6	ounces
Rice, white, long-grain, cooked	2	cup
Broccoli, cooked, chopped	1	cup
Canola oil	1	tbsp
Salt substitute (potassium chloride)	½	tsp
Bone meal powder	2¾	tsp
Salt, iodized (sodium chloride)	1	tsp
Multivitamin & mineral tablet, kids complete	1	each
Zinc, 100 mg tablet	½	tablet

Prepared weight (approximately) = 675 g
Total kcal as prepared = 874 kcal
kcal/g prepared diet = 1.29 kcal/g diet

Nutrient	DM%[a]	As-Fed (g/100 g diet)	ME% (g/100 kcal)	% of total kcal
Protein	31	9.6	7.4	30
Fat	10	3.2	2.5	24
Carbohydrate	48	15.0	11.6	46
Fiber	3.1	1.0	0.7	—
Calcium	1.4	0.4	0.3	

[a]DM%, dry matter percent. If all the water was removed from this diet, this is the percentage of nutrient that would be present.

Diet: Chicken and Pasta

Species: Dog
Life Stage: Puppy (large breed), adult
Special Conditions: Designed for large-breed puppies

Ingredient	Quantity	Measure
Chicken breast, without skin, roasted	4	ounces
Pasta, enriched, cooked	2	cup
Canola oil	2	tsp
Salt substitute (potassium chloride)	½	tsp
Bone meal powder	2½	tsp
Salt, iodized (sodium chloride)	¾	tsp
Multivitamin & mineral tablet, kids complete	1	each
Zinc, 100 mg tablet	½	tablet

Prepared weight (approximately) = 420 g
Total kcal as prepared = 716 kcal
kcal/g prepared diet = 1.70 kcal/g diet

Nutrient	DM%[a]	As-Fed (g/100 g diet)	ME% (g/100 kcal)	% of total kcal
Protein	30	12.2	7.2	29
Fat	9	3.8	2.2	22
Carbohydrate	51	20.8	12.2	49
Fiber	2.9	1.2	0.7	—
Calcium	1.5	0.6	0.4	—

[a]DM%, dry matter percent. If all the water was removed from this diet, this is the percentage of nutrient that would be present.

Diet: Chicken and Potato

Species: Dog
Life Stage: Puppy (large breed), adult
Special Conditions: Designed for large-breed puppies

Ingredient	Quantity	Measure
Chicken breast, without skin, roasted	4	ounces
Potatoes, cooked, diced	2	cup
Canola oil	2	tsp
Salt substitute (potassium chloride)	½	tsp
Bone meal powder	1¾	tsp
Salt, iodized (sodium chloride)	1	tsp
Multivitamin & mineral tablet, kids complete	1	each
Zinc, 100 mg tablet	½	tablet

Prepared weight (approximately) = 451 g
Total kcal as prepared = 545 kcal
kcal/g prepared diet = 1.21 kcal/g diet

Nutrient	DM%[a]	As-Fed (g/100 g diet)	ME% (g/100 kcal)	% of total kcal
Protein	30	9.1	7.5	30
Fat	10	3.0	2.5	24
Carbohydrate	47	14.2	11.7	46
Fiber	4.1	1.2	1.0	—
Calcium	1.4	0.4	0.4	—

[a]DM%, dry matter percent. If all the water was removed from this diet, this is the percentage of nutrient that would be present.

Diet: Ground Beef and Rice

Species: Dog
Life Stage: Puppy (large breed), adult
Special Conditions: Designed for large-breed puppies

Ingredient	Quantity	Measure
Ground beef, 10% fat, pan-browned	6	ounces
Rice, white, long-grain, cooked	2	cup
Canola oil	1	tsp
Salt substitute (potassium chloride)	½	tsp
Bone meal powder	2¾	tsp
Salt, iodized (sodium chloride)	1	tsp
Multivitamin & mineral tablet, kids complete	1	each
Zinc, 100 mg tablet	½	tablet

Prepared weight (approximately) = 510 g
Total kcal as prepared = 847 kcal
kcal/g prepared diet = 1.66 kcal/g diet

Nutrient	DM%[a]	As-Fed (g/100 g diet)	ME% (g/100 kcal)	% of total kcal
Protein	29	11.2	6.7	27
Fat	13	5.1	3.1	30
Carbohydrate	46	17.7	10.6	43
Fiber	0.7	0.3	0.2	—
Calcium	1.5	0.60	0.20	

[a]DM%, dry matter percent. If all the water was removed from this diet, this is the percentage of nutrient that would be present.

Diet: Ground Beef and Pasta

Species: Dog
Life Stage: Puppy (large breed), adult
Special Conditions: Designed for large-breed puppies

Ingredient	Quantity	Measure
Ground beef, 10% fat, pan-browned	7	ounces
Pasta, enriched, cooked	2	cup
Peas, frozen, cooked	1	cup
Canola oil	1	tsp
Salt substitute (potassium chloride)	½	tsp
Bone meal powder	3½	tsp
Salt, iodized (sodium chloride)	1¼	tsp
Multivitamin & mineral tablet, kids complete	1	each
Zinc, 100 mg tablet	½	tablet

Prepared weight (approximately) = 666 g
Total kcal as prepared = 1069 kcal
kcal/g prepared diet = 1.61 kcal/g diet

Nutrient	DM%[a]	As-Fed (g/100 g diet)	ME% (g/100 kcal)	% of total kcal
Protein	33	12.2	7.6	30
Fat	13	4.7	3.0	29
Carbohydrate	44	16.6	10.3	41
Fiber	5.6	2.1	1.3	—
Calcium	1.5	0.6	0.4	

[a]DM%, dry matter percent. If all the water was removed from this diet, this is the percentage of nutrient that would be present.

Diet: Pork and Pasta

Species: Dog
Life Stage: Puppy (large breed), adult
Special Conditions: Designed for large-breed puppies

Ingredient	Quantity	Measure
Pork loin, broiled	5	ounces
Pasta, enriched, cooked	2	cup
Canola oil	1	tsp
Salt substitute (potassium chloride)	½	tsp
Bone meal powder	2½	tsp
Salt, iodized (sodium chloride)	¾	tsp
Multivitamin & mineral tablet, kids complete	1	each
Zinc, 100 mg tablet	½	tablet

Prepared weight (approximately) = 443 g
Total kcal as prepared = 767 kcal
kcal/g prepared diet = 1.73 kcal/g diet

Nutrient	DM%[a]	As-Fed (g/100 g diet)	ME% (g/100 kcal)	% of total kcal
Protein	30	12.2	7.0	28
Fat	11	4.6	2.7	26
Carbohydrate	49	19.7	11.4	46
Fiber	2.8	1.1	0.7	—
Calcium	1.5	0.6	0.4	

[a]DM%, dry matter percent. If all the water was removed from this diet, this is the percentage of nutrient that would be present.

Diet: Tuna and Pasta

Species: Dog
Life Stage: Puppy (large-breed), adult
Special Conditions: Gastric motility disorders

Ingredient	Quantity	Measure
Tuna, in water, canned, drained	6	ounces
Pasta, enriched, cooked	2	cup
Peas, frozen, cooked	½	cup
Canola oil	1	tbsp
Salt substitute (potassium chloride)	½	tsp
Bone meal powder	2¾	tsp
Salt, iodized (sodium chloride)	1	tsp
Multivitamin & mineral tablet, kids complete	1	each
Zinc, 100 mg tablet	½	tablet

Prepared weight (approximately) = 565 g
Total kcal as prepared = 853 kcal
kcal/g prepared diet = 1.51 kcal/g diet

Nutrient	DM%[a]	As-Fed (g/100 g diet)	ME% (g/100 kcal)	% of total kcal
Protein	30	10.8	7.1	29
Fat	11	3.9	2.6	25
Carbohydrate	49	17.5	11.6	46
Fiber	4.7	1.7	1.1	—
Calcium	1.5	0.5	0.34	—

[a]DM%, dry matter percent. If all the water was removed from this diet, this is the percentage of nutrient that would be present.

Diet: Chicken and Pasta

Species: Dog
Life Stage: Adult
Special Conditions: Senior dog

Ingredient	Quantity	Measure
Chicken, breast, without skin, cooked	3	ounces
Pasta, enriched, cooked	3	cup
Broccoli, chopped, cooked	1½	cup
Canola oil	1	tbsp
Salt substitute (potassium chloride)	¾	tsp
Bone meal powder	1¾	tsp
Salt, iodized (sodium chloride)	1	tsp
Multivitamin & mineral tablet, kids complete	1	each
Zinc, 100 mg tablet	½	tablet

Prepared weight (approximately) = 770 g
Total kcal as prepared = 1014 kcal
kcal/g prepared diet = 1.32 kcal/g diet

Nutrient	DM%[a]	As-Fed (g/100 g diet)	ME% (g/100 kcal)	% of total kcal
Protein	23	7.3	5.6	22
Fat	9	2.8	2.2	21
Carbohydrate	60	19.1	14.5	57
Fiber	6.2	2.0	1.5	—

[a]DM%, dry matter percent. If all the water was removed from this diet, this is the percentage of nutrient that would be present.

Diet: Ground Beef and Potato

Species: Dog
Life Stage: Adult
Special Conditions: Senior dog, gastric motility disorders

Ingredient	Quantity	Measure
Ground beef, 10% fat, cooked	4	ounces
Potatoes, diced, cooked	3	cup
Green beans, cooked	1	cup
Canola oil	2	tsp
Salt substitute (potassium chloride)	½	tsp
Bone meal powder	1¼	tsp
Salt, iodized (sodium chloride)	¾	tsp
Kelp, 150 mcg iodine per tablet	1	tablet
Multivitamin & mineral tablet, kids complete	1	each
Zinc, 100 mg tablet	½	tablet

Prepared weight (approximately) = 811 g
Total kcal as prepared = 967 kcal
kcal/g prepared diet = 1.19 kcal/g diet

Nutrient	DM%[a]	As-Fed (g/100 g diet)	ME% (g/100 kcal)	% of total kcal
Protein	23	6.8	5.7	22
Fat	10	3.0	2.5	24
Carbohydrate	56	16.5	13.9	54
Fiber	10.0	2.9	2.5	—

[a]DM%, dry matter percent. If all the water was removed from this diet, this is the percentage of nutrient that would be present.

Diet: Whitefish and Rice

Species: Dog
Life Stage: Adult
Special Conditions: Senior dog, inflammatory bowel disease

Ingredient	Quantity	Measure
Whitefish, fillet, baked or broiled	6	ounces
Rice, white, long-grain, cooked	3	cup
Broccoli, chopped, cooked	1	cup
Canola oil	4	tsp
Salt substitute (potassium chloride)	½	tsp
Bone meal powder	1½	tsp
Salt, iodized (sodium chloride)	¾	tsp
Kelp, 150 mcg iodine per tablet	1	tablet
Multivitamin & mineral tablet, kids complete	1	each
Zinc, 100 mg tablet	½	tablet

Prepared weight (approximately) = 838 g
Total kcal as prepared = 1133 kcal
kcal/g prepared diet = 1.35 kcal/g diet

Nutrient	DM%[a]	As-Fed (g/100 g diet)	ME% (g/100 kcal)	% of total kcal
Protein	22	6.9	5.1	20
Fat	13	4.0	3.0	28
Carbohydrate	55	17.4	12.9	51
Fiber	2.7	0.8	0.6	—

[a]DM%, dry matter percent. If all the water was removed from this diet, this is the percentage of nutrient that would be present.

Diet: Lamb and Rice

Species: Dog
Life Stage: Adult
Special Conditions: Senior dog

Ingredient	Quantity	Measure
Lamb, cooked	5	ounces
Rice, white, long-grain, cooked	3	cup
Broccoli, chopped, cooked	1	cup
Canola oil	1	tsp
Salt substitute (potassium chloride)	½	tsp
Bone meal powder	1¾	tsp
Salt, iodized (sodium chloride)	¾	tsp
Multivitamin & mineral tablet, kids complete	1	each
Kelp, 150 mcg iodine per tablet	1	tablet
Zinc, 100 mg tablet	½	tablet

Prepared weight (approximately) = 796 g
Total kcal as prepared = 1100 kcal
kcal/g prepared diet = 1.38 kcal/g diet

Nutrient	DM%[a]	As-Fed (g/100 g diet)	ME% (g/100 kcal)	% of total kcal
Protein	21	6.6	4.8	19
Fat	13	4.0	2.9	28
Carbohydrate	58	18.3	13.2	53
Fiber	2.8	0.9	0.6	—

[a]DM%, dry matter percent. If all the water was removed from this diet, this is the percentage of nutrient that would be present.

Diet: Cottage Cheese and Rice

Species: Dog
Life Stage: Adult
Special Conditions: Senior dog, gastric motility disorders

Ingredient	Quantity	Measure
Cottage cheese, 1% fat	2	cup
Rice, white, long-grain, cooked	3	cup
Broccoli, chopped, cooked	1	cup
Canola oil	8	tsp
Salt substitute (potassium chloride)	¾	tsp
Bone meal powder	2	tsp
Salt, iodized (sodium chloride)	1	tsp
Multivitamin & mineral tablet, kids complete	1	each
Kelp, 150 mcg iodine per tablet	1	tablet
Zinc, 100 mg tablet	½	tablet

Prepared weight (approximately) = 1142 g
Total kcal as prepared = 1331 kcal
kcal/g prepared diet = 1.16 kcal/g diet

Nutrient	DM%[a]	As-Fed (g/100 g diet)	ME% (g/100 kcal)	% of total kcal
Protein	24	6.3	5.4	21
Fat	14	3.8	3.3	32
Carbohydrate	52	13.8	11.9	47
Fiber	2.3	0.6	0.5	—

[a]DM%, dry matter percent. If all the water was removed from this diet, this is the percentage of nutrient that would be present.

Diet: Tofu and Barley

Species: Dog
Life Stage: Adult
Special Conditions: Senior dog

Ingredient	Quantity	Measure
Tofu, extra firm	12	ounces
Barley, pearled, cooked	2	cup
Peas, green, frozen, cooked	2	cup
Canola oil	2	tsp
Salt substitute (potassium chloride)	½	tsp
Bone meal powder	1¾	tsp
Salt, iodized (sodium chloride)	1	tsp
Multivitamin & mineral tablet, kids complete	1	each
Vitamin B$_{12}$ liquid, 1000 mcg per mL	0.25	mL
Zinc, 100 mg tablet	½	tablet

Prepared weight (approximately) = 1000 g
Total kcal as prepared = 1032 kcal
kcal/g prepared diet = 1.03 kcal/g diet

Nutrient	DM%[a]	As-Fed (g/100 g diet)	ME% (g/100 kcal)	% of total kcal
Protein	23	5.7	5.5	21
Fat	12	3.1	3.0	28
Carbohydrate	56	14.2	137.7	52
Fiber	12.2	3.0	3.0	—

[a]DM%, dry matter percent. If all the water was removed from this diet, this is the percentage of nutrient that would be present.

Diet: Chicken and Potato

Species: Dog
Life Stage: Adult
Special Conditions: Weight loss

Ingredient	Quantity	Measure
Chicken breast, roasted, without skin	6	ounces
Potatoes, diced, cooked	3	cup
Canola oil	1	tbsp
Salt substitute (potassium chloride)	½	tsp
Bone meal powder	2	tsp
Salt, iodized (sodium chloride)	¾	tsp
Multivitamin & mineral tablet, kids complete	1	each
Zinc, 100 mg tablet	½	tablet

Prepared weight (approximately) = 667 g
Total kcal as prepared = 816 kcal
kcal/g prepared diet = 1.22 kcal/g diet

Nutrient	DM%[a]	As-Fed (g/100 g diet)	ME% (g/100 kcal)	% of total kcal
Protein	31	9.2	7.5	30
Fat	10	3.1	2.5	24
Carbohydrate	49	14.3	11.7	46
Fiber	4.3	1.3	1.0	—

[a]DM%, dry matter percent. If all the water was removed from this diet, this is the percentage of nutrient that would be present.

Diet: Chicken and Barley

Species: Dog
Life Stage: Adult
Special Conditions: Weight loss

Ingredient	Quantity	Measure
Chicken breast, without skin, roasted	8	ounces
Barley, pearled, cooked	3	cup
Canola oil	1½	tsp
Salt substitute (potassium chloride)	½	tsp
Bone meal powder	2	tsp
Salt, iodized (sodium chloride)	1¼	tsp
Multivitamin & mineral tablet, kids complete	1	each
Zinc, 100 mg tablet	½	tablet

Prepared weight (approximately) = 723 g
Total kcal as prepared = 1020 kcal
kcal/g prepared diet = 1.41 kcal/g diet

Nutrient	DM%[a]	As-Fed (g/100 g diet)	ME% (g/100 kcal)	% of total kcal
Protein	32	11.2	7.9	32
Fat	7	2.4	1.7	16
Carbohydrate	53	18.5	13.1	52
Fiber	7.1	2.5	1.8	—

[a]DM%, dry matter percent. If all the water was removed from this diet, this is the percentage of nutrient that would be present.

Diet: Chicken, Red Beans, and Pasta

Species: Dog
Life Stage: Adult
Special Conditions: Weight loss

Ingredient	Quantity	Measure
Chicken, breast, without skin, cooked	8	ounces
Pasta, enriched, cooked	2	cup
Beans, red kidney, canned, drained	2	cup
Broccoli, chopped, cooked	1	cup
Canola oil	5	tsp
Salt substitute (potassium chloride)	¾	tsp
Bone meal powder	1	tbsp
Salt, iodized (sodium chloride)	1¼	tsp
Multivitamin & mineral tablet, kids complete	2	each
Zinc, 100 mg tablet	½	tablet

Prepared weight (approximately) = 1223 g
Total kcal as prepared = 1690 kcal
kcal/g prepared diet = 1.38 kcal/g diet

Nutrient	DM%[a]	As-Fed (g/100 g diet)	ME% (g/100 kcal)	% of total kcal
Protein	31	10.4	7.6	30
Fat	9	3.0	2.2	21
Carbohydrate	51	17.2	12.4	49
Fiber	13.6	4.6	3.3	—

[a]DM%, dry matter percent. If all the water was removed from this diet, this is the percentage of nutrient that would be present.

Diet: Ground Beef and Pasta

Species: Dog
Life Stage: Adult
Special Conditions: Weight loss

Ingredient	Quantity	Measure
Ground beef, 10% fat, cooked	6	ounces
Pasta, enriched, cooked	2	cup
Broccoli, chopped, cooked	1	cup
Canola oil	½	tsp
Salt substitute (potassium chloride)	½	tsp
Bone meal powder	2	tsp
Salt, iodized (sodium chloride)	1	tsp
Multivitamin & mineral tablet, kids complete	1	each
Zinc, 100 mg tablet	½	tablet

Prepared weight (approximately) = 625 g
Total kcal as prepared = 913 kcal
kcal/g prepared diet = 1.46 kcal/g diet

Nutrient	DM%[a]	As-Fed (g/100 g diet)	ME% (g/100 kcal)	% of total kcal
Protein	32	10.9	7.5	30
Fat	12	4.2	2.9	27
Carbohydrate	46	15.8	10.8	43
Fiber	4.8	1.6	1.1	—

[a]DM%, dry matter percent. If all the water was removed from this diet, this is the percentage of nutrient that would be present.

Diet: Ground Beef, Red Beans, and Pasta

Species: Dog
Life Stage: Adult
Special Conditions: Weight loss, short bowel syndrome, small intestinal bacterial overgrowth

Ingredient	Quantity	Measure
Ground beef, 10% fat, cooked	10	ounces
Pasta, enriched, cooked	2	cup
Beans, red kidney, canned, drained	2	cup
Carrots, sliced, cooked	1	cup
Canola oil	2	tsp
Salt substitute (potassium chloride)	¾	tsp
Bone meal powder	1	tbsp
Salt, iodized (sodium chloride)	2	tsp
Multivitamin & mineral tablet, kids complete	2	each
Zinc, 100 mg tablet	½	tablet

Prepared weight (approximately) = 1270 g
Total kcal as prepared = 1844 kcal
kcal/g prepared diet = 1.45 kcal/g diet

Nutrient	DM%[a]	As-Fed (g/100 g diet)	ME% (g/100 kcal)	% of total kcal
Protein	31	10.7	7.3	29
Fat	11	3.6	2.6	25
Carbohydrate	49	16.7	11.5	46
Fiber	12.6	4.4	3.0	—

[a]DM%, dry matter percent. If all the water was removed from this diet, this is the percentage of nutrient that would be present.

Diet: Eggs, Barley, and Red Beans

Species: Dog
Life Stage: Adult
Special Conditions: Weight loss

Ingredient	Quantity	Measure
Eggs, hard-boiled	6	each
Barley, cooked	1	cup
Red beans, canned, drained	2	cup
Green beans, cooked	1	cup
Canola oil	1	tsp
Salt substitute (potassium chloride)	¾	tsp
Bone meal powder	2½	tsp
Salt, iodized (sodium chloride)	¾	tsp
Multivitamin & mineral tablet, kids complete	2	each
Zinc, 100 mg tablet	½	tablet

Prepared weight (approximately) = 1196 g
Total kcal as prepared = 1524 kcal
kcal/g prepared diet = 1.27 kcal/g diet

Nutrient	DM%[a]	As-Fed (g/100 g diet)	ME% (g/100 kcal)	% of total kcal
Protein	25	7.8	6.1	24
Fat	11	3.4	2.7	25
Carbohydrate	54	16.6	13.1	51
Fiber	18.3	5.6	4.4	—

[a]DM%, dry matter percent. If all the water was removed from this diet, this is the percentage of nutrient that would be present.

Diet: Tofu, Lentils, and Potato

Species: Dog
Life Stage: Adult
Special Conditions: Weight Loss

Ingredient	Quantity	Measure
Tofu, extra firm	14	ounces
Potatoes, diced, cooked	1½	cup
Lentils, cooked	3	cup
Broccoli, chopped, cooked	1	cup
Canola oil	1	tbsp
Salt substitute (potassium chloride)	¾	tsp
Bone meal powder	1	tbsp
Salt, iodized (sodium chloride)	1½	tsp
Multivitamin & mineral tablet, kids complete	2	each
Zinc, 100 mg tablet	½	tablet
Vitamin B_{12} liquid, 1000 mcg B_{12} per mL	0.25	mL

Prepared weight (approximately) = 1421 g
Total kcal as prepared = 1440 kcal
kcal/g prepared diet = 1.01 kcal/g diet

Nutrient	DM%[a]	As-Fed (g/100 g diet)	ME% (g/100 kcal)	% of total kcal
Protein	27	7.1	7.0	26
Fat	11	?.8	2.8	25
Carbohydrate	51	13.2	13.0	49
Fiber	15.8	4.1	4.0	—

[a]DM%, dry matter percent. If all the water was removed from this diet, this is the percentage of nutrient that would be present.

Diet: Pork and Pasta

Species: Dog
Life Stage: Adult
Special Conditions: Weight loss, lymphangiectasia, protein-losing enteropathy

Ingredient	Quantity	Measure
Pork loin, broiled	4	ounces
Pasta, enriched, cooked	2	cup
Salt substitute (potassium chloride)	¼	tsp
Bone meal powder	1½	tsp
Salt, iodized (sodium chloride)	½	tsp
Multivitamin & mineral tablet, kids complete	1	each
Zinc, 100 mg tablet	½	tablet

Prepared weight (approximately) = 405 g
Total kcal as prepared = 670 kcal
kcal/g prepared diet = 1.66 kcal/g diet

Nutrient	DM%[a]	As-Fed (g/100 g diet)	ME% (g/100 kcal)	% of total kcal
Protein	29	11.5	6.9	28
Fat	8	3.2	2.0	19
Carbohydrate	55	21.6	13.1	53
Fiber	3.2	1.2	0.8	—

[a]DM%, dry matter percent. If all the water was removed from this diet, this is the percentage of nutrient that would be present.

Diet: Rabbit and Quinoa

Species: Dog
Life Stage: Puppy, adult
Special Conditions: Allergy, skin disorders

Ingredient	Quantity	Measure
Rabbit, roasted	6	ounces
Quinoa, cooked	1½	cup
Canola oil	2	tsp
Salt substitute (potassium chloride)	½	tsp
Bone meal powder	2	tsp
Salt, iodized (sodium chloride)	¾	tsp
Multivitamin & mineral tablet, kids complete	1	each
Zinc, 100 mg tablet	½	tablet

Prepared weight (approximately) = 472 g
Total kcal as prepared = 755 kcal
kcal/g prepared diet = 1.60 kcal/g diet

Nutrient	DM%[a]	As-Fed (g/100 g diet)	ME% (g/100 kcal)	% of total kcal
Protein	36	13.0	8.2	32
Fat	17	6.0	3.8	36
Carbohydrate	35	12.7	8.0	32
Fiber	4.6	1.7	1.0	—

[a]DM%, dry matter percent. If all the water was removed from this diet, this is the percentage of nutrient that would be present.

Diet: Venison and Rice

Species: Dog
Life Stage: Adult
Special Conditions: Allergy, pancreatitis (diet provides moderate fat), gastric motility disorders

Ingredient	Quantity	Measure
Venison, roasted	5	ounces
Rice, white, long-grain, cooked	3	cup
Canola oil	4	tsp
Salt substitute (potassium chloride)	½	tsp
Bone meal powder	2	tsp
Salt, iodized (sodium chloride)	1	tsp
Multivitamin & mineral tablet, kids complete	1	each
Zinc, 100 mg tablet	½	tablet

Prepared weight (approximately) = 651 g
Total kcal as prepared = 1009 kcal
kcal/g prepared diet = 1.55 kcal/g diet

Nutrient	DM%[a]	As-Fed (g/100 g diet)	ME% (g/100 kcal)	% of total kcal
Protein	24	8.5	5.5	22
Fat	10	3.8	2.4	24
Carbohydrate	57	20.7	13.3	54
Fiber	0.8	0.3	0.2	—

[a]DM%, dry matter percent. If all the water was removed from this diet, this is the percentage of nutrient that would be present.

Diet: Venison and Quinoa

Species: Dog
Life Stage: Puppy, adult
Special Conditions: Allergy

Ingredient	Quantity	Measure
Venison, roasted	6	ounces
Quinoa, cooked	1½	cup
Canola oil	2	tsp
Salt substitute (potassium chloride)	½	tsp
Bone meal powder	2	tsp
Salt, iodized (sodium chloride)	¾	tsp
Multivitamin & mineral tablet, kids complete	1	each
Zinc, 100 mg tablet	½	tablet

Prepared weight (approximately) = 472 g
Total kcal as prepared = 688 kcal
kcal/g prepared diet = 1.46 kcal/g diet

Nutrient	DM%[a]	As-Fed (g/100 g diet)	ME% (g/100 kcal)	% of total kcal
Protein	39	13.5	9.2	37
Fat	12	4.2	2.9	28
Carbohydrate	37	12.7	8.7	35
Fiber	4.8	1.7	1.1	—

[a]DM%, dry matter percent. If all the water was removed from this diet, this is the percentage of nutrient that would be present.

Diet: Salmon and Couscous

Species: Dog
Life Stage: Adult
Special Conditions: Allergy, skin conditions

Ingredient	Quantity	Measure
Salmon, Atlantic, fillet, baked/broiled	6	ounces
Couscous, cooked	2	cup
Canola oil	1	tbsp
Salt substitute (potassium chloride)	½	tsp
Bone meal powder	2	tsp
Salt, iodized (sodium chloride)	¾	tsp
Multivitamin & mineral tablet, kids complete	1	each
Zinc, 100 mg tablet	½	tablet

Prepared weight (approximately) = 513 g
Total kcal as prepared = 789 kcal
kcal/g prepared diet = 1.54 kcal/g diet

Nutrient	DM%[a]	As-Fed (g/100g diet)	ME% (g/100 kcal)	% of total kcal
Protein	30	10.8	7.0	28
Fat	15	5.5	3.6	35
Carbohydrate	40	14.4	9.4	37
Fiber	2.4	0.9	0.6	—

[a]DM%, dry matter percent. If all the water was removed from this diet, this is the percentage of nutrient that would be present.

Diet: Tofu and Quinoa

Species: Dog
Life Stage: Puppy, adult
Special Conditions: Allergy, skin conditions

Ingredient	Quantity	Measure
Tofu, extra firm	16	ounces
Quinoa, cooked	1½	cup
Canola oil	1	tbsp
Salt substitute (potassium chloride)	½	tsp
Bone meal powder	2	tsp
Salt, iodized (sodium chloride)	¾	tsp
Multivitamin & mineral tablet, kids complete	1	each
Zinc, 100 mg tablet	½	tablet
Vitamin B_{12} liquid, 1000 mcg B_{12} per mL	0.25	mL

Prepared weight (approximately) = 761 g
Total kcal as prepared = 874 kcal
kcal/g prepared diet = 1.15 kcal/g diet

Nutrient	DM%[a]	As-Fed (g/100 g diet)	ME% (g/100 kcal)	% of total kcal
Protein	30	7.5	6.5	24
Fat	24	6.0	5.2	47
Carbohydrate	36	9.1	7.9	29
Fiber	5.0	1.3	1.1	—

[a]DM%, dry matter percent. If all the water was removed from this diet, this is the percentage of nutrient that would be present.

Diet: Tofu, Red Beans, and Rice

Species: Dog
Life Stage: Adult
Special Conditions: Allergy

Ingredient	Quantity	Measure
Tofu, extra firm	12	ounces
Rice, white, long-grain, cooked	1½	cup
Red kidney beans, canned, drained	1	cup
Canola oil	1	tbsp
Salt substitute (potassium chloride)	½	tsp
Bone meal powder	2	tsp
Salt, iodized (sodium chloride)	1	tsp
Multivitamin & mineral tablet, kids complete	1	each
Zinc, 100 mg tablet	½	tablet
Vitamin B_{12} liquid, 1000 mcg B_{12} per mL	0.25	mL

Prepared weight (approximately) = 864 g
Total kcal as prepared = 1048 kcal
kcal/g prepared diet = 1.21 kcal/g diet

Nutrient	DM%[a]	As-Fed (g/100 g diet)	ME% (g/100 kcal)	% of total kcal
Protein	24	6.8	5.6	21
Fat	14	4.1	3.4	31
Carbohydrate	52	15.0	12.4	47
Fiber	10.0	2.9	2.4	—

[a]DM%, dry matter percent. If all the water was removed from this diet, this is the percentage of nutrient that would be present.

Diet: Chicken and Rice

Species: Dog
Life Stage: Adult
Special Conditions: Cancer

Ingredient	Quantity	Measure
Chicken, breast, without skin, cooked	12	ounce
Rice, white, long-grain, cooked	2	cup
Canola oil	6	tbsp
Salt substitute (potassium chloride)	1	tsp
Bone meal powder	3	tsp
Salt, iodized (sodium chloride)	¾	tsp
Multivitamin & mineral tablet, kids complete	2	each
Zinc, 100 mg tablet	½	tablet
Arginine powder, 2.5 g per tsp	½	tsp
Kelp, 150 mcg iodine per tablet	2	tablet
Fish oil, 900 mg omega-3 per tablet	3	tablet

Prepared weight (approximately) = 779 g
Total kcal as prepared = 1768 kcal
kcal/g prepared diet = 2.27 kcal/g diet

Nutrient	DM%[a]	As-Fed (g/100 g diet)	ME% (g/100 kcal)	% of total kcal
Protein	33	14.6	6.4	25
Fat	30	13.0	5.7	55
Carbohydrate	27	11.7	5.2	20
Fiber	0.4	0.16	0.07	—
Arginine	2.4	0.45	0.47	—
Omega-3 fatty acids	5.4	2.4	1.0	—

[a]DM%, dry matter percent. If all the water was removed from this diet, this is the percentage of nutrient that would be present.

Diet: Chicken and Pasta

Species: Dog
Life Stage: Adult
Special Conditions: Cancer

Ingredient	Quantity	Measure
Chicken, breast, without skin, cooked	16	ounce
Pasta, enriched, cooked	2	cup
Canola oil	7	tbsp
Salt substitute (potassium chloride)	1	tsp
Bone meal powder	3¾	tsp
Salt, iodized (sodium chloride)	1	tsp
Multivitamin & mineral tablet, kids complete	2	each
Zinc, 100 mg tablet	½	tablet
Arginine powder, 2.5 g per tsp	½	tsp
Kelp, 150 mcg iodine per tablet	3	tablet
Fish oil, 900 mg omega-3 per tablet	6	tablet

Prepared weight (approximately) = 883 g
Total kcal as prepared = 2155 kcal
kcal/g prepared diet = 2.44 kcal/g diet

Nutrient	DM%[a]	As-Fed (g/100g diet)	ME% (g/100kcal)	% of total kcal
Protein	38	17.8	7.3	28
Fat	30	14.2	5.8	55
Carbohydrate	21	10.0	4.1	16
Fiber	1.2	0.57	0.23	—
Arginine	2.5	1.2	0.48	—
Omega-3 fatty acids	5.8	2.7	1.1	—

[a]DM%, dry matter percent. If all the water was removed from this diet, this is the percentage of nutrient that would be present.

Diet: Ground Beef and Rice

Species: Dog
Life Stage: Adult
Special Conditions: Cancer

Ingredient	Quantity	Measure
Ground beef, 10% fat, cooked	16	ounce
Rice, white, long-grain, cooked	2	cup
Canola oil	6	tbsp
Salt substitute (potassium chloride)	1	tsp
Bone meal powder	3¾	tsp
Salt, iodized (sodium chloride)	1	tsp
Multivitamin & mineral tablet, kids complete	2	each
Zinc, 100 mg tablet	½	tablet
Arginine powder, 2.5 g per tsp	½	tsp
Kelp, 150 mcg iodine per tablet	3	tablet
Fish oil, 900 mg omega-3 per tablet	6	tablet

Prepared weight (approximately) = 905 g
Total kcal as prepared = 2295 kcal
kcal/g prepared diet = 2.54 kcal/g diet

Nutrient	DM%[a]	As-Fed (g/100 g diet)	ME% (g/100 kcal)	% of total kcal
Protein	32	15.2	6.0	23
Fat	35	16.4	6.5	61
Carbohydrate	22	10.1	4.0	15
Fiber	0.3	0.14	0.06	—
Arginine	2.4	1.1	0.45	—
Omega-3 fatty acids	5.0	2.4	0.9	—

[a]DM%, dry matter percent. If all the water was removed from this diet, this is the percentage of nutrient that would be present.

Diet: Ground Beef and Pasta

Species: Dog
Life Stage: Adult
Special Conditions: Cancer

Ingredient	Quantity	Measure
Ground beef, 10% fat, cooked	16	ounce
Pasta, enriched, cooked	2	cup
Canola oil	6	tbsp
Salt substitute (potassium chloride)	1	tsp
Bone meal powder	3¾	tsp
Salt, iodized (sodium chloride)	1	tsp
Multivitamin & mineral tablet, kids complete	2	each
Zinc, 100 mg tablet	½	tablet
Arginine powder, 2.5 g per tsp	½	tsp
Kelp, 150 mcg iodine per tablet	3	tablet
Fish oil, 900 mg omega-3 per tablet	6	tablet

Prepared weight (approximately) = 869 g
Total kcal as prepared = 2327 kcal
kcal/g prepared diet = 2.68 kcal/g diet

Nutrient	DM%[a]	As-Fed (g/100g diet)	ME% (g/100 kcal)	% of total kcal
Protein	34	16.7	6.3	24
Fat	35	17.3	6.5	61
Carbohydrate	21	10.2	3.8	15
Fiber	1.2	0.58	0.22	—
Arginine	2.3	1.2	0.43	—
Omega-3 fatty acids	5.0	2.5	0.9	—

[a]DM%, dry matter percent. If all the water was removed from this diet, this is the percentage of nutrient that would be present.

Diet: Pork and Potato

Species: Dog
Life Stage: Adult
Special Conditions: Cancer

Ingredient	Quantity	Measure
Pork, loin, broiled	14	ounce
Potatoes, diced, cooked	2	cup
Canola oil	6	tbsp
Salt substitute (potassium chloride)	1	tsp
Bone meal powder	3¾	tsp
Salt, iodized (sodium chloride)	1	tsp
Multivitamin & mineral tablet, kids complete	2	each
Zinc, 100 mg tablet	½	tablet
Arginine powder, 2.5 g per tsp	½	tsp
Kelp, 150 mcg iodine per tablet	3	tablet
Fish oil, 900 mg omega-3 per tablet	6	tablet

Prepared weight (approximately) = 845 g
Total kcal as prepared = 1894 kcal
kcal/g prepared diet = 2.24 kcal/g diet

Nutrient	DM%[a]	As-Fed (g/100g diet)	ME% (g/100kcal)	% of total kcal
Protein	31	13.2	5.9	23
Fat	37	15.4	6.9	64
Carbohydrate	18	7.7	3.4	13
Fiber	1.6	0.66	0.3	—
Arginine	2.4	1.0	0.44	—
Omega-3 fatty acids	5.9	2.5	1.1	—

[a]DM%, dry matter percent. If all the water was removed from this diet, this is the percentage of nutrient that would be present.

Diet: Whitefish and Quinoa

Species: Dog
Life Stage: Adult
Special Conditions: Cancer

Ingredient	Quantity	Measure
Whitefish, fillet, baked or broiled	20	ounce
Quinoa, cooked	2½	cup
Canola oil	6	tbsp
Salt substitute (potassium chloride)	1	tsp
Bone meal powder	3¾	tsp
Salt, iodized (sodium chloride)	1	tsp
Multivitamin & mineral tablet, kids complete	2	each
Zinc, 100 mg tablet	½	tablet
Arginine powder, 2.5 g per tsp	½	tsp
Kelp, 150 mcg iodine per tablet	3	tablet

Prepared weight (approximately) = 1156 g
Total kcal as prepared = 2281 kcal
kcal/g prepared diet = 1.97 kcal/g diet

Nutrient	DM%[a]	As-Fed (g/100 g diet)	ME% (g/100 kcal)	% of total kcal
Protein	35	13.8	7.0	27
Fat	30	11.7	5.9	56
Carbohydrate	22	8.7	4.4	17
Fiber	2.8	1.1	0.6	—
Arginine	2.4	1.0	0.49	—
Omega-3 fatty acids	8.0	3.1	1.6	—

[a]DM%, dry matter percent. If all the water was removed from this diet, this is the percentage of nutrient that would be present.

Diet: Chicken and Barley

Species: Dog
Life Stage: Adult
Special Conditions: Diabetes mellitus, short bowel syndrome, small intestinal bacterial overgrowth

Ingredient	Quantity	Measure
Chicken, breast, without skin, cooked	6	ounce
Barley, pearled, cooked	3	cup
Beans, red kidney, canned, drained	1	cup
Broccoli, chopped, cooked	1	cup
Canola oil	2	tbsp
Salt substitute (potassium chloride)	½	tsp
Bone meal powder	2½	tsp
Salt, iodized (sodium chloride)	1¾	tsp
Multivitamin & mineral tablet, kids complete	1	each
Zinc, 100 mg tablet	½	tablet

Prepared weight (approximately) = 1104 g
Total kcal as prepared = 1468 kcal
kcal/g prepared diet = 1.33 kcal/g diet

Nutrient	DM%[a]	As-Fed (g/100 g diet)	ME% (g/100 kcal)	% of total kcal
Protein	24	7.8	5.8	23
Fat	11	3.4	2.6	24
Carbohydrate	57	18.2	13.7	53
Fiber	12.9	4.2	3.1	—

[a]DM%, dry matter percent. If all the water was removed from this diet, this is the percentage of nutrient that would be present.

Diet: Ground Beef and Potato

Species: Dog
Life Stage: Adult
Special Conditions: Diabetes mellitus, short bowel syndrome, small intestinal bacterial overgrowth

Ingredient	Quantity	Measure
Ground beef, 10% fat, cooked	5	ounce
Potatoes, diced, cooked	3	cup
Beans, black, canned, drained	2	cup
Canola oil	1	tbsp
Salt substitute (potassium chloride)	½	tsp
Bone meal powder	2½	tsp
Salt, iodized (sodium chloride)	1½	tsp
Multivitamin & mineral tablet, kids complete	1	each
Zinc, 100 mg tablet	½	tablet

Prepared weight (approximately) = 989 g
Total kcal as prepared = 1315 kcal
kcal/g prepared diet = 1.33 kcal/g diet

Nutrient	DM%[a]	As-Fed (g/100 g diet)	ME% (g/100 kcal)	% of total kcal
Protein	25	8.0	6.0	24
Fat	10	3.4	2.5	24
Carbohydrate	55	17.8	13.5	52
Fiber	12.0	3.9	2.9	—

[a]DM%, dry matter percent. If all the water was removed from this diet, this is the percentage of nutrient that would be present.

Diet: Eggs and Pasta

Species: Dog
Life Stage: Adult
Special Conditions: Diabetes mellitus, short bowel syndrome, small intestinal bacterial overgrowth

Ingredient	Quantity	Measure
Eggs, large, hard-boiled	5	each
Pasta, enriched, cooked	2	cup
Beans, red kidney, canned, drained	1½	cup
Canola oil	1	tbsp
Salt substitute (potassium chloride)	1	tsp
Bone meal powder	2¼	tsp
Salt, iodized (sodium chloride)	1½	tsp
Multivitamin & mineral tablet, kids complete	1	each
Zinc, 100 mg tablet	½	tablet

Prepared weight (approximately) = 951 g
Total kcal as prepared = 1411 kcal
kcal/g prepared diet = 1.48 kcal/g diet

Nutrient	DM%[a]	As-Fed (g/100 g diet)	ME% (g/100 kcal)	% of total kcal
Protein	23	8.0	5.4	21
Fat	14	4.7	3.2	30
Carbohydrate	53	18.2	12.3	48
Fiber	12.0	4.1	2.8	—

[a]DM%, dry matter percent. If all the water was removed from this diet, this is the percentage of nutrient that would be present.

Diet: Tofu and Pasta

Species: Dog
Life Stage: Adult
Special Conditions: Diabetes mellitus, short bowel syndrome, small
intestinal bacterial overgrowth

Ingredient	Quantity	Measure
Tofu, extra firm	12	ounce
Pasta, enriched, cooked	2	cup
Beans, red kidney, canned, drained	1	cup
Canola oil	1	tbsp
Salt substitute (potassium chloride)	¾	tsp
Bone meal powder	2	tsp
Salt, iodized (sodium chloride)	1	tsp
Kelp, 150 mcg iodine per tablet	1	tablet
Multivitamin & mineral tablet, kids complete	1	each
Zinc, 100 mg tablet	½	tablet
Vitamin B_{12} liquid, 1000 mcg B_{12} per mL	0.25	mL

Prepared weight (approximately) = 914 g
Total kcal as prepared = 1182 kcal
kcal/g prepared diet = 1.29 kcal/g diet

Nutrient	DM%[a]	As-Fed (g/100 g diet)	ME% (g/100 kcal)	% of total kcal
Protein	24	7.5	5.8	22
Fat	13	4.1	3.2	30
Carbohydrate	52	16.4	12.6	48
Fiber	10.1	3.2	2.5	—

[a]DM%, dry matter percent. If all the water was removed from this diet, this is the
percentage of nutrient that would be present.

Diet: Chicken and Pasta

Species: Dog
Life Stage: Adult
Special Conditions: Insulinoma

Ingredient	Quantity	Measure
Chicken, breast, without skin, cooked	6	ounce
Pasta, enriched, cooked	3	cup
Canola oil	4	tbsp
Salt substitute (potassium chloride)	¾	tsp
Bone meal powder	1	tbsp
Salt, iodized (sodium chloride)	1¾	tsp
Multivitamin & mineral tablet, kids complete	2	each
Zinc, 100 mg tablet	½	tablet

Prepared weight (approximately) = 674 g
Total kcal as prepared = 1448 kcal
kcal/g prepared diet = 2.14 kcal/g diet

Nutrient	DM%[a]	As-Fed (g/100 g diet)	ME% (g/100 kcal)	% of total kcal
Protein	26	11.4	5.3	21
Fat	22	9.8	4.6	43
Carbohydrate	44	19.6	9.1	36
Fiber	2.5	1.1	0.5	—

[a]DM%, dry matter percent. If all the water was removed from this diet, this is the percentage of nutrient that would be present.

Diet: Ground Beef and Rice

Species: Dog
Life Stage: Adult
Special Conditions: Insulinoma

Ingredient	Quantity	Measure
Ground beef, 25% fat, cooked	9	ounce
Rice, white, long-grain, cooked	3	cup
Canola oil	2	tbsp
Salt substitute (potassium chloride)	¾	tsp
Bone meal powder	2¾	tsp
Salt, iodized (sodium chloride)	1½	tsp
Multivitamin & mineral tablet, kids complete	1	each
Zinc, 100 mg tablet	½	tablet

Prepared weight (approximately) = 780 g
Total kcal as prepared = 1575 kcal
kcal/g prepared diet = 2.02 kcal/g diet

Nutrient	DM%[a]	As-Fed (g/100 g diet)	ME% (g/100 kcal)	% of total kcal
Protein	25	10.2	5.0	20
Fat	24	9.7	4.8	46
Carbohydrate	43	17.2	8.6	34
Fiber	0.6	0.2	0.1	—

[a]DM%, dry matter percent. If all the water was removed from this diet, this is the percentage of nutrient that would be present.

Diet: Chicken and Potato

Species: Dog
Life Stage: Adult
Special Conditions: Lipid disorders requiring a low-fat diet, lymphangiectasia, protein-losing enteropathy. This diet is NOT balanced or complete and should be fed only under the direct supervision of your veterinarian.

Ingredient	Quantity	Measure
Chicken, breast, without skin, cooked	6	ounces
Potatoes, diced, cooked	3	cup
Canola oil	¾	tsp
Salt substitute (potassium chloride)	¼	tsp
Bone meal powder	1½	tsp
Salt, iodized (sodium chloride)	½	tsp
Multivitamin & mineral tablet, kids complete	1	each
Zinc, 100 mg tablet	½	tablet

Prepared weight (approximately) = 653 g
Total kcal as prepared = 723 kcal
kcal/g prepared diet = 1.11 kcal/g diet

Nutrient	DM%[a]	As-Fed (g/100 g diet)	ME% (g/100 kcal)	% of total kcal
Protein	34	9.4	8.5	34
Fat	5	1.5	1.4	13
Carbohydrate	52	14.6	13.2	53
Fiber	4.6	1.3	1.2	—

[a]DM%, dry matter percent. If all the water was removed from this diet, this is the percentage of nutrient that would be present.

Diet: Pork and Rice

Species: Dog
Life Stage: Adult
Special Conditions: Lipid disorders requiring a low-fat diet; This diet is NOT balanced or complete and should be fed only under the direct supervision of your veterinarian.

Ingredient	Quantity	Measure
Pork, loin, broiled	8	ounces
Rice, white, long-grain, cooked	2	cup
Pasta, enriched, cooked	2	cup
Salt substitute (potassium chloride)	½	tsp
Bone meal powder	2	tsp
Salt, iodized (sodium chloride)	1½	tsp
Multivitamin & mineral tablet, kids complete	1	each
Zinc, 100 mg tablet	½	tablet

Prepared weight (approximately) = 843 g
Total kcal as prepared = 1304 kcal
kcal/g prepared diet = 1.56 kcal/g diet

Nutrient	DM%[a]	As-Fed (g/100 g diet)	ME% (g/100 kcal)	% of total kcal
Protein	27	10.1	6.5	27
Fat	8	2.9	1.9	18
Carbohydrate	57	20.9	13.5	55
Fiber	2	0.8	0.5	—

[a]DM%, dry matter percent. If all the water was removed from this diet, this is the percentage of nutrient that would be present.

Diet: Whitefish and Rice

Species: Dog
Life Stage: Adult
Special Conditions: Lipid disorders requiring a low-fat diet, lymphangiectasia, protein-losing enteropathy. This diet is NOT balanced or complete and should only be fed under the direct supervision of your veterinarian.

Ingredient	Quantity	Measure
Whitefish, fillet, baked or broiled	8	ounces
Rice, white, long-grain, cooked	3	cup
Salt substitute (potassium chloride)	½	tsp
Bone meal powder	1¾	tsp
Salt, iodized (sodium chloride)	1¼	tsp
Multivitamin & mineral tablet, kids complete	1	each
Zinc, 100 mg tablet	½	tablet

Prepared weight (approximately) = 718 g
Total kcal as prepared = 1010 kcal
kcal/g prepared diet = 1.41 kcal/g diet

Nutrient	DM%[a]	As-Fed (g/100 g diet)	ME% (g/100 kcal)	% of total kcal
Protein	28	9.5	6.8	28
Fat	7	2.6	1.8	18
Carbohydrate	55	18.7	13.3	54
Fiber	0.8	0.3	0.19	—

[a]DM%, dry matter percent. If all the water was removed from this diet, this is the percentage of nutrient that would be present.

Diet: Chicken and Potato

Species: Dog
Life Stage: Puppy, Adult
Special Conditions: Megaesophagus, obstructive swallowing disorders

Ingredient	Quantity	Measure
Chicken, breast, without skin, cooked	7	ounces
Potatoes, diced, cooked	2	cup
Canola oil	10	tsp
Salt substitute (potassium chloride)	½	tsp
Bone meal powder	3½	tsp
Salt, iodized (sodium chloride)	1½	tsp
Multivitamin & mineral tablet, kids complete	2	each
Zinc, 100 mg tablet	½	tablet

Prepared weight (approximately) = 583 g
Total kcal as prepared = 1020 kcal
kcal/g prepared diet = 1.75 kcal/g diet

Nutrient	DM%[a]	As-Fed (g/100 g diet)	ME% (g/100 kcal)	% of total kcal
Protein	31	11.6	6.6	25
Fat	25	9.3	5.3	50
Carbohydrate	30	11.1	6.4	25
Fiber	2.6	1.0	0.6	—

[a]DM%, dry matter percent. If all the water was removed from this diet, this is the percentage of nutrient that would be present.

Diet: Ground Beef and Pasta

Species: Dog
Life Stage: Adult
Special Conditions: Megaesophagus, obstructive swallowing disorders

Ingredient	Quantity	Measure
Ground beef, 10% fat, cooked	9	ounces
Pasta, enriched, cooked	3	cup
Canola oil	11	tsp
Salt substitute (potassium chloride)	¾	tsp
Bone meal powder	1	tbsp
Salt, iodized (sodium chloride)	2	tsp
Multivitamin & mineral tablet, kids complete	2	each
Zinc, 100 mg tablet	½	tablet

Prepared weight (approximately) = 756 g
Total kcal as prepared = 1712 kcal
kcal/g prepared diet = 2.27 kcal/g diet

Nutrient	DM%[a]	As-Fed (g/100 g diet)	ME% (g/100 kcal)	% of total kcal
Protein	28	12.8	5.7	22
Fat	25	11.4	5.0	48
Carbohydrate	38	17.4	7.7	30
Fiber	2.2	1.0	0.4	—

[a]DM%, dry matter percent. If all the water was removed from this diet, this is the percentage of nutrient that would be present.

Diet: Eggs and Rice

Species: Dog
Life Stage: Adult
Special Conditions: Megaesophagus, obstructive swallowing disorders

Ingredient	Quantity	Measure
Eggs, large, hard-boiled	7	each
Rice, white, long-grain, cooked	2	cup
Sardines, in tomato sauce, canned	4	each
Canola oil	8	tsp
Salt substitute (potassium chloride)	¾	tsp
Bone meal powder	2¾	tsp
Salt, iodized (sodium chloride)	1½	tsp
Multivitamin & mineral tablet, kids complete	2	each
Zinc, 100 mg tablet	½	tablet

Prepared weight (approximately) = 880 g
Total kcal as prepared = 1574 kcal
kcal/g prepared diet = 1.79 kcal/g diet

Nutrient	DM%[a]	As-Fed (g/100 g diet)	ME% (g/100 kcal)	% of total kcal
Protein	28	9.6	5.4	21
Fat	30	10.4	5.8	55
Carbohydrate	32	10.9	6.1	24
Fiber	0.5	0.2	0.1	—

[a]DM%, dry matter percent. If all the water was removed from this diet, this is the percentage of nutrient that would be present.

Diet: Cottage Cheese and Rice

Species: Dog
Life Stage: Adult
Special Conditions: Esophagitis, exocrine pancreatic insufficiency, gastric motility disorders

Ingredient	Quantity	Measure
Cottage cheese, 2% fat	2	cup
Rice, white, long-grain, cooked	2	cup
Canola oil	1	tbsp
Salt substitute (potassium chloride)	¾	tsp
Bone meal powder	2	tsp
Salt, iodized (sodium chloride)	1	tsp
Multivitamin & mineral tablet, kids complete	1	each
Zinc, 100 mg tablet	½	tablet

Prepared weight (approximately) = 800 g
Total kcal as prepared = 928 kcal
kcal/g prepared diet = 1.16 kcal/g diet

Nutrient	DM%[a]	As-Fed (g/100 g diet)	ME% (g/100 kcal)	% of total kcal
Protein	28	7.8	6.7	27
Fat	12	3.2	2.8	27
Carbohydrate	49	13.3	11.5	46
Fiber	0.6	0.2	0.1	

[a]DM%, dry matter percent. If all the water was removed from this diet, this is the percentage of nutrient that would be present.

Diet: Rabbit and Rice

Species: Dog
Life Stage: Adult
Special Conditions: Gastritis, exocrine pancreatic insufficiency, gastric motility disorders

Ingredient	Quantity	Measure
Rabbit, domestic, cooked	4	ounces
Rice, white, long-grain, cooked	3	cup
Canola oil	2½	tsp
Salt substitute (potassium chloride)	¾	tsp
Bone meal powder	1¾	tsp
Salt, iodized (sodium chloride)	⅜	tsp
Multivitamin & mineral tablet, kids complete	1	each
Zinc, 100 mg tablet	½	tablet
Kelp, 150 mcg iodine per tablet	2	tablet

Prepared weight (approximately) = 623 g
Total kcal as prepared = 947 kcal
kcal/g prepared diet = 1.52 kcal/g diet

Nutrient	DM%[a]	As-Fed (g/100 g diet)	ME% (g/100 kcal)	% of total kcal
Protein	20	7.4	4.8	20
Fat	10	3.6	2.3	23
Carbohydrate	59	21.6	14.2	58
Fiber	0.8	0.3	0.2	—

[a]DM%, dry matter percent. If all the water was removed from this diet, this is the percentage of nutrient that would be present.

Diet: Venison and Rice

Species: Dog
Life Stage: Adult
Special Conditions: Gastritis

Ingredient	Quantity	Measure
Venison, cooked	4	ounces
Rice, white, long-grain, cooked	3	cup
Canola oil	1	tbsp
Salt substitute (potassium chloride)	¾	tsp
Bone meal powder	1¾	tsp
Salt, iodized (sodium chloride)	⅜	tsp
Multivitamin & mineral tablet, kids complete	1	each
Zinc, 100 mg tablet	½	tablet
Kelp, 150 mcg iodine per tablet	2	tablet

Prepared weight (approximately) = 625 g
Total kcal as prepared = 923 kcal
kcal/g prepared diet = 1.48 kcal/g diet

Nutrient	DM%[a]	As-Fed (g/100 g diet)	ME% (g/100 kcal)	% of total kcal
Protein	21	7.5	5.1	21
Fat	8	3.0	2.0	20
Carbohydrate	59	21.5	14.6	59
Fiber	0.8	0.3	0.2	—

[a]DM%, dry matter percent. If all the water was removed from this diet, this is the percentage of nutrient that would be present.

Diet: Pork and Rice

Species: Dog
Life Stage: Adult
Special Conditions: Gastritis, exocrine pancreatic insufficiency, gastric motility disorders

Ingredient	Quantity	Measure
Pork loin, broiled	4	ounces
Rice, white, long-grain, cooked	3	cup
Canola oil	2	tsp
Salt substitute (potassium chloride)	¾	tsp
Bone meal powder	1¾	tsp
Salt, iodized (sodium chloride)	⅜	tsp
Multivitamin & mineral tablet, kids complete	1	each
Zinc, 100 mg tablet	½	tablet
Kelp, 150 mcg iodine per tablet	2	tablet

Prepared weight (approximately) = 620 g
Total kcal as prepared = 926 kcal
kcal/g prepared diet = 1.49 kcal/g diet

Nutrient	DM%[a]	As-Fed (g/100 g diet)	ME% (g/100 kcal)	% of total kcal
Protein	19	6.9	4.6	19
Fat	9	3.4	2.3	22
Carbohydrate	60	21.7	14.5	59
Fiber	0.9	0.3	0.2	—

[a]DM%, dry matter percent. If all the water was removed from this diet, this is the percentage of nutrient that would be present.

Diet: Chicken and Rice

Species: Dog
Life Stage: Adult
Special Conditions: Enteritis, exocrine pancreatic insufficiency, gastric motility disorders

Ingredient	Quantity	Measure
Chicken, breast, without skin, cooked	5	ounces
Rice, white, long-grain, cooked	3	cup
Canola oil	2	tbsp
Salt substitute (potassium chloride)	¾	tsp
Bone meal powder	1¾	tsp
Salt, iodized (sodium chloride)	⅜	tsp
Multivitamin & mineral tablet, kids complete	1	each
Zinc, 100 mg tablet	½	tablet
Kelp, 150 mcg iodine per tablet	3	tablet

Prepared weight (approximately) = 672 g
Total kcal as prepared = 1102 kcal
kcal/g prepared diet = 1.64 kcal/g diet

Nutrient	DM%[a]	As-Fed (g/100 g diet)	ME% (g/100 kcal)	% of total kcal
Protein	22	8.4	5.1	21
Fat	13	5.1	3.1	30
Carbohydrate	53	20.0	12.2	49
Fiber	0.7	0.3	0.2	—

[a]DM%, dry matter percent. If all the water was removed from this diet, this is the percentage of nutrient that would be present.

Diet: Ground Beef and Rice

Species: Dog
Life Stage: Adult
Special Conditions: Enteritis, exocrine pancreatic insufficiency, gastric motility disorders

Ingredient	Quantity	Measure
Ground beef, 10% fat, cooked	6	ounces
Rice, white, long-grain, cooked	3	cup
Canola oil	3½	tsp
Salt substitute (potassium chloride)	¾	tsp
Bone meal powder	2	tsp
Salt, iodized (sodium chloride)	⅜	tsp
Multivitamin & mineral tablet, kids complete	1	each
Zinc, 100 mg tablet	½	tablet
Kelp, 150 mcg iodine per tablet	2	tablet

Prepared weight (approximately) = 685 g
Total kcal as prepared = 1156 kcal
kcal/g prepared diet = 1.69 kcal/g diet

Nutrient	DM%[a]	As-Fed (g/100 g diet)	ME% (g/100 kcal)	% of total kcal
Protein	23	8.9	5.3	21
Fat	15	5.6	3.3	32
Carbohydrate	52	19.7	11.6	47
Fiber	0.7	0.3	0.2	—

[a]DM%, dry matter percent. If all the water was removed from this diet, this is the percentage of nutrient that would be present.

Diet: Eggs and Rice

Species: Dog
Life Stage: Adult
Special Conditions: Enteritis, exocrine pancreatic insufficiency

Ingredient	Quantity	Measure
Eggs, hard-boiled	8	each
Rice, white, long-grain, cooked	3	cup
Salt substitute (potassium chloride)	¾	tsp
Bone meal powder	1¾	tsp
Salt, iodized (sodium chloride)	¼	tsp
Multivitamin & mineral tablet, kids complete	1	each
Zinc, 100 mg tablet	½	tablet
Kelp, 150 mcg iodine per tablet	3	tablet

Prepared weight (approximately) = 902 g
Total kcal as prepared = 1240 kcal
kcal/g prepared diet = 1.38 kcal/g diet

Nutrient	DM%[a]	As-Fed (g/100 g diet)	ME% (g/100 kcal)	% of total kcal
Protein	23	7.0	5.1	20
Fat	16	4.8	3.5	34
Carbohydrate	50	15.4	11.2	45
Fiber	0.7	0.2	0.2	—

[a]DM%, dry matter percent. If all the water was removed from this diet, this is the percentage of nutrient that would be present.

Diet: Cottage Cheese and Rice

Species: Dog
Life Stage: Adult
Special Conditions: Enteritis, inflammatory bowel disease, gastric motility disorders

Ingredient	Quantity	Measure
Cottage cheese, 2% fat	2	cup
Rice, white, long-grain, cooked	3	cup
Canola oil	5	tsp
Salt substitute (potassium chloride)	¾	tsp
Bone meal powder	1¾	tsp
Multivitamin & mineral tablet, kids complete	1	each
Zinc, 100 mg tablet	½	tablet
Kelp, 150 mcg iodine per tablet	3	tablet

Prepared weight (approximately) = 975 g
Total kcal as prepared = 1215 kcal
kcal/g prepared diet = 1.25 kcal/g diet

Nutrient	DM%[a]	As-Fed (g/100 g diet)	ME% (g/100 kcal)	% of total kcal
Protein	23	6.8	5.4	22
Fat	12	3.7	2.9	29
Carbohydrate	53	15.5	12.4	50
Fiber	0.6	0.2	0.2	—

[a]DM%, dry matter percent. If all the water was removed from this diet, this is the percentage of nutrient that would be present.

Diet: Whitefish and Couscous

Species: Dog
Life Stage: Adult
Special Conditions: Colitis, gastritis, gastric motility disorders

Ingredient	Quantity	Measure
Whitefish, fillet, cooked	3	ounces
Couscous, cooked	3	cup
Canola oil	1	tbsp
Salt substitute (potassium chloride)	½	tsp
Bone meal powder	1¾	tsp
Salt, iodized (sodium chloride)	⅜	tsp
Multivitamin & mineral tablet, kids complete	1	each
Zinc, 100 mg tablet	½	tablet
Kelp, 150 mcg iodine per tablet	2	tablet

Prepared weight (approximately) = 592 g
Total kcal as prepared = 802 kcal
kcal/g prepared diet = 1.35 kcal/g diet

Nutrient	DM%[a]	As-Fed (g/100 g diet)	ME% (g/100 kcal)	% of total kcal
Protein	19	6.5	4.8	19
Fat	11	3.6	2.6	26
Carbohydrate	57	18.6	13.8	55
Fiber	3.4	1.1	0.8	

[a]DM%, dry matter percent. If all the water was removed from this diet, this is the percentage of nutrient that would be present.

Diet: Rabbit and Potato

Species: Dog
Life Stage: Adult
Special Conditions: Inflammatory bowel disease, gastric motility disorders

Ingredient	Quantity	Measure
Rabbit, domestic, cooked	4	ounce
Potatoes, diced, cooked	3	cup
Canola oil	4	tsp
Bone meal powder	2	tsp
Salt, iodized (sodium chloride)	1	tsp
Multivitamin & mineral tablet, kids complete	1	each
Zinc, 100 mg tablet	½	tablet

Prepared weight (approximately) = 614 g
Total kcal as prepared = 800 kcal
kcal/g prepared diet = 1.30 kcal/g diet

Nutrient	DM%[a]	As-Fed (g/100 g diet)	ME% (g/100 kcal)	% of total kcal
Protein	22	6.8	5.2	20
Fat	15	4.6	3.5	33
Carbohydrate	51	15.5	11.9	45
Fiber	4.5	1.4	1.0	—

[a]DM%, dry matter percent. If all the water was removed from this diet, this is the percentage of nutrient that would be present.

Diet: Pork and Rice

Species: Dog
Life Stage: Adult
Special Conditions: Inflammatory bowel disease, gastric motility disorders

Ingredient	Quantity	Measure
Pork loin, broiled	6	ounce
Rice, white, long-grain, cooked	3	cup
Canola oil	4	tsp
Salt substitute (potassium chloride)	¾	tsp
Bone meal powder	2	tsp
Salt, iodized (sodium chloride)	1	tsp
Multivitamin & mineral tablet, kids complete	1	each
Zinc, 100 mg tablet	½	tablet

Prepared weight (approximately) = 681 g
Total kcal as prepared = 1121 kcal
kcal/g prepared diet = 1.65 kcal/g diet

Nutrient	DM%[a]	As-Fed (g/100 g diet)	ME% (g/100 kcal)	% of total kcal
Protein	23	8.5	5.3	21
Fat	14	5.2	3.2	31
Carbohydrate	54	19.8	12.2	48
Fiber	0.8	0.3	0.2	—

[a]DM%, dry matter percent. If all the water was removed from this diet, this is the percentage of nutrient that would be present.

Diet: Salmon and Couscous

Species: Dog
Lifestage: Adult
Special Conditions: Inflammatory bowel disease, gastric motility disorders

Ingredient	Quantity	Measure
Salmon, Atlantic, fillet, baked/broiled	4	ounces
Couscous, cooked	3	cup
Canola oil	4	tsp
Salt substitute (potassium chloride)	½	tsp
Bone meal powder	2	tsp
Salt, iodized (sodium chloride)	1	tsp
Multivitamin & mineral tablet, kids complete	1	each
Zinc, 100 mg tablet	½	tablet

Prepared weight (approximately) = 620 g
Total kcal as prepared = 903 kcal
kcal/g prepared diet = 1.46 kcal/g diet

Nutrient	DM%[a]	As-Fed (g/100 g diet)	ME% (g/100 kcal)	% of total kcal
Protein	22	7.5	5.2	21
Fat	14	4.6	3.2	31
Carbohydrate	52	17.8	12.2	49
Fiber	3.1	1.1	0.7	—

[a]DM%, dry matter percent. If all the water was removed from this diet, this is the percentage of nutrient that would be present.

Diet: Chicken and Rice

Species: Dog
Life Stage: Adult
Special Conditions: Short bowel syndrome, small intestinal bacterial overgrowth, exocrine pancreatic insufficiency, gastric motility disorders, colitis, inflammatory bowel disease, gastritis

Ingredient	Quantity	Measure
Chicken, breast, without skin, cooked	4	ounces
Rice, white, long-grain, cooked	2	cup
Beans, red kidney, canned, drained	2	cup
Canola oil	7	tsp
Salt substitute (potassium chloride)	1	tsp
Bone meal powder	2½	tsp
Salt, iodized (sodium chloride)	1¾	tsp
Multivitamin & mineral tablet, kids complete	2	each
Zinc, 100 mg tablet	½	tablet

Prepared weight (approximately) = 1001 g
Total kcal as prepared = 1499 kcal
kcal/g prepared diet = 1.50 kcal/g diet

Nutrient	DM%[a]	As-Fed (g/100 g diet)	ME% (g/100 kcal)	% of total kcal
Protein	23	8.1	5.4	21
Fat	11	4.0	2.7	26
Carbohydrate	56	20.1	13.4	53
Fiber	13.0	4.7	3.1	—

[a]DM%, dry matter percent. If all the water was removed from this diet, this is the percentage of nutrient that would be present.

Diet: Chicken and Quinoa

Species: Dog
Life Stage: Adult
Special Conditions: Colitis, skin conditions

Ingredient	Quantity	Measure
Chicken, breast, without skin, cooked	5	ounces
Quinoa, cooked	3	cup
Canola oil	5	tsp
Salt substitute (potassium chloride)	½	tsp
Bone meal powder	1¾	tsp
Salt, iodized (sodium chloride)	⅜	tsp
Multivitamin & mineral tablet, kids complete	1	each
Zinc, 100 mg tablet	½	tablet
Kelp, 150 mcg iodine per tablet	3	tablet

Prepared weight (approximately) = 747 g
Total kcal as prepared = 1110 kcal
kcal/g prepared diet = 1.49 kcal/g diet

Nutrient	DM%[a]	As-Fed (g/100 g diet)	ME% (g/100 kcal)	% of total kcal
Protein	27	9.2	6.2	24
Fat	15	5.2	3.5	34
Carbohydrate	46	16.0	10.7	42
Fiber	6.0	2.1	1.4	—

[a]DM%, dry matter percent. If all the water was removed from this diet, this is the percentage of nutrient that would be present.

Diet: Pork and Barley

Species: Dog
Life Stage: Adult
Special Conditions: Colitis

Ingredient	Quantity	Measure
Pork loin, broiled	8	ounces
Barley, pearled, cooked	3	cup
Canola oil	4	tsp
Salt substitute (potassium chloride)	¾	tsp
Bone meal powder	2	tsp
Salt, iodized (sodium chloride)	⅜	tsp
Multivitamin & mineral tablet, kids complete	1	each
Zinc, 100 mg tablet	½	tablet
Kelp, 150 mcg iodine per tablet	2	tablet

Prepared weight (approximately) = 741 g
Total kcal as prepared = 1195 kcal
kcal/g prepared diet = 1.61 kcal/g diet

Nutrient	DM%[a]	As-Fed (g/100 g diet)	ME% (g/100 kcal)	% of total kcal
Protein	26	9.6	5.9	23
Fat	15	5.6	3.5	33
Carbohydrate	49	18.1	11.2	44
Fiber	6.5	2.4	1.5	—

[a]DM%, dry matter percent. If all the water was removed from this diet, this is the percentage of nutrient that would be present.

Diet: Tuna and Rice

Species: Dog
Life Stage: Adult
Special Conditions: Colitis, exocrine pancreatic insufficiency, skin conditions

Ingredient	Quantity	Measure
Tuna, with water, canned, drained	6	ounces
Rice, white, long-grain, cooked	2	cup
Canola oil	1	tbsp
Salt substitute (potassium chloride)	½	tsp
Bone meal powder	1¾	tsp
Salt, iodized (sodium chloride)	⅛	tsp
Multivitamin & mineral tablet, kids complete	1	each
Zinc, 100 mg tablet	½	tablet
Kelp, 150 mcg iodine per tablet	2	tablet

Prepared weight (approximately) = 521 g
Total kcal as prepared = 756 kcal
kcal/g prepared diet = 1.45 kcal/g diet

Nutrient	DM%[a]	As-Fed (g/100 g diet)	ME% (g/100 kcal)	% of total kcal
Protein	27	9.3	6.4	26
Fat	11	3.8	2.6	26
Carbohydrate	50	17.3	11.9	48
Fiber	0.7	0.2	0.2	—

[a]DM%, dry matter percent. If all the water was removed from this diet, this is the percentage of nutrient that would be present.

Diet: Tofu and Rice

Species: Dog
Life Stage: Adult
Special Conditions: Colitis, inflammatory bowel disease, gastric motility disorders

Ingredient	Quantity	Measure
Tofu, extra firm	12	ounces
Rice, white, long-grain, cooked	2	cup
Canola oil	1	tsp
Salt substitute (potassium chloride)	¾	tsp
Bone meal powder	1¾	tsp
Salt, iodized (sodium chloride)	⅜	tsp
Multivitamin & mineral tablet, kids complete	1	each
Zinc, 100 mg tablet	½	tablet
Kelp, 150 mcg iodine per tablet	2	tablet

Prepared weight (approximately) = 684 g
Total kcal as prepared = 766 kcal
kcal/g prepared diet = 1.12 kcal/g diet

Nutrient	DM%[a]	As-Fed (g/100 g diet)	ME% (g/100 kcal)	% of total kcal
Protein	22	6.2	5.5	21
Fat	13	3.7	3.3	31
Carbohydrate	51	14.2	12.7	48
Fiber	1.4	0.4	0.3	—

[a]DM%, dry matter percent. If all the water was removed from this diet, this is the percentage of nutrient that would be present.

Diet: Turkey and Pasta

Species: Dog
Life Stage: Adult
Special Conditions: Lymphangiectasia, protein-losing enteropathy, gastric motility disorders

Ingredient	Quantity	Measure
Turkey, white meat, without skin, cooked	6	ounces
Pasta, enriched, cooked	3	cup
Canola oil	1	tsp
Salt substitute (potassium chloride)	½	tsp
Bone meal powder	1½	tsp
Salt, iodized (sodium chloride)	1	tsp
Multivitamin & mineral tablet, kids complete	1	each
Zinc, 100 mg tablet	½	tablet

Prepared weight (approximately) = 610 g
Total kcal as prepared = 976 kcal
kcal/g prepared diet = 1.60 kcal/g diet

Nutrient	DM%[a]	As-Fed (g/100 g diet)	ME% (g/100 kcal)	% of total kcal
Protein	32	12.3	7.7	31
Fat	6	2.3	1.4	14
Carbohydrate	55	21.4	13.4	54
Fiber	3.2	1.2	0.8	—

[a]DM%, dry matter percent. If all the water was removed from this diet, this is the percentage of nutrient that would be present.

Diet: Whitefish and Pasta

Species: Dog
Life Stage: Adult
Special Conditions: Lymphangiectasia, protein-losing enteropathy, gastric motility disorders

Ingredient	Quantity	Measure
Whitefish, fillet, baked or broiled	8	ounces
Pasta, enriched, cooked	3	cup
Salt substitute (potassium chloride)	½	tsp
Bone meal powder	1¾	tsp
Salt, iodized (sodium chloride)	1¼	tsp
Multivitamin & mineral tablet, kids complete	1	each
Zinc, 100 mg tablet	½	tablet

Prepared weight (approximately) = 664 g
Total kcal as prepared = 1058 kcal
kcal/g prepared diet = 1.59 kcal/g diet

Nutrient	DM%[a]	As-Fed (g/100 g diet)	ME% (g/100 kcal)	% of total kcal
Protein	31	12.0	7.5	31
Fat	8	3.2	2.0	19
Carbohydrate	51	19.7	12.4	50
Fiber	3.0	1.1	0.7	—

[a]DM%, dry matter percent. If all the water was removed from this diet, this is the percentage of nutrient that would be present.

Diet: Lamb and Rice

Species: Dog
Life Stage: Adult
Special Conditions: Gastritis

Ingredient	Quantity	Measure
Lamb, cooked	4	ounces
Rice, white, long-grain, cooked	3	cup
Canola oil	1	tsp
Salt substitute (potassium chloride)	¾	tsp
Bone meal powder	1¾	tsp
Salt, iodized (sodium chloride)	⅜	tsp
Multivitamin & mineral tablet, kids complete	1	each
Zinc, 100 mg tablet	½	tablet
Kelp, 150 mcg iodine per tablet	2	tablet

Prepared weight (approximately) = 616 g
Total kcal as prepared = 969 kcal
kcal/g prepared diet = 1.57 kcal/g diet

Nutrient	DM%[a]	As-Fed (g/100 g diet)	ME% (g/100 kcal)	% of total kcal
Protein	18.3	6.8	4.3	17
Fat	11.6	4.3	2.7	27
Carbohydrate	59.0	21.9	13.9	56
Fiber	0.8	0.3	0.2	—

[a]DM%, dry matter percent. If all the water was removed from this diet, this is the percentage of nutrient that would be present.

Diet: Chicken and Rice

Species: Dog
Life Stage: Adult
Special Conditions: Low sodium for heart conditions

Ingredient	Quantity	Measure
Chicken, breast, without skin, cooked	4	ounces
Rice, white, long-grain, cooked	3	cup
Canola oil	4	tsp
Kelp tablets, 150 mcg iodine per tablet	2	each
Salt substitute (potassium chloride)	½	tsp
Bone meal powder	1¾	tsp
Salt, iodized (sodium chloride)	⅛	tsp
Multivitamin & mineral tablet, kids complete	1	each
Zinc, 100 mg tablet	½	tablet

Prepared weight (approximately) = 627 g
Total kcal as prepared = 973 kcal
kcal/g prepared diet = 1.55 kcal/g diet

Nutrient	DM%[a]	As-Fed (g/100 g diet)	ME% (g/100 kcal)	% of total kcal
Protein	21	7.6	4.9	20
Fat	10	3.8	2.5	24
Carbohydrate	59	21.5	13.8	56
Fiber	0.0	0.30	0.2	
Sodium	0.17	0.06	0.04	—

[a]DM%, dry matter percent. If all the water was removed from this diet, this is the percentage of nutrient that would be present.

Diet: Ground Beef and Potato

Species: Dog
Life Stage: Adult
Special Conditions: Low sodium for heart conditions

Ingredient	Quantity	Measure
Ground beef, 10% fat, cooked	6	ounces
Potatoes, diced, cooked	3	cup
Canola oil	2	tsp
Kelp tablets, 150 mcg iodine per tablet	2	each
Salt substitute (potassium chloride)	½	tsp
Bone meal powder	2	tsp
Salt, iodized (sodium chloride)	⅛	tsp
Multivitamin & mineral tablet, kids complete	1	each
Zinc, 100 mg tablet	½	tablet

Prepared weight (approximately) = 669 g
Total kcal as prepared = 885 kcal
kcal/g prepared diet = 1.32 kcal/g diet

Nutrient	DM%[a]	As-Fed (g/100 g diet)	ME% (g/100 kcal)	% of total kcal
Protein	27	8.5	6.5	25
Fat	14	4.5	3.4	33
Carbohydrate	46	14.2	10.8	42
Fiber	4.0	1.3	1.0	—
Sodium	0.22	0.07	0.05	—

[a]DM%, dry matter percent. If all the water was removed from this diet, this is the percentage of nutrient that would be present.

Diet: Tofu and Pasta

Species: Dog
Life Stage: Adult
Special Conditions: Low sodium for heart conditions, skin conditions

Ingredient	Quantity	Measure
Tofu, extra firm	12	ounces
Pasta, enriched, cooked	2	cup
Canola oil	2	tsp
Kelp tablets, 150 mcg iodine per tablet	2	each
Salt substitute (potassium chloride)	½	tsp
Bone meal powder	1½	tsp
Salt, iodized (sodium chloride)	⅛	tsp
Multivitamin & mineral tablet, kids complete	1	each
Zinc, 100 mg tablet	½	tablet
Vitamin B_{12} liquid, 1000 mcg B_{12} per mL	0.25	mL

Prepared weight (approximately) = 650 g
Total kcal as prepared = 839 kcal
kcal/g prepared diet = 1.29 kcal/g diet

Nutrient	DM%[a]	As-Fed (g/100 g diet)	ME% (g/100 kcal)	% of total kcal
Protein	25	7.7	6.0	23
Fat	16	4.9	3.8	25
Carbohydrate	47	14.5	11.2	42
Fiber	3.2	1.0	0.8	—
Sodium	0.16	0.05	0.04	—

[a]DM%, dry matter percent. If all the water was removed from this diet, this is the percentage of nutrient that would be present.

Diet: Pork and Sweet Potato

Species: Dog
Life Stage: Adult
Special Conditions: Low sodium for heart conditions, esophagitis, skin conditions

Ingredient	Quantity	Measure
Pork loin, broiled	4	ounces
Sweet potatoes, cooked	½	cup
Potatoes, white, cooked	1½	cup
Canola oil	2	tsp
Kelp tablets, 150 mcg iodine per tablet	1	each
Bone meal powder	1½	tsp
Multivitamin & mineral tablet, kids complete	1	each
Zinc, 100 mg tablet	½	tablet

Prepared weight (approximately) = 469 g
Total kcal as prepared = 603 kcal
kcal/g prepared diet = 1.29 kcal/g diet

Nutrient	DM%[a]	As-Fed (g/100 g diet)	ME% (g/100 kcal)	% of total kcal
Protein	26	7.8	6.1	24
Fat	14	4.3	3.3	32
Carbohydrate	49	14.7	11.4	44
Fiber	5.3	1.6	1.2	—
Sodium	0.07	0.02	0.02	—

[a]DM%, dry matter percent. If all the water was removed from this diet, this is the percentage of nutrient that would be present.

Diet: Whitefish and Barley

Species: Dog
Life Stage: Adult
Special Conditions: Low sodium for heart conditions

Ingredient	Quantity	Measure
Whitefish, baked/broiled	6	ounces
Barley, pearled, cooked	3	cup
Canola oil	1	tbsp
Kelp tablets, 150 mcg iodine per tablet	2	each
Salt substitute (potassium chloride)	¼	tsp
Bone meal powder	1½	tsp
Salt, iodized (sodium chloride)	⅛	tsp
Multivitamin & mineral tablet, kids complete	1	each
Zinc, 100 mg tablet	½	tablet

Prepared weight (approximately) = 674 g
Total kcal as prepared = 999 kcal
kcal/g prepared diet = 1.48 kcal/g diet

Nutrient	DM%[a]	As-Fed (g/100 g diet)	ME% (g/100 kcal)	% of total kcal
Protein	22	7.8	5.2	20
Fat	12	4.3	2.9	27
Carbohydrate	56	19.9	134.0	52
Fiber	7.5	2.7	1.8	—
Sodium	0.17	0.06	0.04	—

[a]DM%, dry matter percent. If all the water was removed from this diet, this is the percentage of nutrient that would be present.

Diet: Lamb and Pasta

Species: Dog
Life Stage: Adult
Special Conditions: Low sodium for heart conditions

Ingredient	Quantity	Measure
Lamb, cooked	4	ounces
Pasta, enriched, cooked	3	cup
Canola oil	1½	tsp
Kelp tablets, 150 mcg iodine per tablet	2	each
Salt substitute (potassium chloride)	½	tsp
Bone meal powder	1¾	tsp
Salt, iodized (sodium chloride)	⅛	tsp
Multivitamin & mineral tablet, kids complete	1	each
Zinc, 100 mg tablet	½	tablet

Prepared weight (approximately) = 561 g
Total kcal as prepared = 1037 kcal
kcal/g prepared diet = 1.85 kcal/g diet

Nutrient	DM%[a]	As-Fed (g/100 g diet)	ME% (g/100 kcal)	% of total kcal
Protein	22	9.5	5.1	20
Fat	13	5.6	3.0	29
Carbohydrate	55	23.3	12.6	50
Fiber	3.2	1.4	0.7	—
Sodium	0.16	0.07	0.04	—

[a]DM%, dry matter percent. If all the water was removed from this diet, this is the percentage of nutrient that would be present.

Diet: Chicken and Rice

Species: Dog
Life Stage: Puppy, adult
Special Conditions: Low sodium for heart conditions. This diet is NOT complete and balanced for a puppy (low sodium) and should only be fed under the supervision of your veterinarian.

Ingredient	Quantity	Measure
Chicken, breast, without skin, cooked	10	ounces
Rice, white, long-grain, cooked	3	cup
Canola oil	3	tbsp
Kelp tablets, 150 mcg iodine per tablet	3	each
Salt substitute (potassium chloride)	¾	tsp
Bone meal powder	5	tsp
Salt, iodized (sodium chloride)	⅛	tsp
Multivitamin & mineral tablet, kids complete	1	each
Zinc, 100 mg tablet	½	tablet

Prepared weight (approximately) = 836 g
Total kcal as prepared = 1460 kcal
kcal/g prepared diet = 1.75 kcal/g diet

Nutrient	DM%[a]	As-Fed (g/100 g diet)	ME% (g/100 kcal)	% of total kcal
Protein	31	12.0	6.9	28
Fat	16	6.4	3.7	36
Carbohydrate	41	16.1	9.2	37
Fiber	0.6	0.23	0.1	—
Sodium	0.16	0.06	0.04	—

[a]DM%, dry matter percent. If all the water was removed from this diet, this is the percentage of nutrient that would be present.

Diet: Ground Beef and Potato

Species: Dog
Life Stage: Puppy, adult
Special Conditions: Low sodium for heart conditions. This diet is NOT complete and balanced for a puppy (low sodium) and should only be fed under the supervision of your veterinarian.

Ingredient	Quantity	Measure
Ground beef, 10% fat, cooked	12	ounces
Potatoes, diced, cooked	3	cup
Canola oil	1	tbsp
Kelp tablets, 150 mcg iodine per tablet	3	each
Salt substitute (potassium chloride)	½	tsp
Bone meal powder	4	tsp
Salt, iodized (sodium chloride)	⅛	tsp
Multivitamin & mineral tablet, kids complete	1	each
Zinc, 100 mg tablet	½	tablet

Prepared weight (approximately) = 855 g
Total kcal as prepared = 1317 kcal
kcal/g prepared diet = 1.54 kcal/g diet

Nutrient	DM%[a]	As-Fed (g/100 g diet)	ME% (g/100 kcal)	% of total kcal
Protein	36	12.4	8.0	31
Fat	19	6.5	4.2	40
Carbohydrate	32	11.1	7.2	28
Fiber	2.9	1.0	0.6	—
Sodium	0.21	0.07	0.05	—

[a]DM%, dry matter percent. If all the water was removed from this diet, this is the percentage of nutrient that would be present.

Diet: Chicken and Rice

Species: Dog
Life Stage: Adult
Special Conditions: Liver disease. This diet should be used under the supervision of your veterinarian.

Ingredient	Quantity	Measure
Chicken, breast, without skin, cooked	5	ounce
Rice, white, long-grain, cooked	2	cup
Broccoli, chopped, cooked	2	cup
Canola oil	7	tsp
Salt substitute (potassium chloride)	¼	tsp
Bone meal powder	2	tsp
Salt, iodized (sodium chloride)	⅛	tsp
Multivitamin & mineral tablet, kids complete	1	each
Zinc, 100 mg tablet	½	tablet
Arginine powder, 2.5 g per tsp	¼	tsp
Kelp, 150 mcg iodine per tablet	2	tablet

Prepared weight (approximately) = 824 g
Total kcal as prepared = 1047 kcal
kcal/g prepared diet = 1.27 kcal/g diet

Nutrient	DM%[a]	As-Fed (g/100 g diet)	ME% (g/100 kcal)	% of total kcal
Protein	25	7.3	5.7	22
Fat	17	4.8	3.8	36
Carbohydrate	48	13.6	10.7	42
Fiber	4.9	1.4	1.1	—
Arginine	2.0	0.56	0.44	—

[a]DM%, dry matter percent. If all the water was removed from this diet, this is the percentage of nutrient that would be present.

Diet: Chicken and Pasta

Species: Dog
Life Stage: Adult
Special Conditions: Liver disease. This diet should be used under the supervision of your veterinarian.

Ingredient	Quantity	Measure
Chicken, breast, without skin, cooked	6	ounce
Pasta, enriched, cooked	2	cup
Peas, frozen, cooked	2	cup
Canola oil	8	tsp
Salt substitute (potassium chloride)	¾	tsp
Bone meal powder	2	tsp
Salt, iodized (sodium chloride)	⅛	tsp
Multivitamin & mineral tablet, kids complete	1	each
Zinc, 100 mg tablet	½	tablet
Arginine powder, 2.5 g per tsp	¼	tsp
Kelp, 150 mcg iodine per tablet	3	tablet

Prepared weight (approximately) = 836 g
Total kcal as prepared = 1307 kcal
kcal/g prepared diet = 1.56 kcal/g diet

Nutrient	DM%[a]	As-Fed (g/100 g diet)	ME% (g/100 kcal)	% of total kcal
Protein	29	10.2	6.5	26
Fat	16	5.6	3.6	34
Carbohydrate	45	15.9	10.2	40
Fiber	7.6	2.7	1.7	—
Arginine	2.0	0.68	0.43	—

[a]DM%, dry matter percent. If all the water was removed from this diet, this is the percentage of nutrient that would be present.

Diet: Ground Beef and Pasta

Species: Dog
Life Stage: Adult
Special Conditions: Liver disease. This diet should be used under the supervision of your veterinarian.

Ingredient	Quantity	Measure
Ground beef, 10% fat, cooked	5	ounce
Pasta, enriched, cooked	2	cup
Broccoli, chopped, cooked	1½	cup
Canola oil	1	tbsp
Salt substitute (potassium chloride)	¼	tsp
Bone meal powder	2	tsp
Multivitamin & mineral tablet, kids complete	1	each
Zinc, 100 mg tablet	½	tablet
Arginine powder, 2.5 g per tsp	¼	tsp
Kelp, 150 mcg iodine per tablet	2	tablet

Prepared weight (approximately) = 690 g
Total kcal as prepared = 978 kcal
kcal/g prepared diet = 1.42 kcal/g diet

Nutrient	DM%[a]	As-Fed (g/100 g diet)	ME% (g/100 kcal)	% of total kcal
Protein	28	9.0	6.4	25
Fat	15	5.0	3.5	33
Carbohydrate	47	15.1	10.7	42
Fiber	5.7	1.8	1.3	—
Arginine	2.0	0.61	0.43	—

[a]DM%, dry matter percent. If all the water was removed from this diet, this is the percentage of nutrient that would be present.

Diet: Ground Beef and Potato

Species: Dog
Life Stage: Adult
Special Conditions: Liver disease. This diet should be used under the supervision of your veterinarian.

Ingredient	Quantity	Measure
Ground beef, 10% fat, cooked	5	ounce
Potatoes, diced, cooked	2	cup
Green beans, cooked	½	cup
Canola oil	5	tsp
Salt substitute (potassium chloride)	⅛	tsp
Bone meal powder	2	tsp
Salt, iodized (sodium chloride)	⅛	tsp
Multivitamin & mineral tablet, kids complete	1	each
Zinc, 100 mg tablet	½	tablet
Arginine powder, 2.5 g per tsp	¼	tsp
Kelp, 150 mcg iodine per tablet	2	tablet

Prepared weight (approximately) = 599 g
Total kcal as prepared = 914 kcal
kcal/g prepared diet = 1.53 kcal/g diet

Nutrient	DM%[a]	As-Fed (g/100 g diet)	ME% (g/100 kcal)	% of total kcal
Protein	26	8.9	5.8	23
Fat	20	6.9	4.5	42
Carbohydrate	41	13.9	9.1	35
Fiber	6.6	2.2	1.4	—
Arginine	2.0	0.66	0.43	—

[a]DM%, dry matter percent. If all the water was removed from this diet, this is the percentage of nutrient that would be present.

Diet: Eggs and Rice

Species: Dog
Life Stage: Adult
Special Conditions: Liver disease. This diet should be used under the supervision of your veterinarian.

Ingredient	Quantity	Measure
Eggs, large, hard-boiled	8	each
Rice, white, long-grain, cooked	1½	cup
Broccoli, chopped, cooked	1½	cup
Canola oil	1	tsp
Salt substitute (potassium chloride)	¼	tsp
Bone meal powder	2	tsp
Multivitamin & mineral tablet, kids complete	1	each
Zinc, 100 mg tablet	½	tablet
Arginine powder, 2.5 g per tsp	¼	tsp
Kelp, 150 mcg iodine per tablet	2	tablet

Prepared weight (approximately) = 896 g
Total kcal as prepared = 1055 kcal
kcal/g prepared diet = 1.18 kcal/g diet

Nutrient	DM%[a]	As-Fed (g/100 g diet)	ME% (g/100 kcal)	% of total kcal
Protein	27	6.9	5.9	23
Fat	21	5.4	4.6	44
Carbohydrate	39	9.9	8.4	33
Fiber	3.8	0.97	0.8	—
Arginine	2.0	0.52	0.44	—

[a]DM%, dry matter percent. If all the water was removed from this diet, this is the percentage of nutrient that would be present.

Diet: Tofu and Rice

Species: Dog
Life Stage: Adult
Special Conditions: Liver disease. This diet should be used under the supervision of your veterinarian.

Ingredient	Quantity	Measure
Tofu, extra firm	16	ounce
Rice, white, long-grain, cooked	1½	cup
Broccoli, chopped, cooked	1	cup
Canola oil	4	tsp
Salt substitute (potassium chloride)	¼	tsp
Bone meal powder	2	tsp
Salt, iodized (sodium chloride)	⅛	tsp
Multivitamin & mineral tablet, kids complete	1	each
Zinc, 100 mg tablet	½	tablet
Arginine powder, 2.5 g per tsp	¼	tsp
Kelp, 150 mcg iodine per tablet	2	tablet
Vitamin B_{12} liquid, 1000 mcg B_{12} per mL	0.25	mL

Prepared weight (approximately) = 887 g
Total kcal as prepared = 945 kcal
kcal/g prepared diet = 1.06 kcal/g diet

Nutrient	DM%[a]	As-Fed (g/100 g diet)	ME% (g/100 kcal)	% of total kcal
Protein	25	6.2	5.8	21
Fat	21	5.2	4.9	44
Carbohydrate	41	9.9	9.3	34
Fiber	3.6	0.89	0.8	—
Arginine	2.0	0.50	0.47	—

[a]DM%, dry matter percent. If all the water was removed from this diet, this is the percentage of nutrient that would be present.

Diet: Tofu and Pasta

Species: Dog
Life Stage: Adult
Special Conditions: Liver disease. This diet should be used under the supervision of your veterinarian.

Ingredient	Quantity	Measure
Tofu, extra firm	16	ounce
Pasta, enriched, cooked	1½	cup
Canola oil	4	tsp
Salt substitute (potassium chloride)	½	tsp
Salt, iodized (sodium chloride)	⅛	tsp
Bone meal powder	1¾	tsp
Multivitamin & mineral tablet, kids complete	1	each
Vitamin B_{12}, 1000 mcg B_{12} per mL	0.25	mL
Zinc, 100 mg tablet	½	tablet
Arginine powder, 2.5 g per tsp	¼	tsp
Kelp, 150 mcg iodine per tablet	2	tablet

Prepared weight (approximately) = 704 g
Total kcal as prepared = 914 kcal
kcal/g prepared diet = 1.30 kcal/g diet

Nutrient	DM%[a]	As-Fed (g/100 g diet)	ME% (g/100 kcal)	% of total kcal
Protein	28	8.1	6.3	23
Fat	23	6.7	5.2	46
Carbohydrate	37	10.6	8.2	30
Fiber	2.7	0.8	0.6	—
Arginine	2.0	0.57	0.44	—

[a]DM%, dry matter percent. If all the water was removed from this diet, this is the percentage of nutrient that would be present.

Diet: Chicken and Rice

Species: Dog
Lifestage: Adult
Special Conditions: Liver disease (hepatic encephalopathy). This diet
should be used under the supervision of your veterinarian.

Ingredient	Quantity	Measure
Chicken, breast, without skin, cooked	2	ounce
Rice, white, long-grain, cooked	2	cup
Broccoli, chopped, cooked	1	cup
Canola oil	7	tsp
Salt substitute (potassium chloride)	½	tsp
Bone meal powder	2	tsp
Salt, iodized (sodium chloride)	⅛	tsp
Multivitamin & mineral tablet, kids complete	1	each
Zinc, 100 mg tablet	½	tablet
Arginine powder, 2.5 g per tsp	¼	tsp
Kelp, 150 mcg iodine per tablet	2	tablet

Prepared weight (approximately) = 584 g
Total kcal as prepared = 852 kcal
kcal/g prepared diet = 1.46 kcal/g diet

Nutrient	DM%[a]	As-Fed (g/100 g diet)	ME% (g/100 kcal)	% of total kcal
Protein	16	5.1	3.5	14
Fat	19	6.2	4.3	40
Carbohydrate	53	17.4	11.9	46
Fiber	3.4	1.1	0.8	—
Arginine	1.4	0.46	0.32	—

[a]DM%, dry matter percent. If all the water was removed from this diet, this is the
percentage of nutrient that would be present.

Diet: Tofu and Rice

Species: Dog
Life Stage: Adult
Special Conditions: Liver disease (hepatic encephalopathy). This diet should be used under the supervision of your veterinarian.

Ingredient	Quantity	Measure
Tofu, extra firm	8	ounce
Rice, white, long-grain, cooked	2	cup
Canola oil	7	tsp
Salt substitute (potassium chloride)	½	tsp
Bone meal powder	2	tsp
Salt, iodized (sodium chloride)	⅛	tsp
Multivitamin & mineral tablet, kids complete	1	each
Zinc, 100 mg tablet	½	tablet
Arginine powder, 2.5 g per tsp	½	tsp
Kelp, 150 mcg iodine per tablet	2	tablet
Vitamin B_{12} liquid, 1000 mcg B_{12} per mL	0.25	mL

Prepared weight (approximately) = 598 g
Total kcal as prepared = 910 kcal
kcal/g prepared diet = 1.52 kcal/g diet

Nutrient	DM%[a]	As-Fed (g/100 g diet)	ME% (g/100 kcal)	% of total kcal
Protein	16	5.2	3.4	13
Fat	24	7.8	5.1	47
Carbohydrate	48	15.8	10.4	40
Fiber	1.1	0.36	0.2	—
Arginine	1.8	0.58	0.38	—

[a]DM%, dry matter percent. If all the water was removed from this diet, this is the percentage of nutrient that would be present.

Diet: Tofu and Rice

Species: Dog
Life Stage: Adult
Special Conditions: Liver disease (diet has restricted copper). This diet should be used under the supervision of your veterinarian.

Ingredient	Quantity	Measure
Tofu, extra firm	16	ounce
Rice, white, long-grain, cooked	1½	cup
Canola oil	4	tsp
Salt substitute (potassium chloride)	½	tsp
Bone meal powder	2	tsp
Salt, iodized (sodium chloride)	⅛	tsp
Multivitamin & mineral tablet, kids complete	½	each
Zinc, 100 mg tablet	½	tablet
Iron, 18 mg iron per tablet	1	tablet
Arginine powder, 2.5 g per tsp	¼	tsp
Kelp, 150 mcg iodine per tablet	2	tablet
Vitamin B_{12} liquid, 1000 mcg B_{12} per mL	0.25	mL

Prepared weight (approximately) = 732 g
Total kcal as prepared = 888 kcal
kcal/g prepared diet = 1.21 kcal/g diet

Nutrient	DM%[a]	As-Fed (g/100 g diet)	ME% (g/100 kcal)	% of total kcal
Protein	26	7.0	5.8	21
Fat	23	6.3	5.2	47
Carbohydrate	38	10.4	8.6	32
Fiber	1.4	0.38	0.3	—
Arginine	2.1	0.57	0.47	—
Copper		0.28 mg	0.23 mg	—

[a]DM%, dry matter percent. If all the water was removed from this diet, this is the percentage of nutrient that would be present.

Diet: Chicken and Rice

Species: Dog
Life Stage: Adult
Special Conditions: Pancreatitis diet with low fat, exocrine pancreatic insufficiency, lymphangiectasia, protein-losing enteropathy

Ingredient	Quantity	Measure
Chicken, breast, without skin, cooked	4	ounce
Rice, white, long-grain, cooked	2	cup
Canola oil	2	tsp
Salt substitute (potassium chloride)	½	tsp
Bone meal powder	1½	tsp
Salt, iodized (sodium chloride)	½	tsp
Multivitamin & mineral tablet, kids complete	1	each
Zinc, 100 mg tablet	½	tablet

Prepared weight (approximately) = 451 g
Total kcal as prepared = 685 kcal
kcal/g prepared diet = 1.52 kcal/g diet

Nutrient	DM%[a]	As-Fed (g/100 g diet)	ME% (g/100 kcal)	% of total kcal
Protein	27	9.7	6.4	26
Fat	9	3.2	2.1	21
Carbohydrate	56	20.0	13.2	54
Fiber	0.8	0.3	0.2	—

[a]DM%, dry matter percent. If all the water was removed from this diet, this is the percentage of nutrient that would be present.

Diet: Cottage Cheese and Rice

Species: Dog
Life Stage: Adult
Special Conditions: Pancreatitis diet with low fat, exocrine pancreatic insufficiency, lymphangiectasia, protein-losing enteropathy

Ingredient	Quantity	Measure
Cottage cheese, 1% fat	1	cup
Rice, white, long-grain, cooked	3	cup
Canola oil	2	tsp
Salt substitute (potassium chloride)	¾	tsp
Bone meal powder	2	tsp
Salt, iodized (sodium chloride)	1	tsp
Multivitamin & mineral tablet, kids complete	1	each
Zinc, 100 mg tablet	½	tablet

Prepared weight (approximately) = 727 g
Total kcal as prepared = 866 kcal
kcal/g prepared diet = 1.19 kcal/g diet

Nutrient	DM%[a]	As-Fed (g/100 g diet)	ME% (g/100 kcal)	% of total kcal
Protein	19	5.6	4.7	19
Fat	6	1.8	1.5	15
Carbohydrate	65	19.4	16.3	66
Fiber	0.9	0.3	0.2	—

[a]DM%, dry matter percent. If all the water was removed from this diet, this is the percentage of nutrient that would be present.

Diet: Pork and Potato

Species: Dog
Life Stage: Adult
Special Conditions: Pancreatitis diet with low fat, lymphangiectasia, protein-losing enteropathy. This diet is NOT balanced and complete (low fat) and should only be used under the supervision of your veterinarian.

Ingredient	Quantity	Measure
Pork loin, broiled	5	ounce
Potatoes, diced, cooked	3	cup
Salt substitute (potassium chloride)	½	tsp
Bone meal powder	1½	tsp
Salt, iodized (sodium chloride)	¾	tsp
Multivitamin & mineral tablet, kids complete	1	each
Zinc, 100 mg tablet	½	tablet

Prepared weight (approximately) = 624 g
Total kcal as prepared = 691 kcal
kcal/g prepared diet = 1.11 kcal/g diet

Nutrient	DM%[a]	As-Fed (g/100 g diet)	ME% (g/100 kcal)	% of total kcal
Protein	27	7.4	6.7	27
Fat	8	2.2	2.0	19
Carbohydrate	55	15.3	13.8	55
Fiber	4.8	1.3	1.2	—

[a]DM%, dry matter percent. If all the water was removed from this diet, this is the percentage of nutrient that would be present.

Diet: Chicken and Rice

Species: Dog
Life Stage: Adult
Special Conditions: Pancreatitis diet with moderate fat, exocrine pancreatic insufficiency, skin conditions

Ingredient	Quantity	Measure
Chicken, breast, without skin, cooked	4	ounce
Rice, white, long-grain, cooked	2	cup
Canola oil	1	tbsp
Salt substitute (potassium chloride)	½	tsp
Bone meal powder	1¾	tsp
Salt, iodized (sodium chloride)	½	tsp
Multivitamin & mineral tablet, kids complete	1	each
Zinc, 100 mg tablet	½	tablet

Prepared weight (approximately) = 457 g
Total kcal as prepared = 726 kcal
kcal/g prepared diet = 1.59 kcal/g diet

Nutrient	DM%[a]	As-Fed (g/100 g diet)	ME% (g/100 kcal)	% of total kcal
Protein	26	9.6	6.0	24
Fat	11	4.2	2.6	26
Carbohydrate	54	19.7	12.4	50
Fiber	0.8	0.3	0.2	—

[a]DM%, dry matter percent. If all the water was removed from this diet, this is the percentage of nutrient that would be present.

Diet: Eggs and Rice

Species: Dog
Life Stage: Adult
Special Conditions: Pancreatitis diet with moderate fat, gastric motility disorders, exocrine pancreatic insufficiency

Ingredient	Quantity	Measure
Eggs, whole, large, hard-boiled	5	each
Rice, white, long-grain, cooked	2	cup
Salt substitute (potassium chloride)	½	tsp
Bone meal powder	2	tsp
Salt, iodized (sodium chloride)	¾	tsp
Multivitamin & mineral tablet, kids complete	1	each
Zinc, 100 mg tablet	½	tablet

Prepared weight (approximately) = 581 g
Total kcal as prepared = 802 kcal
kcal/g prepared diet = 1.38 kcal/g diet

Nutrient	DM%[a]	As-Fed (g/100 g diet)	ME% (g/100 kcal)	% of total kcal
Protein	22	6.9	5.0	20
Fat	15	4.7	3.4	33
Carbohydrate	52	16.0	11.2	47
Fiber	0.7	0.2	0.2	—

[a]DM%, dry matter percent. If all the water was removed from this diet, this is the percentage of nutrient that would be present.

Diet: Cottage Cheese and Rice

Species: Dog
Life Stage: Adult
Special Conditions: Pancreatitis diet with moderate fat, exocrine pancreatic insufficiency

Ingredient	Quantity	Measure
Cottage cheese, 1% fat	1½	cup
Rice, white, long-grain, cooked	3	cup
Canola oil	5	tsp
Salt substitute (potassium chloride)	¾	tsp
Bone meal powder	2	tsp
Salt, iodized (sodium chloride)	1	tsp
Multivitamin & mineral tablet, kids complete	1	each
Zinc, 100 mg tablet	½	tablet

Prepared weight (approximately) = 854 g
Total kcal as prepared = 1070 kcal
kcal/g prepared diet = 1.25 kcal/g diet

Nutrient	DM%[a]	As-Fed (g/100 g diet)	ME% (g/100 kcal)	% of total kcal
Protein	22	6.4	5.1	20
Fat	11	3.3	2.6	26
Carbohydrate	57	16.8	13.4	54
Fiber	0.8	0.2	0.2	—

[a]DM%, dry matter percent. If all the water was removed from this diet, this is the percentage of nutrient that would be present.

Diet: Pork and Potato

Species: Dog
Lifestage: Adult
Special Conditions: Pancreatitis diet with moderate fat, skin conditions

Ingredient	Quantity	Measure
Pork loin, broiled	5	ounce
Potatoes, diced, cooked	3	cup
Canola oil	1½	tsp
Salt substitute (potassium chloride)	½	tsp
Bone meal powder	1½	tsp
Salt, iodized (sodium chloride)	¾	tsp
Multivitamin & mineral tablet, kids complete	1	each
Zinc, 100 mg tablet	½	tablet

Prepared weight (approximately) = 631 g
Total kcal as prepared = 752 kcal
kcal/g prepared diet = 1.19 kcal/g diet

Nutrient	DM%[a]	As-Fed (g/100 g diet)	ME% (g/100 kcal)	% of total kcal
Protein	26	7.4	6.2	24
Fat	11	3.3	2.7	26
Carbohydrate	53	15.1	12.7	50
Fiber	4.7	1.3	1.1	

[a]DM%, dry matter percent. If all the water was removed from this diet, this is the percentage of nutrient that would be present.

Diet: Chicken and Rice

Species: Dog
Life Stage: Adult
Special Conditions: Renal disease (moderate protein, low sodium, low phosphorus). This diet is NOT complete and balanced and should only be used in dogs with renal failure under the supervision of your veterinarian.

Ingredient	Quantity	Measure
Chicken breast, skinless, cooked	3	ounce
Rice, white, long-grain, cooked	3	cup
Egg, large, hard-boiled	1	each
Canola oil	4	tsp
Salt substitute (potassium chloride)	½	tsp
Baking soda (calcium carbonate)	½	tsp
Salt, iodized (sodium chloride)	¼	tsp
Multivitamin & mineral tablet, kids complete	1	each
Zinc, 100 mg tablet	½	tablet

Prepared weight (approximately) = 636 g
Total kcal as prepared = 1003 kcal
kcal/g prepared diet = 1.58 kcal/g diet

Nutrient	DM%[a]	As-Fed (g/100 g diet)	ME% (g/100 kcal)	% of total kcal
Protein	21	7.1	4.5	18
Fat	13	4.4	2.8	28
Carbohydrate	62	21.2	13.5	54
Fiber	0.9	0.3	0.2	—
Phosphorus	0.2	0.09	0.05	—
Sodium	0.3	0.11	0.07	—

[a]DM%, dry matter percent. If all the water was removed from this diet, this is the percentage of nutrient that would be present.

Diet: Ground Beef and Rice

Species: Dog
Life Stage: Adult
Special Conditions: Renal disease (low phosphorus). This diet is NOT complete and balanced and should only be used in dogs with renal failure under the supervision of your veterinarian.

Ingredient	Quantity	Measure
Ground beef, 25% fat, cooked	4	ounce
Rice, white, long-grain, cooked	3	cup
Egg, large, hard-boiled	1	each
Canola oil	2	tsp
Salt substitute (potassium chloride)	½	tsp
Baking soda (calcium carbonate)	½	tsp
Salt, iodized (sodium chloride)	½	tsp
Multivitamin & mineral tablet, kids complete	1	each
Zinc, 100 mg tablet	½	tablet

Prepared weight (approximately) = 657 g
Total kcal as prepared = 1095 kcal
kcal/g prepared diet = 1.67 kcal/g diet

Nutrient	DM%[a]	As-Fed (g/100 g diet)	ME% (g/100 kcal)	% of total kcal
Protein	21	7.4	4.5	18
Fat	16	5.6	3.4	33
Carbohydrate	58	20.6	12.3	49
Fiber	0.8	0.3	0.2	—
Phosphorus	0.2	0.09	0.05	—
Sodium	0.6	0.21	0.12	—

[a]DM%, dry matter percent. If all the water was removed from this diet, this is the percentage of nutrient that would be present.

Diet: Salmon and Potato

Species: Dog
Life Stage: Adult
Special Conditions: Renal disease (moderate protein, low sodium, low phosphorus). This diet is NOT complete and balanced and should only be used in dogs with renal failure under the supervision of your veterinarian.

Ingredient	Quantity	Measure
Salmon, wild, fillet, baked or broiled	3	ounce
Potatoes, diced, cooked	3	cup
Canola oil	1	tbsp
Salt substitute (potassium chloride)	¼	tsp
Baking soda (calcium carbonate)	½	tsp
Salt, iodized (sodium chloride)	⅛	tsp
Multivitamin & mineral tablet, kids complete	1	each
Zinc, 100 mg tablet	½	tablet

Prepared weight (approximately) = 573 g
Total kcal as prepared = 690 kcal
kcal/g prepared diet = 1.20 kcal/g diet

Nutrient	DM%[a]	As-Fed (g/100 g diet)	ME% (g/100 kcal)	% of total kcal
Protein	19	5.3	4.4	17
Fat	13	3.7	3.1	29
Carbohydrate	59	16.6	13.8	54
Fiber	5.2	1.5	1.2	—
Phosphorus	0.3	0.08	0.07	—
Sodium	0.2	0.06	0.05	—

[a]DM%, dry matter percent. If all the water was removed from this diet, this is the percentage of nutrient that would be present.

Diet: Chicken and Potato

Species: Dog
Life Stage: Adult
Special Conditions: Renal disease (low protein, low sodium, low phosphorus). This diet is NOT complete and balanced and should only be used in dogs with renal failure under the supervision of your veterinarian.

Ingredient	Quantity	Measure
Chicken breast, skinless, cooked	2	ounce
Potatoes, cooked in skin, diced	4	cup
Canola oil	4	tsp
Salt substitute (potassium chloride)	½	tsp
Baking soda (calcium carbonate)	½	tsp
Salt, iodized (sodium chloride)	⅛	tsp
Multivitamin & mineral tablet, kids complete	½	each
Zinc, 100 mg tablet	½	tablet
Iron, 18 mg tablet	1	tablet
Vitamin B$_{12}$ liquid	0.25	mL

Prepared weight (approximately) = 707 g
Total kcal as prepared = 804 kcal
kcal/g prepared diet = 1.14 kcal/g diet

Nutrient	DM%[a]	As-Fed (g/100 g diet)	ME% (g/100 kcal)	% of total kcal
Protein	15	4.1	3.6	14
Fat	11	3.0	2.7	25
Carbohydrate	67	17.9	15.7	61
Fiber	5.9	1.6	1.4	—
Phosphorus	0.2	0.06	0.05	—
Sodium	0.2	0.05	0.04	—

[a]DM%, dry matter percent. If all the water was removed from this diet, this is the percentage of nutrient that would be present.

Diet: Ground Beef and Potato

Species: Dog
Life Stage: Adult
Special Conditions: Renal disease (low protein, low sodium, low phosphorus). This diet is NOT complete and balanced and should only be used in dogs with renal failure under the supervision of your veterinarian.

Ingredient	Quantity	Measure
Ground beef, 25% fat, cooked	2	ounce
Potatoes, diced, cooked	4	cup
Canola oil	4	tsp
Salt substitute (potassium chloride)	½	tsp
Baking soda (calcium carbonate)	½	tsp
Salt, iodized (sodium chloride)	⅛	tsp
Multivitamin & mineral tablet, kids complete	½	each
Zinc, 100 mg tablet	½	tablet
Iron, 18 mg iron per tablet	1	tablet

Prepared weight (approximately) = 707 g
Total kcal as prepared = 867 kcal
kcal/g prepared diet = 1.23 kcal/g diet

Nutrient	DM%[a]	As-Fed (g/100 g diet)	ME% (g/100 kcal)	% of total kcal
Protein	14	3.8	3.1	12
Fat	15	4.2	3.4	32
Carbohydrate	64	17.8	14.6	56
Fiber	5.7	1.6	1.3	—
Phosphorus	0.2	0.06	0.05	—
Sodium	0.2	0.05	0.04	—

[a]DM%, dry matter percent. If all the water was removed from this diet, this is the percentage of nutrient that would be present.

Diet: Ground Beef and Tapioca

Species: Dog
Life Stage: Adult
Special Conditions: Renal disease (low protein, low phosphorus). This diet is NOT complete and balanced and should only be used in dogs with renal failure under the supervision of your veterinarian.

Ingredient	Quantity	Measure
Ground beef, 25% fat, cooked	2	ounce
Tapioca pudding, fat-free snack cup	4	each
Canola oil	1	tbsp
Salt substitute (potassium chloride)	½	tsp
Bone meal powder	⅛	tsp
Multivitamin & mineral tablet, kids complete	½	each
Zinc, 100 mg tablet	½	tablet
Iron, 18 mg iron per tablet	1	tablet

Prepared weight (approximately) = 528 g
Total kcal as prepared = 683 kcal
kcal/g prepared diet = 1.29 kcal/g diet

Nutrient	DM%[a]	As-Fed (g/100 g diet)	ME% (g/100 kcal)	% of total kcal
Protein	13	3.6	2.8	11
Fat	17	4.6	3.6	35
Carbohydrate	64	17.5	13.6	54
Fiber	0.1	0.01	0.0	—
Phosphorus	0.2	0.04	0.03	—
Sodium	0.7	0.18	0.14	—

[a]DM%, dry matter percent. If all the water was removed from this diet, this is the percentage of nutrient that would be present.

Diet: Eggs and Rice

Species: Dog
Life Stage: Adult
Special Conditions: Renal disease (low protein, low sodium, low phosphorus). This diet is NOT complete and balanced and should only be used in dogs with renal failure under the supervision of your veterinarian.

Ingredient	Quantity	Measure
Eggs, hard-boiled	1	each
Rice, white, long-grain, cooked	3	cup
Canola oil	4	tsp
Salt substitute (potassium chloride)	½	tsp
Baking Soda (calcium carbonate)	¼	tsp
Salt, iodized (sodium chloride)	⅛	tsp
Multivitamin & mineral tablet, kids complete	1	each
Zinc, 100 mg tablet	½	tablet

Prepared weight (approximately) = 549 g
Total kcal as prepared = 863 kcal
kcal/g prepared diet = 1.57 kcal/g diet

Nutrient	DM%[a]	As-Fed (g/100 g diet)	ME% (g/100 kcal)	% of total kcal
Protein	10	3.5	2.2	9
Fat	13	4.6	2.9	28
Carbohydrate	72	24.6	15.7	63
Fiber	1.0	0.4	0.2	—
Phosphorus	0.2	0.06	0.04	—
Sodium	0.2	0.07	0.04	—

[a]DM%, dry matter percent. If all the water was removed from this diet, this is the percentage of nutrient that would be present.

Diet: Eggs and Potato

Species: Dog
Life Stage: Adult
Special Conditions: Renal disease (low protein, low sodium, low phosphorus). This diet is NOT complete and balanced and should only be used in dogs with renal failure under the supervision of your veterinarian.

Ingredient	Quantity	Measure
Eggs, hard-boiled	1	each
Potatoes, cooked in skin, diced	3	cup
Canola oil	4	tsp
Salt substitute (potassium chloride)	½	tsp
Baking soda (calcium carbonate)	¼	tsp
Salt, iodized (sodium chloride)	⅛	tsp
Multivitamin & mineral tablet, kids complete	½	each
Zinc, 100 mg tablet	½	tablet
Iron, 18 mg tablet	1	tablet

Prepared weight (approximately) = 543 g
Total kcal as prepared = 652 kcal
kcal/g prepared diet = 1.20 kcal/g diet

Nutrient	DM%[a]	As-Fed (g/100 g diet)	ME% (g/100 kcal)	% of total kcal
Protein	10	2.8	2.3	9
Fat	17	4.5	3.8	35
Carbohydrate	66	17.6	14.6	56
Fiber	5.8	1.6	1.3	—
Phosphorus	0.2	0.06	0.05	—
Sodium	0.3	0.07	0.06	—

[a]DM%, dry matter percent. If all the water was removed from this diet, this is the percentage of nutrient that would be present.

Diet: Tofu and Rice

Species: Dog
Life Stage: Adult
Special Conditions: Renal disease (low protein, low sodium, low phosphorus). This diet is NOT complete and balanced, and should only be used in dogs with renal failure under the supervision of your veterinarian.

Ingredient	Quantity	Measure
Tofu, extra firm	4	ounce
Rice, white, long-grain, cooked	3	cup
Canola oil	4	tsp
Salt substitute (potassium chloride)	½	tsp
Baking soda (calcium carbonate)	¼	tsp
Salt, iodized (sodium chloride)	⅛	tsp
Multivitamin & mineral tablet, kids complete	1	each
Zinc, 100 mg tablet	½	tablet

Prepared weight (approximately) = 613 g
Total kcal as prepared = 889 kcal
kcal/g prepared diet = 1.45 kcal/g diet

Nutrient	DM%[a]	As-Fed (g/100 g diet)	ME% (g/100 kcal)	% of total kcal
Protein	12	3.9	2.7	10
Fat	14	4.3	3.0	29
Carbohydrate	70	22.3	15.4	61
Fiber	1.2	0.4	0.3	—
Phosphorus	0.2	0.07	0.05	—
Sodium	0.2	0.05	0.04	—

[a]DM%, dry matter percent. If all the water was removed from this diet, this is the percentage of nutrient that would be present.

Diet: Chicken and Rice

Species: Dog
Life Stage: Adult
Special Conditions: To prevent recurrence of struvite urinary stones.
This diet is NOT complete and balanced. Use only under the supervision of your veterinarian. Urinary pH must be monitored.

Ingredient	Quantity	Measure
Chicken, breast, without skin, cooked	5	ounce
Rice, white, long-grain, cooked	3	cup
Canola oil	5	tsp
Salt substitute (potassium chloride)	½	tsp
Bone meal powder	1	tsp
Baking soda (calcium carbonate)	¼	tsp
Salt, iodized (sodium chloride)	¾	tsp
Multivitamin & mineral tablet, kids complete	1	each
Zinc, 100 mg tablet	½	tablet

Prepared weight (approximately) = 652 g
Total kcal as prepared = 1061 kcal
kcal/g prepared diet = 1.63 kcal/g diet

Nutrient	DM%[a]	As-Fed (g/100 g diet)	ME% (g/100 kcal)	% of total kcal
Protein	24	8.7	5.3	20
Fat	13	4.6	2.8	25
Carbohydrate	66	23.8	14.6	55
Fiber	0.9	0.33	0.2	—
Phosphorus	0.46	0.16	0.10	—

[a]DM%, dry matter percent. If all the water was removed from this diet, this is the percentage of nutrient that would be present.

Diet: Ground Beef and Rice

Species: Dog
Life Stage: Adult
Special Conditions: To prevent recurrence of struvite urinary stones. This diet is NOT complete and balanced. Use only under the supervision of your veterinarian. Urinary pH must be monitored.

Ingredient	Quantity	Measure
Ground beef, 25% fat, cooked	5	ounce
Rice, white, long-grain, cooked	3	cup
Canola oil	2	tsp
Salt substitute (potassium chloride)	¼	tsp
Bone meal powder	1¼	tsp
Salt, iodized (sodium chloride)	¾	tsp
Multivitamin & mineral tablet, kids complete	1	each
Zinc, 100 mg tablet	½	tablet

Prepared weight (approximately) = 637 g
Total kcal as prepared = 1095 kcal
kcal/g prepared diet = 1.72 kcal/g diet

Nutrient	DM%[a]	As-Fed (g/100 g diet)	ME% (g/100 kcal)	% of total kcal
Protein	21	7.8	4.6	18
Fat	15	5.7	3.3	32
Carbohydrate	57	21.1	12.3	49
Fiber	0.8	0.30	0.2	—
Phosphorus	0.50	0.18	0.11	—

[a]DM%, dry matter percent. If all the water was removed from this diet, this is the percentage of nutrient that would be present.

Diet: Tofu and Rice

Species: Dog
Life Stage: Adult
Special Conditions: To prevent recurrence of struvite urinary stones. This diet is NOT complete and balanced. Use only under the supervision of your veterinarian. Urinary pH must be monitored.

Ingredient	Quantity	Measure
Tofu, extra firm	14	ounce
Rice, white, long-grain, cooked	3	cup
Canola oil	1	tbsp
Salt substitute (potassium chloride)	½	tsp
Bone meal powder	¾	tsp
Salt, iodized (sodium chloride)	¾	tsp
Multivitamin & mineral tablet, kids complete	1	each
Zinc, 100 mg tablet	½	tablet

Prepared weight (approximately) = 897 g
Total kcal as prepared = 1105 kcal
kcal/g prepared diet = 1.23 kcal/g diet

Nutrient	DM%[a]	As-Fed (g/100 g diet)	ME% (g/100 kcal)	% of total kcal
Protein	21	5.8	4.7	18
Fat	15	4.3	3.5	32
Carbohydrate	57	15.9	12.9	50
Fiber	1.4	0.39	0.3	—
Phosphorus	0.47	0.13	0.11	—

[a]DM%, dry matter percent. If all the water was removed from this diet, this is the percentage of nutrient that would be present.

Diet: Chicken and Rice

Species: Dog
Life Stage: Adult
Special Conditions: To prevent recurrence of oxalate urinary stones. This diet is NOT complete and balanced (low protein). Use only under the supervision of your veterinarian. Urinary pH must be monitored.

Ingredient	Quantity	Measure
Chicken, breast, without skin, cooked	2	ounce
Rice, white, long-grain, cooked	3	cup
Canola oil	5	tsp
Salt substitute (potassium chloride)	½	tsp
Bone meal powder	2	tsp
Salt, iodized (sodium chloride)	¼	tsp
Multivitamin & mineral tablet, kids complete	1	each
Zinc, 100 mg tablet	½	tablet

Prepared weight (approximately) = 566 g
Total kcal as prepared = 920 kcal
kcal/g prepared diet = 1.62 kcal/g diet

Nutrient	DM%[a]	As-Fed (g/100 g diet)	ME% (g/100 kcal)	% of total kcal
Protein	15	5.4	3.3	13
Fat	13	4.7	2.9	28
Carbohydrate	66	23.8	14.6	59
Fiber	0.9	0.33	0.2	—
Phosphorus	0.68	0.24	0.15	—

[a]DM%, dry matter percent. If all the water was removed from this diet, this is the percentage of nutrient that would be present.

Diet: Eggs and Rice

Species: Dog
Life Stage: Adult
Special Conditions: To prevent recurrence of oxalate urinary stones. This diet is NOT complete and balanced (low protein). Use only under the supervision of your veterinarian. Urinary pH must be monitored.

Ingredient	Quantity	Measure
Eggs, large, hard-boiled	1	each
Rice, white, long-grain, cooked	3	cup
Canola oil	4	tsp
Salt substitute (potassium chloride)	½	tsp
Bone meal powder	1¾	tsp
Salt, iodized (sodium chloride)	⅛	tsp
Multivitamin & mineral tablet, kids complete	1	each
Zinc, 100 mg tablet	½	tablet

Prepared weight (approximately) = 554 g
Total kcal as prepared = 863 kcal
kcal/g prepared diet = 1.56 kcal/g diet

Nutrient	DM%[a]	As-Fed (g/100 g diet)	ME% (g/100 kcal)	% of total kcal
Protein	10	3.4	2.2	9
Fat	13	4.6	2.9	28
Carbohydrate	70	24.4	15.7	63
Fiber	1.0	0.34	0.20	—
Phosphorus	0.6	0.22	0.20	—

[a]DM%, dry matter percent. If all the water was removed from this diet, this is the percentage of nutrient that would be present.

Diet: Chicken and Potato

Species: Dog
Life Stage: Adult
Special Conditions: To prevent recurrence of urate or cystine urinary stones. This diet is NOT complete and balanced (low protein). Use only under the supervision of your veterinarian. Urinary pH must be monitored.

Ingredient	Quantity	Measure
Chicken, breast, without skin, cooked	2	ounce
Potatoes, diced, cooked	3	cup
Canola oil	1	tbsp
Salt substitute (potassium chloride)	¼	tsp
Bone meal powder	1¾	tsp
Salt, iodized (sodium chloride)	¾	tsp
Multivitamin & mineral tablet, kids complete	1	each
Zinc, 100 mg tablet	½	tablet

Prepared weight (approximately) = 552 g
Total kcal as prepared = 629 kcal
kcal/g prepared diet = 1.14 kcal/g diet

Nutrient	DM%[a]	As-Fed (g/100 g diet)	ME% (g/100 kcal)	% of total kcal
Protein	17	4.8	4.2	16
Fat	11	3.0	2.6	25
Carbohydrate	61	17.2	15.2	59
Fiber	5.5	1.5	1.3	—
Phosphorus	0.8	0.23	0.20	—

[a]DM%, dry matter percent. If all the water was removed from this diet, this is the percentage of nutrient that would be present.

Diet: Tofu and Rice

Species: Dog
Life Stage: Adult
Special Conditions: To prevent recurrence of urate or cystine urinary stones. This diet is NOT complete and balanced (low protein). Use only under the supervision of your veterinarian. Urinary pH must be monitored.

Ingredient	Quantity	Measure
Tofu, extra firm	6	ounce
Rice, white, long-grain, cooked	2	cup
Canola oil	4	tsp
Salt substitute (potassium chloride)	½	tsp
Bone meal powder	2	tsp
Salt, iodized (sodium chloride)	¾	tsp
Multivitamin & mineral tablet, kids complete	1	each
Vitamin B_{12} liquid, 1000 mcg B_{12} per mL	0.25	mL
Zinc, 100 mg tablet	½	tablet

Prepared weight (approximately) = 520 g
Total kcal as prepared = 735 kcal
kcal/g prepared diet = 1.41 kcal/g diet

Nutrient	DM%[a]	As-Fed (g/100 g diet)	ME% (g/100 kcal)	% of total kcal
Protein	15	4.9	3.4	13
Fat	18	5.7	4.0	38
Carbohydrate	56	18.0	12.7	49
Fiber	1.2	0.4	0.3	—
Phosphorus	0.8	0.27	0.19	—

[a]DM%, dry matter percent. If all the water was removed from this diet, this is the percentage of nutrient that would be present.

Cat Diet Recipes

Diets for Healthy Cats

Adults

Kittens, Gestation, and Lactation

Senior

Weight Loss

Diets for Cats with Special Conditions

Allergy

Cancer

Endocrine

Diabetes Mellitus

Idiopathic Hypercalcemia

Insulinoma

Lipid Disorders

Gastrointestinal

Gastritis

Gastric Mobility Disorders

Heart

Liver

Pancreas

Exocrine Pancreatic Insufficiency

Pancreatitis

Renal

Urinary Stones

Struvite Stone Prevention

Oxalate Stone Prevention

Diet: Chicken and Rice

Species: Cat
Life Stage: Adult
Special Conditions: Skin conditions, insulinoma

Ingredient	Quantity	Measure
Chicken, breast, without skin, cooked	6	ounces
Rice, white, long-grain, cooked	½	cup
Canola oil	5	tsp
Salt substitute (potassium chloride)	¼	tsp
Bone meal powder	¾	tsp
Salt, iodized (sodium chloride)	⅛	tsp
Multivitamin & mineral tablet, kids complete	1	each
Taurine powder, 1000 mg per ¼ tsp	¼	tsp

Prepared weight (approximately) = 280 g
Total kcal as prepared = 594 kcal
kcal/g prepared diet = 2.12 kcal/g diet

Nutrient	DM%[a]	As-Fed (g/100 g diet)	ME% (g/100 kcal)	% of total kcal
Protein	48	19.6	9.2	37
Fat	26	10.6	5.0	48
Carbohydrate	20	8.3	3.9	15
Fiber	0.3	0.1	0.1	—

[a]DM%, dry matter percent. If all the water was removed from this diet, this is the percentage of nutrient that would be present.

Diet: Turkey and Rice

Species: Cat
Life Stage: Adult
Special Conditions: Skin conditions, insulinoma

Ingredient	Quantity	Measure
Turkey, white meat, without skin, roasted	6	ounces
Rice, white, long-grain, cooked	½	cup
Canola oil	5	tsp
Salt substitute (potassium chloride)	¼	tsp
Bone meal powder	¾	tsp
Salt, iodized (sodium chloride)	⅛	tsp
Multivitamin & mineral tablet, kids complete	1	each
Taurine powder, 1000 mg per ¼ tsp	¼	tsp

Prepared weight (approximately) = 280 g
Total kcal as prepared = 580 kcal
kcal/g prepared diet = 2.07 kcal/g diet

Nutrient	DM%[a]	As-Fed (g/100 g diet)	ME% (g/100 kcal)	% of total kcal
Protein	47	19.0	9.1	36
Fat	26	10.4	5.0	48
Carbohydrate	21	8.3	4.0	16
Fiber	0.3	0.1	0.1	—

[a]DM%, dry matter percent. If all the water was removed from this diet, this is the percentage of nutrient that would be present.

Diet: Ground Beef and Rice

Species: Cat
Life Stage: Adult
Special Conditions: Skin conditions, insulinoma

Ingredient	Quantity	Measure
Ground beef, 10% fat, cooked	6	ounces
Rice, white, long-grain, cooked	½	cup
Canola oil	1	tbsp
Salt substitute (potassium chloride)	⅛	tsp
Bone meal powder	1	tsp
Salt, iodized (sodium chloride)	⅛	tsp
Multivitamin & mineral tablet, kids complete	½	each
Taurine powder, 1000 mg per ¼ tsp	¼	tsp

Prepared weight (approximately) = 269 g
Total kcal as prepared = 620 kcal
kcal/g prepared diet = 2.30 kcal/g diet

Nutrient	DM%[a]	As-Fed (g/100 g diet)	ME% (g/100 kcal)	% of total kcal
Protein	44	18.8	8.2	32
Fat	30	12.9	5.6	54
Carbohydrate	20	8.4	3.7	14
Fiber	0.3	0.1	0.1	—

[a]DM%, dry matter percent. If all the water was removed from this diet, this is the percentage of nutrient that would be present.

Diet: Lamb and Rice

Species: Cat
Life Stage: Adult
Special Conditions: Skin conditions

Ingredient	Quantity	Measure
Lamb, cooked	5	ounces
Rice, white, long-grain, cooked	½	cup
Canola oil	1½	tsp
Salt substitute (potassium chloride)	¼	tsp
Bone meal powder	¾	tsp
Salt, iodized (sodium chloride)	⅛	tsp
Multivitamin & mineral tablet, kids complete	½	each
Taurine powder, 1000 mg per ¼ tsp	¼	tsp

Prepared weight (approximately) = 234 g
Total kcal as prepared = 551 kcal
kcal/g prepared diet = 2.35 kcal/g diet

Nutrient	DM%[a]	As-Fed (g/100 g diet)	ME% (g/100 kcal)	% of total kcal
Protein	38	16.4	7.0	27
Fat	33	14.0	5.9	57
Carbohydrate	23	9.7	4.1	16
Fiber	0.3	0.1	0.1	—

[a]DM%, dry matter percent. If all the water was removed from this diet, this is the percentage of nutrient that would be present.

Diet: Tuna and Rice

Species: Cat
Life Stage: Adult
Special Conditions: Skin conditions, insulinoma

Ingredient	Quantity	Measure
Tuna, in oil, canned, drained	4	ounces
Egg, large, hard-boiled	1	each
Rice, white, long-grain, cooked	½	cup
Canola oil	1	tbsp
Salt substitute (potassium chloride)	¼	tsp
Bone meal powder	¾	tsp
Salt, iodized (sodium chloride)	⅛	tsp
Multivitamin & mineral tablet, kids complete	½	each
Taurine powder, 1000 mg per ¼ tsp	¼	tsp

Prepared weight (approximately) = 263 g
Total kcal as prepared = 531 kcal
kcal/g prepared diet = 2.02 kcal/g diet

Nutrient	DM%[a]	As-Fed (g/100 g diet)	ME% (g/100 kcal)	% of total kcal
Protein	40	15.8	7.8	31
Fat	28	11.0	5.4	52
Carbohydrate	23	8.9	4.4	17
Fiber	0.3	0.1	0.06	—

[a]DM%, dry matter percent. If all the water was removed from this diet, this is the percentage of nutrient that would be present.

Diet: Whitefish and Rice

Species: Cat
Life Stage: Adult
Special Conditions: Skin conditions, insulinoma

Ingredient	Quantity	Measure
Whitefish, fillet, baked or broiled	6	ounces
Rice, white, long-grain, cooked	½	cup
Canola oil	1	tbsp
Salt substitute (potassium chloride)	⅛	tsp
Bone meal powder	¾	tsp
Salt, iodized (sodium chloride)	⅛	tsp
Multivitamin & mineral tablet, kids complete	½	each
Taurine powder, 1000 mg per ¼ tsp	¼	tsp

Prepared weight (approximately) = 269 g
Total kcal as prepared = 521 kcal
kcal/g prepared diet = 1.94 kcal/g diet

Nutrient	DM%[a]	As-Fed (g/100 g diet)	ME% (g/100 kcal)	% of total kcal
Protein	42	16.3	8.4	33
Fat	26	10.0	5.2	50
Carbohydrate	22	8.5	4.4	17
Fiber	0.3	0.1	0.06	—

[a]DM%, dry matter percent. If all the water was removed from this diet, this is the percentage of nutrient that would be present.

Diet: Salmon and Rice

Species: Cat
Life Stage: Adult
Special Conditions: Skin conditions, insulinoma

Ingredient	Quantity	Measure
Salmon, wild, fillet, baked	4	ounces
Egg, large, hard-boiled	1	each
Rice, white, long-grain, cooked	½	cup
Canola oil	1	tbsp
Salt substitute (potassium chloride)	⅛	tsp
Bone meal powder	¾	tsp
Salt, iodized (sodium chloride)	⅛	tsp
Multivitamin & mineral tablet, kids complete	½	each
Taurine powder, 1000 mg per ¼ tsp	¼	tsp

Prepared weight (approximately) = 262 g
Total kcal as prepared = 512 kcal
kcal/g prepared diet = 1.96 kcal/g diet

Nutrient	DM%[a]	As-Fed (g/100 g diet)	ME% (g/100 kcal)	% of total kcal
Protein	36	14.2	7.3	29
Fat	28	11.0	5.6	53
Carbohydrate	23	8.9	4.6	18
Fiber	0.3	0.1	0.06	—

[a]DM%, dry matter percent. If all the water was removed from this diet, this is the percentage of nutrient that would be present.

Diet: Tofu and Eggs

Species: Cat
Life Stage: Adult
Special Conditions: NOTE: This diet is not strictly vegetarian as it contains eggs.

Ingredient	Quantity	Measure
Tofu, extra firm	10	ounces
Eggs, large, hard-boiled	3	each
Canola oil	1½	tsp
Salt substitute (potassium chloride)	¼	tsp
Bone meal powder	¾	tsp
Salt, iodized (sodium chloride)	⅛	tsp
Multivitamin & mineral tablet, kids complete	½	each
Taurine powder, 1000 mg per ¼ tsp	¼	tsp

Prepared weight (approximately) = 449 g
Total kcal as prepared = 556 kcal
kcal/g prepared diet = 1.24 kcal/g diet

Nutrient	DM%[a]	As-Fed (g/100 g diet)	ME% (g/100 kcal)	% of total kcal
Protein	44	10.4	8.4	31
Fat	37	8.8	7.1	63
Carbohydrate	8	1.9	1.5	6
Fiber	1.1	0.2	0.2	—

[a]DM%, dry matter percent. If all the water was removed from this diet, this is the percentage of nutrient that would be present.

Diet: Chicken and Rice

Species: Cat
Life Stage: Kitten, adult
Special Conditions: Gestation, lactation, skin conditions

Ingredient	Quantity	Measure
Chicken, breast, without skin, cooked	6	ounces
Rice, white, long-grain, cooked	½	cup
Canola oil	5	tsp
Salt substitute (potassium chloride)	¼	tsp
Bone meal powder	1½	tsp
Salt, iodized (sodium chloride)	⅛	tsp
Multivitamin & mineral tablet, kids complete	1	each
Taurine powder, 1000 mg per ¼ tsp	¼	tsp

Prepared weight (approximately) = 282 g
Total kcal as prepared = 594 kcal
kcal/g prepared diet = 2.11 kcal/g diet

Nutrient	DM%[a]	As-Fed (g/100 g diet)	ME% (g/100 kcal)	% of total kcal
Protein	47	19.5	9.2	37
Fat	25	10.5	5.0	48
Carbohydrate	20	8.3	3.9	15
Fiber	0.3	0.1	0.1	—

[a]DM%, dry matter percent. If all the water was removed from this diet, this is the percentage of nutrient that would be present.

Diet: Turkey and Rice

Species: Cat
Life Stage: Kitten, adult
Special Conditions: Gestation, lactation, skin conditions

Ingredient	Quantity	Measure
Turkey, light meat, without skin, roasted	6	ounces
Rice, white, long-grain, cooked	½	cup
Canola oil	5	tsp
Salt substitute (potassium chloride)	¼	tsp
Bone meal powder	1½	tsp
Salt, iodized (sodium chloride)	⅛	tsp
Multivitamin & mineral tablet, kids complete	1	each
Taurine powder, 1000 mg per ¼ tsp	¼	tsp

Prepared weight (approximately) = 282 g
Total kcal as prepared = 580 kcal
kcal/g prepared diet = 2.06 kcal/g diet

Nutrient	DM%[a]	As-Fed (g/100 g diet)	ME% (g/100 kcal)	% of total kcal
Protein	46	18.8	9.1	36
Fat	25	10.3	5.0	48
Carbohydrate	20	8.3	4.0	16
Fiber	0.3	0.1	0.1	—

[a]DM%, dry matter percent. If all the water was removed from this diet, this is the percentage of nutrient that would be present.

Diet: Ground Beef and Rice

Species: Cat
Life Stage: Kitten, adult
Special Conditions: Gestation, lactation, skin conditions, insulinoma

Ingredient	Quantity	Measure
Ground beef, 10% fat, cooked	6	ounces
Rice, white, long-grain, cooked	½	cup
Canola oil	1	tbsp
Salt substitute (potassium chloride)	⅛	tsp
Bone meal powder	1½	tsp
Salt, iodized (sodium chloride)	⅛	tsp
Multivitamin & mineral tablet, kids complete	1	each
Taurine powder, 1000 mg per ¼ tsp	¼	tsp

Prepared weight (approximately) = 272 g
Total kcal as prepared = 622 kcal
kcal/g prepared diet = 2.29 kcal/g diet

Nutrient	DM%[a]	As-Fed (g/100 g diet)	ME% (g/100 kcal)	% of total kcal
Protein	43	18.6	8.1	32
Fat	29	12.8	5.6	53
Carbohydrate	20	8.6	3.7	15
Fiber	0.3	0.1	0.1	—

[a]DM%, dry matter percent. If all the water was removed from this diet, this is the percentage of nutrient that would be present.

Diet: Lamb and Rice

Species: Cat
Life Stage: Kitten, adult
Special Conditions: Gestation, lactation, skin conditions

Ingredient	Quantity	Measure
Lamb, cooked	7	ounces
Rice, white, long-grain, cooked	½	cup
Canola oil	1¼	tsp
Salt substitute (potassium chloride)	¼	tsp
Bone meal powder	2	tsp
Salt, iodized (sodium chloride)	⅛	tsp
Multivitamin & mineral tablet, kids complete	1	each
Vitamin K, 100 mcg per tablet	1	tablet
Taurine powder, 1000 mg per ¼ tsp	¼	tsp

Prepared weight (approximately) = 295 g
Total kcal as prepared = 696 kcal
kcal/g prepared diet = 2.36 kcal/g diet

Nutrient	DM%[a]	As-Fed (g/100 g diet)	ME% (g/100 kcal)	% of total kcal
Protein	40	17.9	7.6	30
Fat	32	14.2	6.0	57
Carbohydrate	18	7.9	3.3	13
Fiber	0.2	0.1	0.1	—

[a]DM%, dry matter percent. If all the water was removed from this diet, this is the percentage of nutrient that would be present.

Diet: Tuna and Rice

Species: Cat
Life Stage: Kitten, adult
Special Conditions: Gestation, lactation, skin conditions, insulinoma

Ingredient	Quantity	Measure
Tuna, in oil, canned, drained	5	ounces
Egg, large, hard-boiled	1	each
Rice, white, long-grain, cooked	½	cup
Canola oil	1	tbsp
Salt substitute (potassium chloride)	¼	tsp
Bone meal powder	1½	tsp
Salt, iodized (sodium chloride)	⅛	tsp
Multivitamin & mineral tablet, kids complete	1	each
Taurine powder, 1000 mg per ¼ tsp	¼	tsp

Prepared weight (approximately) = 294 g
Total kcal as prepared = 589 kcal
kcal/g prepared diet = 2.00 kcal/g diet

Nutrient	DM%[a]	As-Fed (g/100 g diet)	ME% (g/100 kcal)	% of total kcal
Protein	42	17.0	8.4	33
Fat	26	10.6	5.3	51
Carbohydrate	20	8.1	4.0	16
Fiber	0.3	0.1	0.1	—

[a]DM%, dry matter percent. If all the water was removed from this diet, this is the percentage of nutrient that would be present.

Diet: Whitefish and Rice

Species: Cat
Life Stage: Kitten, adult
Special Conditions: Gestation, lactation, skin conditions, insulinoma

Ingredient	Quantity	Measure
Whitefish, fillet, baked or broiled	6	ounces
Rice, white, long-grain, cooked	½	cup
Canola oil	1	tbsp
Salt substitute (potassium chloride)	⅛	tsp
Bone meal powder	1¼	tsp
Salt, iodized (sodium chloride)	⅛	tsp
Multivitamin & mineral tablet, kids complete	1	each
Taurine powder, 1000 mg per ¼ tsp	¼	tsp

Prepared weight (approximately) = 271 g
Total kcal as prepared = 523 kcal
kcal/g prepared diet = 1.93 kcal/g diet

Nutrient	DM%[a]	As-Fed (g/100 g diet)	ME% (g/100 kcal)	% of total kcal
Protein	41	16.1	8.4	33
Fat	25	10.0	5.2	49
Carbohydrate	22	8.6	4.4	18
Fiber	0.3	0.1	0.1	—

[a]DM%, dry matter percent. If all the water was removed from this diet, this is the percentage of nutrient that would be present.

Diet: Salmon and Rice

Species: Cat
Life Stage: Kitten, adult
Special Conditions: Gestation, lactation, skin conditions, insulinoma

Ingredient	Quantity	Measure
Salmon, wild, fillet, baked	6	ounces
Egg, large, hard-boiled	1	each
Rice, white, long-grain, cooked	½	cup
Canola oil	1	tbsp
Salt substitute (potassium chloride)	⅛	tsp
Bone meal powder	1½	tsp
Salt, iodized (sodium chloride)	⅛	tsp
Multivitamin & mineral tablet, kids complete	1	each
Taurine powder, 1000 mg per ¼ tsp	¼	tsp

Prepared weight (approximately) = 322 g
Total kcal as prepared = 618 kcal
kcal/g prepared diet = 1.92 kcal/g diet

Nutrient	DM%[a]	As-Fed (g/100 g diet)	ME% (g/100 kcal)	% of total kcal
Protein	40	16.1	8.4	33
Fat	26	10.4	5.4	52
Carbohydrate	18	7.4	3.9	15
Fiber	0.2	0.1	0.1	—

[a]DM%, dry matter percent. If all the water was removed from this diet, this is the percentage of nutrient that would be present.

Diet: Mackerel and Rice

Species: Cat
Life Stage: Kitten, adult
Special Conditions: Gestation, lactation, skin conditions, insulinoma

Ingredient	Quantity	Measure
Mackerel, jack, canned, drained	5	ounces
Egg, large, hard-boiled	1	each
Rice, white, long-grain, cooked	½	cup
Canola oil	1	tbsp
Salt substitute (potassium chloride)	¼	tsp
Bone meal powder	1	tsp
Salt, iodized (sodium chloride)	⅛	tsp
Multivitamin & mineral tablet, kids complete	½	each
Taurine powder, 1000 mg per ¼ tsp	¼	tsp

Prepared weight (approximately) = 292 g
Total kcal as prepared = 527 kcal
kcal/g prepared diet = 1.81 kcal/g diet

Nutrient	DM%[a]	As-Fed (g/100 g diet)	ME% (g/100 kcal)	% of total kcal
Protein	40	14.2	7.8	31
Fat	28	9.8	5.4	52
Carbohydrate	23	8.0	4.4	17
Fiber	0.3	0.1	0.1	—

[a]DM%, dry matter percent. If all the water was removed from this diet, this is the percentage of nutrient that would be present.

Diet: Sardines and Rice

Species: Cat
Life Stage: Kitten, adult
Special Conditions: Gestation, lactation, skin conditions, insulinoma

Ingredient	Quantity	Measure
Sardines, in oil, canned, drained	5	ounces
Egg, large, hard-boiled	1	each
Rice, white, long-grain, cooked	½	cup
Canola oil	1½	tsp
Salt substitute (potassium chloride)	⅛	tsp
Bone meal powder	¾	tsp
Salt, iodized (sodium chloride)	⅛	tsp
Multivitamin & mineral tablet, kids complete	½	each
Taurine powder, 1000 mg per ¼ tsp	¼	tsp

Prepared weight (approximately) = 283 g
Total kcal as prepared = 539 kcal
kcal/g prepared diet = 1.90 kcal/g diet

Nutrient	DM%[a]	As-Fed (g/100 g diet)	ME% (g/100 kcal)	% of total kcal
Protein	40	15.3	8.0	32
Fat	27	10.2	5.3	51
Carbohydrate	22	8.2	4.3	17
Fiber	0.3	0.1	0.06	—

[a]DM%, dry matter percent. If all the water was removed from this diet, this is the percentage of nutrient that would be present.

Diet: Chicken and Rice

Species: Cat
Life Stage: Adult
Special Conditions: Senior cats

Ingredient	Quantity	Measure
Chicken, breast, without skin, cooked	4	ounces
Rice, white, long-grain, cooked	½	cup
Canola oil	1	tbsp
Salt substitute (potassium chloride)	¼	tsp
Bone meal powder	⅔	tsp
Salt, iodized (sodium chloride)	⅛	tsp
Multivitamin & mineral tablet, kids complete	½	each
Taurine powder, 1000 mg per ¼ tsp	¼	tsp

Prepared weight (approximately) = 212 g
Total kcal as prepared = 416 kcal
kcal/g prepared diet = 1.96 kcal/g diet

Nutrient	DM%[a]	As-Fed (g/100 g diet)	ME% (g/100 kcal)	% of total kcal
Protein	45	17.6	9.0	36
Fat	22	8.6	4.4	42
Carbohydrate	27	10.7	5.5	22
Fiber	0.4	0.2	0.08	—

[a]DM%, dry matter percent. If all the water was removed from this diet, this is the percentage of nutrient that would be present.

Diet: Ground Beef and Rice

Species: Cat
Life Stage: Adult
Special Conditions: Senior cats

Ingredient	Quantity	Measure
Ground beef, 10% fat, cooked	3	ounces
Rice, white, long-grain, cooked	½	cup
Canola oil	½	tsp
Salt substitute (potassium chloride)	⅛	tsp
Bone meal powder	½	tsp
Salt, iodized (sodium chloride)	⅛	tsp
Multivitamin & mineral tablet, kids complete	½	each
Vitamin K, 100 mcg per tablet	1	tablet
Taurine powder, 1000 mg per ¼ tsp	¼	tsp

Prepared weight (approximately) = 172 g
Total kcal as prepared = 321 kcal
kcal/g prepared diet = 1.86 kcal/g diet

Nutrient	DM%[a]	As-Fed (g/100 g diet)	ME% (g/100 kcal)	% of total kcal
Protein	39	15.3	8.2	33
Fat	19	7.4	4.0	39
Carbohydrate	34	13.2	7.1	28
Fiber	0.5	0.2	0.1	—

[a]DM%, dry matter percent. If all the water was removed from this diet, this is the percentage of nutrient that would be present.

Diet: Tuna and Rice

Species: Cat
Life Stage: Adult
Special Conditions: Senior cats

Ingredient	Quantity	Measure
Tuna, canned, in oil, drained	3	ounces
Egg, large, hard-boiled	1	each
Rice, white, long-grain, cooked	½	cup
Canola oil	1½	tsp
Salt substitute (potassium chloride)	¼	tsp
Bone meal powder	¼	tsp
Baking soda (calcium carbonate)	¼	tsp
Salt, iodized (sodium chloride)	⅛	tsp
Multivitamin & mineral tablet, kids complete	½	each
Taurine powder, 1000 mg per ¼ tsp	¼	tsp

Prepared weight (approximately) = 227 g
Total kcal as prepared = 413 kcal
kcal/g prepared diet = 1.82 kcal/g diet

Nutrient	DM%[a]	As-Fed (g/100 g diet)	ME% (g/100 kcal)	% of total kcal
Protein	39	14.6	8.0	32
Fat	23	8.6	4.7	46
Carbohydrate	28	10.3	5.7	22
Fiber	0.4	0.1	0.08	—

[a]DM%, dry matter percent. If all the water was removed from this diet, this is the percentage of nutrient that would be present.

Diet: Whitefish and Rice

Species: Cat
Life Stage: Adult
Special Conditions: Senior cats

Ingredient	Quantity	Measure
Whitefish, fillet, baked	4	ounces
Rice, white, long-grain, cooked	½	cup
Canola oil	2	tsp
Salt substitute (potassium chloride)	⅛	tsp
Bone meal powder	⅛	tsp
Baking soda (calcium carbonate)	¼	tsp
Salt, iodized (sodium chloride)	⅛	tsp
Multivitamin & mineral tablet, kids complete	½	each
Taurine powder, 1000 mg per ¼ tsp	¼	tsp

Prepared weight (approximately) = 206 g
Total kcal as prepared = 382 kcal
kcal/g prepared diet = 1.85 kcal/g diet

Nutrient	DM%[a]	As-Fed (g/100 g diet)	ME% (g/100 kcal)	% of total kcal
Protein	38	14.5	7.8	31
Fat	23	8.8	4.7	45
Carbohydrate	29	11.0	6.0	24
Fiber	0.4	0.2	0.08	—

[a]DM%, dry matter percent. If all the water was removed from this diet, this is the percentage of nutrient that would be present.

Diet: Salmon and Rice

Species: Cat
Life Stage: Adult
Special Conditions: Senior cats

Ingredient	Quantity	Measure
Salmon, wild, fillet, baked	4	ounces
Egg, large, hard-boiled	½	each
Rice, white, long-grain, cooked	½	cup
Canola oil	2	tsp
Salt substitute (potassium chloride)	⅛	tsp
Bone meal powder	⅓	tsp
Baking soda (calcium carbonate)	¼	tsp
Salt, iodized (sodium chloride)	⅛	tsp
Multivitamin & mineral tablet, kids complete	½	each
Taurine powder, 1000 mg per ¼ tsp	¼	tsp

Prepared weight (approximately) = 232 g
Total kcal as prepared = 432 kcal
kcal/g prepared diet = 1.86 kcal/g diet

Nutrient	DM%[a]	As-Fed (g/100 g diet)	ME% (g/100 kcal)	% of total kcal
Protein	37	14.7	7.9	31
Fat	23	9.2	5.0	48
Carbohydrate	25	9.9	5.3	21
Fiber	0.4	0.1	0.08	—

[a]DM%, dry matter percent. If all the water was removed from this diet, this is the percentage of nutrient that would be present.

Diet: Chicken and Barley

Species: Cat
Life Stage: Adult
Special Conditions: Weight loss, gastric motility disorders, idiopathic hypercalcemia

Ingredient	Quantity	Measure
Chicken, breast, without skin, cooked	6	ounces
Barley, pearled, cooked	½	cup
Lentils, cooked	½	cup
Canola oil	2	tsp
Salt substitute (potassium chloride)	⅛	tsp
Bone meal powder	¾	tsp
Salt, iodized (sodium chloride)	⅛	tsp
Multivitamin & mineral tablet, kids complete	1	each
Taurine powder, 1000 mg per ¼ tsp	¼	tsp

Prepared weight (approximately) = 364 g
Total kcal as prepared = 579 kcal
kcal/g prepared diet = 1.59 kcal/g diet

Nutrient	DM%[a]	As-Fed (g/100 g diet)	ME% (g/100 kcal)	% of total kcal
Protein	49	17.5	11.0	43
Fat	12	4.4	2.8	27
Carbohydrate	33	11.9	7.4	30
Fiber	8	3.0	1.9	—

[a]DM%, dry matter percent. If all the water was removed from this diet, this is the percentage of nutrient that would be present.

Diet: Ground Beef and Lentils

Species: Cat
Life Stage: Adult
Special Conditions: Weight loss, gastric motility disorders, idiopathic hypercalcemia

Ingredient	Quantity	Measure
Ground beef, 5% fat, cooked	8	ounces
Lentils, cooked	1	cup
Canola oil	½	tsp
Salt substitute (potassium chloride)	⅛	tsp
Bone meal powder	1	tsp
Salt, iodized (sodium chloride)	⅛	tsp
Multivitamin & mineral tablet, kids complete	1	each
Vitamin K, 100 mcg per tablet	1	tablet
Taurine powder, 1000 mg per ¼ tsp	¼	tsp

Prepared weight (approximately) = 435 g
Total kcal as prepared = 692 kcal
kcal/g prepared diet = 1.59 kcal/g diet

Nutrient	DM%[a]	As-Fed (g/100 g diet)	ME% (g/100 kcal)	% of total kcal
Protein	54	19.3	12.1	48
Fat	13	4.7	2.9	28
Carbohydrate	26	9.4	5.9	24
Fiber	10	3.6	2.3	—

[a]DM%, dry matter percent. If all the water was removed from this diet, this is the percentage of nutrient that would be present.

Diet: Lamb and Lentils

Species: Cat
Life Stage: Adult
Special Conditions: Weight loss, gastric motility disorders, short bowel syndrome, small intestinal bacterial overgrowth, idiopathic hypercalcemia

Ingredient	Quantity	Measure
Lamb, cooked	4	ounces
Lentils, cooked	1	cup
Salt substitute (potassium chloride)	⅛	tsp
Bone meal powder	1	tsp
Salt, iodized (sodium chloride)	⅛	tsp
Multivitamin & mineral tablet, kids complete	1	each
Vitamin K, 100 mcg vitamin K per tablet	1	tablet
Taurine powder, 1000 mg per ¼ tsp	¼	tsp

Prepared weight (approximately) = 320 g
Total kcal as prepared = 541 kcal
kcal/g prepared diet = 1.69 kcal/g diet

Nutrient	DM%[a]	As-Fed (g/100 g diet)	ME% (g/100 kcal)	% of total kcal
Protein	39	14.6	8.6	34
Fat	17.9	6.6	3.9	37
Carbohydrate	34.5	12.8	7.6	29
Fiber	13.2	4.9	2.9	—

[a] DM%, dry matter percent. If all the water was removed from this diet, this is the percentage of nutrient that would be present.

Diet: Whitefish and Lentils

Species: Cat
Life Stage: Adult
Special Conditions: Weight loss, gastric motility disorders, short bowel syndrome, small intestinal bacterial overgrowth, idiopathic hypercalcemia

Ingredient	Quantity	Measure
Whitefish, fillet, baked or broiled	8	ounces
Lentils, cooked	1	Cup
Canola oil	1	tsp
Salt substitute (potassium chloride)	⅛	tsp
Bone meal powder	1	tsp
Salt, iodized (sodium chloride)	⅛	tsp
Multivitamin & mineral tablet, kids complete	1	each
Vitamin K, 100 mcg vitamin K per tablet	1	tablet
Taurine powder, 1000 mg per ¼ tsp	¼	tsp

Prepared weight (approximately) = 438 g
Total kcal as prepared = 665 kcal
kcal/g prepared diet = 1.52 kcal/g diet

Nutrient	DM%[a]	As-Fed (g/100 g diet)	ME% (g/100 kcal)	% of total kcal
Protein	48	16.8	11.0	44
Fat	15	5.1	3.4	32
Carbohydrate	27	9.3	6.1	24
Fiber	10	3.6	2.4	—

[a]DM%, dry matter percent. If all the water was removed from this diet, this is the percentage of nutrient that would be present.

Diet: Tuna and Lentils

Species: Cat
Life Stage: Adult
Special Conditions: Weight loss, gastric motility disorders, idiopathic hypercalcemia

Ingredient	Quantity	Measure
Tuna, canned, in water, drained	5	ounces
Egg, large, hard-boiled	1	each
Lentils, cooked	1	cup
Canola oil	1½	tsp
Salt substitute (potassium chloride)	¼	tsp
Bone meal powder	1	tsp
Salt, iodized (sodium chloride)	⅛	tsp
Multivitamin & mineral tablet, kids complete	1	each
Vitamin K, 100 mcg vitamin K per tablet	1	tablet
Taurine powder, 1000 mg per ¼ tsp	¼	tsp

Prepared weight (approximately) = 406 g
Total kcal as prepared = 555 kcal
kcal/g prepared diet = 1.37 kcal/g diet

Nutrient	DM%[a]	As-Fed (g/100 g diet)	ME% (g/100 kcal)	% of total kcal
Protein	45	14.2	10.4	41
Fat	14	4.3	3.1	30
Carbohydrate	33	10.2	7.5	29
Fiber	12	3.9	2.8	—

[a]DM%, dry matter percent. If all the water was removed from this diet, this is the percentage of nutrient that would be present.

Diet: Salmon and Barley

Species: Cat
Life Stage: Adult
Special Conditions: Weight loss, lymphangiectasia, protein-losing enteropathy, gastric motility disorders, idiopathic hypercalcemia

Ingredient	Quantity	Measure
Salmon, wild, fillet, baked	6	ounces
Egg, large, hard-boiled	½	each
Barley, pearled, cooked	1	cup
Canola oil	½	tsp
Salt substitute (potassium chloride)	⅛	tsp
Bone meal powder	1	tsp
Salt, iodized (sodium chloride)	⅛	tsp
Multivitamin & mineral tablet, kids complete	1	each
Vitamin K, 100 mcg vitamin K per tablet	1	tablet
Taurine powder, 1000 mg per ¼ tsp	¼	tsp

Prepared weight (approximately) = 363 g
Total kcal as prepared = 566 kcal
kcal/g prepared diet = 1.56 kcal/g diet

Nutrient	DM%[a]	As-Fed (g/100g diet)	ME% (g/100 kcal)	% of total kcal
Protein	37	13.8	8.8	35
Fat	14	5.4	3.4	33
Carbohydrate	34	12.6	8.1	32
Fiber	4	1.6	1.0	—

[a]DM%, dry matter percent. If all the water was removed from this diet, this is the percentage of nutrient that would be present.

Diet: Rabbit and Rice

Species: Cat
Life Stage: Kitten, adult
Special Conditions: Allergy, gestation, lactation

Ingredient	Quantity	Measure
Rabbit, domestic, cooked	6	ounces
Rice, white, long-grain, cooked	½	cup
Canola oil	5	tsp
Salt substitute (potassium chloride)	⅛	tsp
Bone meal powder	1¾	tsp
Salt, iodized (sodium chloride)	⅛	tsp
Multivitamin & mineral tablet, kids complete	1	each
Taurine powder, 1000 mg per ¼ tsp	¼	tsp

Prepared weight (approximately) = 282 g
Total kcal as prepared = 648 kcal
kcal/g prepared diet = 2.30 kcal/g diet

Nutrient	DM%[a]	As-Fed (g/100 g diet)	ME% (g/100 kcal)	% of total kcal
Protein	41	18.3	8.0	31
Fat	30	13.2	5.7	55
Carbohydrate	19	8.2	3.6	14
Fiber	0.2	0.1	0.1	—

[a]DM%, dry matter percent. If all the water was removed from this diet, this is the percentage of nutrient that would be present.

Diet: Rabbit and Quinoa

Species: Cat
Life Stage: Kitten, adult
Special Conditions: Allergy, gestation, lactation

Ingredient	Quantity	Measure
Rabbit, domestic, cooked	5	ounces
Quinoa, cooked	¼	cup
Canola oil	5	tsp
Salt substitute (potassium chloride)	⅛	tsp
Bone meal powder	1¼	tsp
Salt, iodized (sodium chloride)	⅛	tsp
Multivitamin & mineral tablet, kids complete	1	each
Taurine powder, 1000 mg per ¼ tsp	¼	tsp

Prepared weight (approximately) = 219 g
Total kcal as prepared = 545 kcal
kcal/g prepared diet = 2.48 kcal/g diet

Nutrient	DM%[a]	As-Fed (g/100 g diet)	ME% (g/100 kcal)	% of total kcal
Protein	43	19.7	7.9	31
Fat	35	16.2	6.5	62
Carbohydrate	11	5.0	2.0	8
Fiber	1.3	0.6	0.2	—

[a]DM%, dry matter percent. If all the water was removed from this diet, this is the percentage of nutrient that would be present.

Diet: Venison and Rice

Species: Cat
Life Stage: Kitten, adult
Special Conditions: Allergy, gestation, lactation

Ingredient	Quantity	Measure
Venison, roasted	6	ounces
Rice, white, long-grain, cooked	½	cup
Canola oil	5	tsp
Salt substitute (potassium chloride)	⅛	tsp
Bone meal powder	1½	tsp
Salt, iodized (sodium chloride)	⅛	tsp
Multivitamin & mineral tablet, kids complete	1	each
Taurine powder, 1000 mg per ¼ tsp	¼	tsp

Prepared weight (approximately) = 281 g
Total kcal as prepared = 582 kcal
kcal/g prepared diet = 2.07 kcal/g diet

Nutrient	DM%[a]	As-Fed (g/100 g diet)	ME% (g/100 kcal)	% of total kcal
Protein	47	19.1	9.2	36
Fat	25	10.3	5.0	48
Carbohydrate	20	8.3	4.0	16
Fiber	0.3	0.1	0.1	—

[a]DM%, dry matter percent. If all the water was removed from this diet, this is the percentage of nutrient that would be present.

Diet: Venison and Quinoa

Species: Cat
Life Stage: Kitten, adult
Special Conditions: Allergy, gestation, lactation

Ingredient	Quantity	Measure
Venison, roasted	5	ounces
Quinoa, cooked	¼	cup
Canola oil	5	tsp
Salt substitute (potassium chloride)	⅛	tsp
Bone meal powder	1¼	tsp
Salt, iodized (sodium chloride)	⅛	tsp
Multivitamin & mineral tablet, kids complete	1	each
Taurine powder, 1000 mg per ¼ tsp	¼	tsp

Prepared weight (approximately) = 219 g
Total kcal as prepared = 490 kcal
kcal/g prepared diet = 2.23 kcal/g diet

Nutrient	DM%[a]	As-Fed (g/100g diet)	ME% (g/100 kcal)	% of total kcal
Protein	48	20.5	9.2	36
Fat	31	13.2	5.9	55
Carbohydrate	12	5.0	2.2	9
Fiber	1.4	0.6	0.3	—

[a]DM%, dry matter percent. If all the water was removed from this diet, this is the percentage of nutrient that would be present.

Diet: Chicken and Rice

Species: Cat
Life Stage: Adult
Special Conditions: Cancer

Ingredient	Quantity	Measure
Chicken, breast, without skin, cooked	6	ounces
Rice, white, long-grain, cooked	½	cup
Canola oil	2	tbsp
Salt substitute (potassium chloride)	¼	tsp
Bone meal powder	1	tsp
Salt, iodized (sodium chloride)	⅛	tsp
Multivitamin & mineral tablet, kids complete	1	each
Vitamin K, 100 mcg vitamin K per tablet	1	tablet
Arginine powder, 2.5 g per tsp	¼	tsp
Fish oil, 900 mg omega-3 per tablet	1	tablet
Taurine powder, 1000 mg per ¼ tsp	¼	tsp

Prepared weight (approximately) = 288 g
Total kcal as prepared = 650 kcal
kcal/g prepared diet = 2.26 kcal/g diet

Nutrient	DM%[a]	As-Fed (g/100 g diet)	ME% (g/100 kcal)	% of total kcal
Protein	45	19.1	8.4	33
Fat	29	12.4	5.5	53
Carbohydrate	19	8.1	3.6	14
Fiber	0.3	0.1	0.05	—
Arginine	3.3	1.4	0.6	—
Omega-3 fatty acids	5.1	2.2	1.0	—

[a]DM%, dry matter percent. If all the water was removed from this diet, this is the percentage of nutrient that would be present.

Diet: Ground Beef and Rice

Species: Cat
Life Stage: Adult
Special Conditions: Cancer

Ingredient	Quantity	Measure
Ground beef, 10% fat, cooked	8	ounces
Rice, white, long-grain, cooked	¼	cup
Canola oil	4	tsp
Salt substitute (potassium chloride)	⅛	tsp
Bone meal powder	1	tsp
Salt, iodized (sodium chloride)	⅛	tsp
Multivitamin & mineral tablet, kids complete	1	each
Vitamin K, 100 mcg vitamin K per tablet	1	tablet
Arginine powder, 2.5 g per tsp	¼	tsp
Fish oil, 900 mg omega-3 per tablet	1	tablet
Taurine powder, 1000 mg per ¼ tsp	¼	tsp

Prepared weight (approximately) = 295 g
Total kcal as prepared = 757 kcal
kcal/g prepared diet = 2.56 kcal/g diet

Nutrient	DM%[a]	As-Fed (g/100 g diet)	ME% (g/100 kcal)	% of total kcal
Protein	49	22.3	8.7	34
Fat	35	16.1	6.3	60
Carbohydrate	9	4.1	1.6	6
Fiber	0.1	0.05	0.02	—
Arginine	3.6	1.6	0.6	—
Omega-3 fatty acids	3.4	1.6	0.6	—

[a]DM%, dry matter percent. If all the water was removed from this diet, this is the percentage of nutrient that would be present.

Diet: Tuna and Rice

Species: Cat
Life Stage: Adult
Special Conditions: Cancer

Ingredient	Quantity	Measure
Tuna, canned, in water, drained	8	ounces
Egg, large, hard-boiled	1	each
Rice, white, long-grain, cooked	¼	cup
Canola oil	2	tbsp
Salt substitute (potassium chloride)	¼	tsp
Bone meal powder	1	tsp
Salt, iodized (sodium chloride)	⅛	tsp
Multivitamin & mineral tablet, kids complete	1	each
Vitamin K, 100 mcg vitamin K per tablet	1	tablet
Arginine powder, 2.5 g per tsp	¼	tsp
Fish oil, 900 mg omega-3 per tablet	1	tablet
Taurine powder, 1000 mg per ¼ tsp	¼	tsp

Prepared weight (approximately) = 355 g
Total kcal as prepared = 686 kcal
kcal/g prepared diet = 1.93 kcal/g diet

Nutrient	DM%[a]	As-Fed (g/100 g diet)	ME% (g/100 kcal)	% of total kcal
Protein	49	17.2	8.9	35
Fat	33	11.8	6.1	58
Carbohydrate	10	3.6	1.9	7
Fiber	0.1	0.04	0.02	—
Arginine	3.5	1.2	0.6	—
Omega-3 fatty acids	8.3	2.9	1.5	—

[a]DM%, dry matter percent. If all the water was removed from this diet, this is the percentage of nutrient that would be present.

Diet: Whitefish and Rice

Species: Cat
Life Stage: Adult
Special Conditions: Cancer

Ingredient	Quantity	Measure
Whitefish, fillet, baked	10	ounces
Rice, white, long-grain, cooked	½	cup
Canola oil	2	tbsp
Salt substitute (potassium chloride)	⅛	tsp
Bone meal powder	½	tsp
Baking soda (calcium carbonate)	½	tsp
Salt, iodized (sodium chloride)	⅛	tsp
Multivitamin & mineral tablet, kids complete	1	each
Vitamin K, 100 mcg vitamin K per tablet	1	tablet
Arginine powder, 2.5 g per tsp	¼	tsp
Fish oil, 900 mg omega-3 per tablet	1	tablet
Taurine powder, 1000 mg per ¼ tsp	¼	tsp

Prepared weight (approximately) = 401 g
Total kcal as prepared = 857 kcal
kcal/g prepared diet = 2.13 kcal/g diet

Nutrient	DM%[a]	As-Fed (g/100g diet)	ME% (g/100 kcal)	% of total kcal
Protein	44	17.9	8.3	33
Fat	31	12.8	6.0	57
Carbohydrate	14	5.8	2.7	10
Fiber	0.2	0.08	0.04	—
Arginine	3.1	1.2	0.6	—
Omega-3 fatty acids	10.2	4.1	1.9	—

[a]DM%, dry matter percent. If all the water was removed from this diet, this is the percentage of nutrient that would be present.

Diet: Chicken and Lentils

Species: Cat
Life Stage: Adult
Special Conditions: Diabetes mellitus, idiopathic hypercalcemia, gastric motility disorders, short bowel syndrome, small intestinal bacterial overgrowth

Ingredient	Quantity	Measure
Chicken, breast, without skin, cooked	5	ounces
Lentils, cooked	1	cup
Canola oil	5	tsp
Salt substitute (potassium chloride)	⅛	tsp
Bone meal powder	1	tsp
Salt, iodized (sodium chloride)	⅛	tsp
Multivitamin & mineral tablet, kids complete	1	each
Vitamin K, 100 mcg vitamin K per tablet	1	tablet
Taurine powder, 1000 mg per ¼ tsp	¼	tsp

Prepared weight (approximately) = 371 g
Total kcal as prepared = 674 kcal
kcal/g prepared diet = 1.81 kcal/g diet

Nutrient	DM%[a]	As-Fed (g/100 g diet)	ME% (g/100 kcal)	% of total kcal
Protein	44	16.7	9.2	36
Fat	21	7.9	4.3	41
Carbohydrate	29	11.0	6.1	24
Fiber	11	4.2	2.3	—

[a]DM%, dry matter percent. If all the water was removed from this diet, this is the percentage of nutrient that would be present.

Diet: Ground Beef and Lentils

Species: Cat
Life Stage: Adult
Special Conditions: Diabetes mellitus, idiopathic hypercalcemia, gastric motility disorders, short bowel syndrome, small intestinal bacterial overgrowth

Ingredient	Quantity	Measure
Ground beef, 10% fat, cooked	7	ounces
Lentils, cooked	1	cup
Canola oil	1½	tsp
Salt substitute (potassium chloride)	⅛	tsp
Bone meal powder	1	tsp
Salt, iodized (sodium chloride)	⅛	tsp
Multivitamin & mineral tablet, kids complete	1	each
Taurine powder, 1000 mg per ¼ tsp	¼	tsp

Prepared weight (approximately) = 411 g
Total kcal as prepared = 752 kcal
kcal/g prepared diet = 1.83 kcal/g diet

Nutrient	DM%[a]	As-Fed (g/100g diet)	ME% (g/100 kcal)	% of total kcal
Protein	48	18.1	9.9	39
Fat	20	7.7	4.2	40
Carbohydrate	26	10.0	5.4	21
Fiber	10	3.8	2.1	—

[a]DM%, dry matter percent. If all the water was removed from this diet, this is the percentage of nutrient that would be present.

Diet: Tuna and Lentils

Species: Cat
Life Stage: Adult
Special Conditions: Diabetes mellitus, idiopathic hypercalcemia, gastric motility disorders, short bowel syndrome, small intestinal bacterial overgrowth

Ingredient	Quantity	Measure
Tuna, canned, in oil, drained	5	ounces
Egg, large, hard-boiled	2	each
Lentils, cooked	1	cup
Canola oil	2	tsp
Salt substitute (potassium chloride)	¼	tsp
Bone meal powder	1	tsp
Salt, iodized (sodium chloride)	⅛	tsp
Multivitamin & mineral tablet, kids complete	1	each
Vitamin K, 100 mcg vitamin K per tablet	1	tablet
Taurine powder, 1000 mg per ¼ tsp	¼	tsp

Prepared weight (approximately) = 458 g
Total kcal as prepared = 752 kcal
kcal/g prepared diet = 1.64 kcal/g diet

Nutrient	DM%[a]	As-Fed (g/100 g diet)	ME% (g/100 kcal)	% of total kcal
Protein	45	15.7	9.5	37
Fat	20	7.1	4.3	41
Carbohydrate	26	9.2	5.6	22
Fiber	9.7	3.4	2.1	—

[a]DM%, dry matter percent. If all the water was removed from this diet, this is the percentage of nutrient that would be present.

Diet: Mackerel and Lentils

Species: Cat
Life Stage: Adult
Special Conditions: Diabetes mellitus, idiopathic hypercalcemia, gastric motility disorders, short bowel syndrome, small intestinal bacterial overgrowth

Ingredient	Quantity	Measure
Mackerel, jack, canned, drained	6	ounces
Eggs, large, hard-boiled	2	each
Lentils, cooked	1	cup
Canola oil	2	tsp
Salt substitute (potassium chloride)	¼	tsp
Bone meal powder	1	tsp
Salt, iodized (sodium chloride)	⅛	tsp
Multivitamin & mineral tablet, kids complete	1	each
Vitamin K, 100 mcg vitamin K per tablet	1	tablet
Taurine powder, 1000 mg per ¼ tsp	¼	tsp

Prepared weight (approximately) = 486 g
Total kcal as prepared = 737 kcal
kcal/g prepared diet = 1.51 kcal/g diet

Nutrient	DM%[a]	As-Fed (g/100 g diet)	ME% (g/100 kcal)	% of total kcal
Protein	45	14.4	9.5	37
Fat	20	6.5	4.3	41
Carbohydrate	27	8.6	5.7	22
Fiber	10	3.2	2.1	—

[a]DM%, dry matter percent. If all the water was removed from this diet, this is the percentage of nutrient that would be present.

Diet: Chicken and Rice

Species: Cat
Life Stage: Adult
Special Conditions: Lipid disorders, lymphangiectasia, protein-losing enteropathy. This diet is NOT complete and balanced and should be used only under the supervision of your veterinarian.

Ingredient	Quantity	Measure
Chicken, breast, without skin, cooked	6	ounces
Rice, white, long-grain, cooked	½	cup
Canola oil	½	tsp
Salt substitute (potassium chloride)	⅛	tsp
Bone meal powder	¾	tsp
Salt, iodized (sodium chloride)	⅛	tsp
Multivitamin & mineral tablet, kids complete	1	each
Vitamin K, 100 mcg vitamin K per tablet	1	tablet
Taurine powder, 1000 mg per ¼ tsp	¼	tsp

Prepared weight (approximately) = 259 g
Total kcal as prepared = 408 kcal
kcal/g prepared diet = 1.58 kcal/g diet

Nutrient	DM%[a]	As-Fed (g/100 g diet)	ME% (g/100 kcal)	% of total kcal
Protein	58	21.2	13.4	55
Fat	9	3.3	2.1	21
Carbohydrate	25	9.0	5.7	24
Fiber	0.3	0.1	0.08	—

[a]DM%, dry matter percent. If all the water was removed from this diet, this is the percentage of nutrient that would be present.

Diet: Chicken and Rice

Species: Cat
Life Stage: Adult
Special Conditions: Enteritis

Ingredient	Quantity	Measure
Chicken, breast, without skin, cooked	6	ounces
Rice, white, long-grain, cooked	½	cup
Canola oil	1	Tbsp
Salt substitute (potassium chloride)	⅛	tsp
Bone meal powder	¾	tsp
Salt, iodized (sodium chloride)	⅛	tsp
Multivitamin & mineral tablet, kids complete	1	each
Vitamin K, 100 mcg vitamin K per tablet	1	tablet
Taurine powder, 1000 mg per ¼ tsp	¼	tsp

Prepared weight (approximately) = 271 g
Total kcal as prepared = 511 kcal
kcal/g prepared diet = 1.89 kcal/g diet

Nutrient	DM%[a]	As-Fed (g/100 g diet)	ME% (g/100 kcal)	% of total kcal
Protein	53	20.3	10.7	43
Fat	20	7.5	4.0	39
Carbohydrate	23	8.6	4.6	18
Fiber	0.3	0.12	0.06	—

[a]DM%, dry matter percent. If all the water was removed from this diet, this is the percentage of nutrient that would be present.

Diet: Ground Beef and Rice

Species: Cat
Life Stage: Adult
Special Conditions: Enteritis

Ingredient	Quantity	Measure
Ground beef, 10% fat, cooked	8	ounces
Rice, white, long-grain, cooked	⅔	cup
Canola oil	½	tsp
Salt substitute (potassium chloride)	⅛	tsp
Bone meal powder	1	tsp
Salt, iodized (sodium chloride)	⅛	tsp
Multivitamin & mineral tablet, kids complete	½	each
Vitamin K, 100 mcg vitamin K per tablet	1	tablet
Taurine powder, 1000 mg per ¼ tsp	¼	tsp

Prepared weight (approximately) = 342 g
Total kcal as prepared = 682 kcal
kcal/g prepared diet = 1.99 kcal/g diet

Nutrient	DM%[a]	As-Fed (g/100 g diet)	ME% (g/100 kcal)	% of total kcal
Protein	49	19.7	9.9	39
Fat	22	8.7	4.4	43
Carbohydrate	22	8.9	4.4	18
Fiber	0.3	0.12	0.06	—

[a]DM%, dry matter percent. If all the water was removed from this diet, this is the percentage of nutrient that would be present.

Diet: Tuna and Rice

Species: Cat
Life Stage: Adult
Special Conditions: Enteritis

Ingredient	Quantity	Measure
Tuna, canned, in oil, drained	4	ounces
Egg, large, hard-boiled	1	each
Rice, white, long-grain, cooked	½	cup
Canola oil	1½	tsp
Salt substitute (potassium chloride)	¼	tsp
Bone meal powder	¾	tsp
Salt, iodized (sodium chloride)	⅛	tsp
Multivitamin & mineral tablet, kids complete	½	each
Taurine powder, 1000 mg per ¼ tsp	¼	tsp

Prepared weight (approximately) = 256 g
Total kcal as prepared = 469 kcal
kcal/g prepared diet = 1.83 kcal/g diet

Nutrient	DM%[a]	As-Fed (g/100 g diet)	ME% (g/100 kcal)	% of total kcal
Protein	43	16.2	8.84	35
Fat	23	8.5	4.7	45
Carbohydrate	24	9.1	5.0	20
Fiber	0.3	0.12	0.06	—

[a]DM%, dry matter percent. If all the water was removed from this diet, this is the percentage of nutrient that would be present.

Diet: Rabbit and Quinoa

Species: Cat
Life Stage: Adult
Special Conditions: Inflammatory bowel disease, colitis, gastritis

Ingredient	Quantity	Measure
Rabbit, domestic, cooked	4	ounces
Quinoa, cooked	¼	cup
Canola oil	1	tsp
Salt substitute (potassium chloride)	⅛	tsp
Bone meal powder	½	tsp
Salt, iodized (sodium chloride)	⅛	tsp
Multivitamin & mineral tablet, kids complete	½	each
Vitamin K, 100 mcg vitamin K per tablet	1	tablet
Taurine powder, 1000 mg per ¼ tsp	¼	tsp

Prepared weight (approximately) = 170 g
Total kcal as prepared = 322 kcal
kcal/g prepared diet = 1.89 kcal/g diet

Nutrient	DM%[a]	As-Fed (g/100 g diet)	ME% (g/100 kcal)	% of total kcal
Protein	51	20.6	10.9	43
Fat	22	8.6	4.6	44
Carbohydrate	15	6.1	3.2	13
Fiber	1.9	0.8	0.4	—

[a]DM%, dry matter percent. If all the water was removed from this diet, this is the percentage of nutrient that would be present.

Diet: Venison and Rice

Species: Cat
Life Stage: Adult
Special Conditions: Inflammatory bowel disease, colitis, gastritis, enteritis, allergy, struvite stone prevention

Ingredient	Quantity	Measure
Venison, cooked	4	ounces
Rice, white, long-grain, cooked	½	cup
Canola oil	1	tbsp
Salt substitute (potassium chloride)	⅛	tsp
Bone meal powder	⅔	tsp
Salt, iodized (sodium chloride)	⅛	tsp
Multivitamin & mineral tablet, kids complete	½	each
Vitamin K, 100 mcg vitamin K per tablet	1	tablet
Taurine powder, 1000 mg per ¼ tsp	¼	tsp

Prepared weight (approximately) = 213 g
Total kcal as prepared = 408 kcal
kcal/g prepared diet = 1.92 kcal/g diet

Nutrient	DM%[a]	As-Fed (g/100 g diet)	ME% (g/100 kcal)	% of total kcal
Protein	43	17.1	8.9	36
Fat	21	8.4	4.4	42
Carbohydrate	27	10.7	5.6	22
Fiber	0.4	0.15	0.08	—

[a]DM%, dry matter percent. If all the water was removed from this diet, this is the percentage of nutrient that would be present.

Diet: Cottage Cheese and Rice

Species: Cat
Life Stage: Adult
Special Conditions: Inflammatory bowel disease, colitis, gastritis, enteritis

Ingredient	Quantity	Measure
Cottage cheese, 1% fat	¾	cup
Eggs, large, hard-boiled	4	each
Rice, white, long-grain, cooked	½	cup
Canola oil	½	tsp
Salt substitute (potassium chloride)	½	tsp
Bone meal powder	1	tsp
Multivitamin & mineral tablet, kids complete	½	each
Vitamin K, 100 mcg vitamin K per tablet	1	tablet
Taurine powder, 1000 mg per ¼ tsp	¼	tsp

Prepared weight (approximately) = 459 g
Total kcal as prepared = 558 kcal
kcal/g prepared diet = 1.21 kcal/g diet

Nutrient	DM%[a]	As-Fed (g/100 g diet)	ME% (g/100 kcal)	% of total kcal
Protein	42	10.5	8.7	35
Fat	22	5.6	4.6	44
Carbohydrate	26	6.5	5.3	21
Fiber	0.3	0.07	0.06	—

[a]DM%, dry matter percent. If all the water was removed from this diet, this is the percentage of nutrient that would be present.

Diet: Pork and Barley

Species: Cat
Life Stage: Adult
Special Conditions: Inflammatory bowel disease, colitis, gastritis, allergy, struvite stone prevention

Ingredient	Quantity	Measure
Pork loin, broiled	5	ounces
Barley, pearled, cooked	½	cup
Canola oil	1	tsp
Salt substitute (potassium chloride)	⅛	tsp
Salt, iodized (sodium chloride)	⅛	tsp
Bone meal powder	¾	tsp
Multivitamin & mineral tablet, kids complete	½	each
Vitamin K, 100 mcg vitamin K per tablet	1	tablet
Taurine powder, 1000 mg per ¼ tsp	¼	tsp

Prepared weight (approximately) = 232 g
Total kcal as prepared = 419 kcal
kcal/g prepared diet = 1.81 kcal/g diet

Nutrient	DM%[a]	As-Fed (g/100 g diet)	ME% (g/100 kcal)	% of total kcal
Protein	45	17.0	9.4	37
Fat	20	7.8	4.3	42
Carbohydrate	26	9.8	5.4	21
Fiber	3.4	1.3	0.7	—

[a]DM%, dry matter percent. If all the water was removed from this diet, this is the percentage of nutrient that would be present.

Diet: Chicken and Rice

Species: Cat
Life Stage: Adult
Special Conditions: Heart disease

Ingredient	Quantity	Measure
Chicken, breast, without skin, cooked	6	ounces
Rice, white, long-grain, cooked	½	cup
Canola oil	5	tsp
Salt substitute (potassium chloride)	⅛	tsp
Salt, iodized (sodium chloride)	⅛	tsp
Bone meal powder	¾	tsp
Multivitamin & mineral tablet, kids complete	1	each
Vitamin K, 100 mcg vitamin K per tablet	1	tablet
Taurine powder, 1000 mg per ¼ tsp	¼	tsp

Prepared weight (approximately) = 280 g
Total kcal as prepared = 594 kcal
kcal/g prepared diet = 2.12 kcal/g diet

Nutrient	DM%[a]	As-Fed (g/100 g diet)	ME% (g/100 kcal)	% of total kcal
Protein	48	19.6	9.2	37
Fat	26	10.6	5.0	48
Carbohydrate	20	8.3	3.9	15
Fiber	0.3	0.1	0.05	—
Sodium	0.37	0.15	0.07	—

[a]DM%, dry matter percent. If all the water was removed from this diet, this is the percentage of nutrient that would be present.

Diet: Ground Beef and Rice

Species: Cat
Life Stage: Adult
Special Conditions: Heart disease

Ingredient	Quantity	Measure
Ground beef, 10% fat, cooked	8	ounces
Rice, white, long-grain, cooked	⅔	cup
Canola oil	4	tsp
Salt substitute (potassium chloride)	⅛	tsp
Salt, iodized (sodium chloride)	⅛	tsp
Bone meal powder	1⅛	tsp
Multivitamin & mineral tablet, kids complete	½	each
Vitamin K, 100 mcg vitamin K per tablet	1	tablet
Taurine powder, 1000 mg per ¼ tsp	¼	tsp

Prepared weight (approximately) = 359 g
Total kcal as prepared = 826 kcal
kcal/g prepared diet = 2.30 kcal/g diet

Nutrient	DM%[a]	As-Fed (g/100 g diet)	ME% (g/100 kcal)	% of total kcal
Protein	44	18.8	8.2	32
Fat	30	12.9	5.6	54
Carbohydrate	20	8.5	3.7	14
Fiber	0.3	0.1	0.05	—
Sodium	0.32	0.14	0.06	—

[a]DM%, dry matter percent. If all the water was removed from this diet, this is the percentage of nutrient that would be present.

Diet: Whitefish and Rice

Species: Cat
Life Stage: Adult
Special Conditions: Heart disease

Ingredient	Quantity	Measure
Whitefish, fillet, baked	8	ounces
Rice, white, long-grain, cooked	⅔	cup
Canola oil	4	tsp
Salt substitute (potassium chloride)	¼	tsp
Salt, iodized (sodium chloride)	⅛	tsp
Bone meal powder	1	tsp
Multivitamin & mineral tablet, kids complete	½	each
Vitamin K, 100 mcg vitamin K per tablet	1	tablet
Taurine powder, 1000 mg per ¼ tsp	¼	tsp

Prepared weight (approximately) = 359 g
Total kcal as prepared = 695 kcal
kcal/g prepared diet = 1.93 kcal/g diet

Nutrient	DM%[a]	As-Fed (g/100 g diet)	ME% (g/100 kcal)	% of total kcal
Protein	42	16.2	8.4	33
Fat	26	10.0	5.2	50
Carbohydrate	22	8.4	4.4	17
Fiber	0.3	0.12	0.06	—
Sodium	0.31	0.12	0.06	—

[a]DM%, dry matter percent. If all the water was removed from this diet, this is the percentage of nutrient that would be present.

Diet: Tofu and Chicken

Species: Cat
Life Stage: Adult
Special Conditions: Liver disease. This diet should be used under the
supervision of your veterinarian.

Ingredient	Quantity	Measure
Tofu, extra firm	5	ounces
Chicken, breast, without skin, cooked	3	ounces
Egg, large, hard-boiled	½	each
Lentils, cooked	¼	cup
Chicken fat	1	tbsp
Canola oil	1	tsp
Salt substitute (potassium chloride)	¼	tsp
Salt, iodized (sodium chloride)	⅛	tsp
Bone meal powder	¾	tsp
Multivitamin & mineral tablet, kids complete	1	each
Arginine powder, 2.5 g per tsp	⅛	tsp
Vitamin K, 100 mcg vitamin K per tablet	1	tablet
Taurine powder, 1000 mg per ¼ tsp	½	tsp

Prepared weight (approximately) = 328 g
Total kcal as prepared = 526 kcal
kcal/g prepared diet = 1.60 kcal/g diet

Nutrient	DM%[a]	As-Fed (g/100 g diet)	ME% (g/100 kcal)	% of total kcal
Protein	46	14.6	9.1	35
Fat	30	9.6	6.0	55
Carbohydrate	14	4.3	2.7	10
Fiber	4.3	1.4	0.8	—
Arginine	3.2	1.0	0.6	—

[a]DM%, dry matter percent. If all the water was removed from this diet, this is the
percentage of nutrient that would be present.

Diet: Tofu and Ground Beef

Species: Cat
Life Stage: Adult
Special Conditions: Liver disease. This diet should be used under the supervision of your veterinarian.

Ingredient	Quantity	Measure
Tofu, extra firm	5	ounces
Ground beef, 10% fat, cooked	3	ounces
Egg, large, hard-boiled	½	each
Lentils, cooked	¼	cup
Canola oil	1½	tsp
Salt substitute (potassium chloride)	¼	tsp
Salt, iodized (sodium chloride)	⅛	tsp
Bone meal powder	¾	tsp
Multivitamin & mineral tablet, kids complete	1	each
Arginine powder, 2.5 g per tsp	⅛	tsp
Vitamin K, 100 mcg vitamin K per tablet	1	tablet
Taurine powder, 1000 mg per ¼ tsp	½	tsp

Prepared weight (approximately) = 318 g
Total kcal as prepared = 487 kcal
kcal/g prepared diet = 1.53 kcal/g diet

Nutrient	DM%[a]	As-Fed (g/100 g diet)	ME% (g/100 kcal)	% of total kcal
Protein	46	14.4	9.4	36
Fat	28	8.9	5.8	53
Carbohydrate	14	4.4	2.9	11
Fiber	4.5	1.4	0.9	—
Arginine	3.3	1.0	0.7	—

[a]DM%, dry matter percent. If all the water was removed from this diet, this is the percentage of nutrient that would be present.

Diet: Tofu and Cottage Cheese

Species: Cat
Life Stage: Adult
Special Conditions: Liver disease. This diet should be used under the supervision of your veterinarian.

Ingredient	Quantity	Measure
Tofu, extra firm	5	ounces
Cottage cheese, 1% fat	½	cup
Eggs, large, hard-boiled	1½	each
Lentils, cooked	¼	cup
Canola oil	1	tsp
Salt substitute (potassium chloride)	¼	tsp
Salt, iodized (sodium chloride)	⅛	tsp
Bone meal powder	¾	tsp
Multivitamin & mineral tablet, kids complete	1	each
Arginine powder, 2.5 g per tsp	⅛	tsp
Vitamin K, 100 mcg vitamin K per tablet	1	tablet
Taurine powder, 1000 mg per ¼ tsp	½	tsp

Prepared weight (approximately) = 393 g
Total kcal as prepared = 429 kcal
kcal/g prepared diet = 1.09 kcal/g diet

Nutrient	DM%[a]	As-Fed (g/100 g diet)	ME% (g/100 kcal)	% of total kcal
Protein	44	10.7	9.8	37
Fat	24	5.6	5.2	47
Carbohydrate	19	4.5	4.1	16
Fiber	4.7	1.1	1.0	—
Arginine	2.9	0.7	0.7	—

[a]DM%, dry matter percent. If all the water was removed from this diet, this is the percentage of nutrient that would be present.

Diet: Tofu and Tuna

Species: Cat
Life Stage: Adult
Special Conditions: Liver disease. This diet should be used under the supervision of your veterinarian.

Ingredient	Quantity	Measure
Tofu, extra firm	5	ounces
Tuna, canned, in water, drained	2	ounces
Egg, large, hard-boiled	½	each
Lentils, cooked	¼	cup
Canola oil	1½	tsp
Salt substitute (potassium chloride)	¼	tsp
Salt, iodized (sodium chloride)	⅛	tsp
Bone meal powder	¾	tsp
Multivitamin & mineral tablet, kids complete	1	each
Arginine powder, 2.5 g per tsp	⅛	tsp
Vitamin K, 100 mcg vitamin K per tablet	1	tablet
Taurine powder, 1000 mg per ¼ tsp	½	tsp

Prepared weight (approximately) = 289 g
Total kcal as prepared = 364 kcal
kcal/g prepared diet = 1.26 kcal/g diet

Nutrient	DM%[a]	As-Fed (g/100 g diet)	ME% (g/100 kcal)	% of total kcal
Protein	44	12.1	9.6	36
Fat	25	6.8	5.4	49
Carbohydrate	18	4.9	3.9	15
Fiber	5.6	1.6	1.2	—
Arginine	3.2	0.9	0.7	—

[a]DM%, dry matter percent. If all the water was removed from this diet, this is the percentage of nutrient that would be present.

Diet: Tofu and Lentils

Species: Cat
Life Stage: Adult
Special Conditions: Liver disease (hepatic encephalopathy). This diet is NOT complete and balanced and should only be used under the direct supervision of your veterinarian.

Ingredient	Quantity	Measure
Tofu, extra firm	4	ounces
Lentils, cooked	¼	cup
Chicken fat	4	tsp
Salt substitute (potassium chloride)	⅛	tsp
Salt, iodized (sodium chloride)	⅛	tsp
Bone meal powder	½	tsp
Multivitamin & mineral tablet, kids complete	½	each
Arginine powder, 2.5 g per tsp	¼	tsp
Vitamin K, 100 mcg vitamin K per tablet	1	tablet
Taurine powder, 1000 mg per ¼ tsp	¼	tsp

Prepared weight (approximately) = 186 g
Total kcal as prepared = 316 kcal
kcal/g prepared diet = 1.70 kcal/g diet

Nutrient	DM%[a]	As-Fed (g/100 g diet)	ME% (g/100 kcal)	% of total kcal
Protein	26	8.4	5.0	18
Fat	40	12.8	7.5	67
Carbohydrate	21	6.8	4.0	15
Fiber	7	2.3	1.4	—
Arginine	2.3	0.8	0.4	—

[a]DM%, dry matter percent. If all the water was removed from this diet, this is the percentage of nutrient that would be present.

Diet: Chicken and Rice

Species: Cat
Life Stage: Adult
Special Conditions: Pancreatitis

Ingredient	Quantity	Measure
Chicken, breast, without skin, cooked	5	ounces
Rice, white, long-grain, cooked	1	cup
Canola oil	1½	tsp
Salt substitute (potassium chloride)	¼	tsp
Salt, iodized (sodium chloride)	⅛	tsp
Bone meal powder	¾	tsp
Multivitamin & mineral tablet, kids complete	½	each
Vitamin K, 100 mcg vitamin K per tablet	1	tablet
Taurine powder, 1000 mg per ¼ tsp	¼	tsp

Prepared weight (approximately) = 314 g
Total kcal as prepared = 503 kcal
kcal/g prepared diet = 1.60 kcal/g diet

Nutrient	DM%[a]	As-Fed (g/100 g diet)	ME% (g/100 kcal)	% of total kcal
Protein	43	15.4	9.6	39
Fat	11	4.0	2.5	25
Carbohydrate	40	14.3	8.9	36
Fiber	0.6	0.2	0.1	—

[a]DM%, dry matter percent. If all the water was removed from this diet, this is the percentage of nutrient that would be present.

Diet: Tuna and Rice

Species: Cat
Life Stage: Adult
Special Conditions: Pancreatitis

Ingredient	Quantity	Measure
Tuna, canned, in water, drained	6	ounces
Eggs, large, hard-boiled	2	each
Rice, white, long-grain, cooked	1	cup
Canola oil	½	tsp
Salt substitute (potassium chloride)	¼	tsp
Salt, iodized (sodium chloride)	⅛	tsp
Bone meal powder	1	tsp
Multivitamin & mineral tablet, kids complete	1	each
Vitamin K, 100 mcg vitamin K per tablet	1	tablet
Taurine powder, 1000 mg per ¼ tsp	¼	tsp

Prepared weight (approximately) = 439 g
Total kcal as prepared = 603 kcal
kcal/g prepared diet = 1.37 kcal/g diet

Nutrient	DM%[a]	As-Fed (g/100 g diet)	ME% (g/100 kcal)	% of total kcal
Protein	43	13.0	9.5	38
Fat	14	4.2	3.1	30
Carbohydrate	35	10.6	7.7	32
Fiber	0.5	0.1	0.1	—

[a]DM%, dry matter percent. If all the water was removed from this diet, this is the percentage of nutrient that would be present.

Diet: Chicken and Rice

Species: Cat
Life Stage: Adult
Special Conditions: Exocrine pancreatic insufficiency

Ingredient	Quantity	Measure
Chicken, breast, without skin, cooked	6	ounces
Rice, white, long-grain, cooked	½	cup
Canola oil	2	tsp
Salt substitute (potassium chloride)	⅛	tsp
Bone meal powder	¾	tsp
Salt, iodized (sodium chloride)	⅛	tsp
Multivitamin & mineral tablet, kids complete	1	each
Vitamin K, 100 mcg vitamin K per tablet	1	tablet
Taurine powder, 1000 mg per ¼ tsp	¼	tsp

Prepared weight (approximately) = 266 g
Total kcal as prepared = 470 kcal
kcal/g prepared diet = 1.77 kcal/g diet

Nutrient	DM%[a]	As-Fed (g/100 g diet)	ME% (g/100 kcal)	% of total kcal
Protein	54	20.6	11.7	47
Fat	15	5.9	3.3	33
Carbohydrate	23	8.8	5.0	20
Fiber	0.3	0.1	0.1	—

[a]DM%, dry matter percent. If all the water was removed from this diet, this is the percentage of nutrient that would be present.

Diet: Chicken and Rice

Species: Cat
Life Stage: Adult
Special Conditions: Renal disease. This diet is NOT complete and balanced and should only be used in cats with renal failure under the direct supervision of your veterinarian.

Ingredient	Quantity	Measure
Chicken, breast, without skin, cooked	3	ounces
Rice, white, long-grain, cooked	⅔	cup
Canola oil	5	tsp
Salt substitute (potassium chloride)	¼	tsp
Salt, iodized (sodium chloride)	⅛	tsp
Bone meal powder	¼	tsp
Baking soda (calcium carbonate)	⅛	tsp
Multivitamin & mineral tablet, kids complete	½	each
Vitamin K, 100 mcg vitamin K per tablet	1	tablet
Taurine powder, 1000 mg per ¼ tsp	¼	tsp

Prepared weight (approximately) = 220 g
Total kcal as prepared = 486 kcal
kcal/g prepared diet = 2.21 kcal/g diet

Nutrient	DM%[a]	As-Fed (g/100 g diet)	ME% (g/100 kcal)	% of total kcal
Protein	32	13.3	6.0	24
Fat	29	12.1	5.5	52
Carbohydrate	33	13.8	6.2	24
Fiber	0.5	0.2	0.09	—
Phosphorus	0.43	0.18	0.08	—
Sodium	0.39	0.16	0.07	—

[a]DM%, dry matter percent. If all the water was removed from this diet, this is the percentage of nutrient that would be present.

Diet: Ground Beef and Rice

Species: Cat
Life Stage: Adult
Special Conditions: Renal disease. This diet is NOT complete and balanced and should only be used in cats with renal failure under the direct supervision of your veterinarian.

Ingredient	Quantity	Measure
Ground beef, 10% fat, cooked	3	ounces
Rice, white, long-grain, cooked	¾	cup
Canola oil	4	tsp
Salt substitute (potassium chloride)	¼	tsp
Salt, iodized (sodium chloride)	⅛	tsp
Bone meal powder	¼	tsp
Baking soda (calcium carbonate)	⅛	tsp
Multivitamin & mineral tablet, kids complete	½	each
Vitamin K, 100 mcg vitamin K per tablet	1	tablet
Taurine powder, 1000 mg per ¼ tsp	¼	tsp

Prepared weight (approximately) = 228 g
Total kcal as prepared = 517 kcal
kcal/g prepared diet = 2.26 kcal/g diet

Nutrient	DM%[a]	As-Fed (g/100 g diet)	ME% (g/100 kcal)	% of total kcal
Protein	28	12.0	5.3	21
Fat	30	12.8	5.7	54
Carbohydrate	35	14.9	6.6	25
Fiber	0.5	0.2	0.09	—
Phosphorus	0.43	0.18	0.08	—
Sodium	0.38	0.16	0.07	—

[a]DM%, dry matter percent. If all the water was removed from this diet, this is the percentage of nutrient that would be present.

Diet: Lamb and Rice

Species: Cat
Life Stage: Adult
Special Conditions: Renal disease. This diet is NOT complete and balanced, and should only be used in cats with renal failure under the direct supervision of your veterinarian.

Ingredient	Quantity	Measure
Lamb, cooked	4	ounces
Rice, white, long-grain, cooked	⅔	cup
Canola oil	4	tsp
Salt substitute (potassium chloride)	¼	tsp
Salt, iodized (sodium chloride)	⅛	tsp
Bone meal powder	¼	tsp
Baking soda (calcium carbonate)	¼	tsp
Multivitamin & mineral tablet, kids complete	½	each
Vitamin K, 100 mcg vitamin K per tablet	1	tablet
Taurine powder, 1000 mg per ¼ tsp	¼	tsp

Prepared weight (approximately) = 245 g
Total kcal as prepared = 612 kcal
kcal/g prepared diet = 2.50 kcal/g diet

Nutrient	DM%[a]	As-Fed (g/100 g diet)	ME% (g/100 kcal)	% of total kcal
Protein	29	13.0	5.2	20
Fat	36	16.1	6.4	61
Carbohydrate	28	12.4	5.0	19
Fiber	0.4	0.2	0.07	—
Phosphorus	0.38	0.17	0.07	—
Sodium	0.35	0.16	0.06	—

[a]DM%, dry matter percent. If all the water was removed from this diet, this is the percentage of nutrient that would be present.

Diet: Tuna and Rice

Species: Cat
Life Stage: Adult
Special Conditions: Renal disease. This diet is NOT complete and balanced, and should only be used in cats with renal failure under the direct supervision of your veterinarian.

Ingredient	Quantity	Measure
Tuna, canned, in water, drained	3	ounces
Rice, white, long-grain, cooked	⅔	cup
Canola oil	4	tsp
Salt substitute (potassium chloride)	¼	tsp
Bone meal powder	¼	tsp
Baking soda (calcium carbonate)	⅛	tsp
Multivitamin & mineral tablet, kids complete	½	each
Vitamin K, 100 mcg vitamin K per tablet	1	tablet
Taurine powder, 1000 mg per ¼ tsp	¼	tsp

Prepared weight (approximately) = 215 g
Total kcal as prepared = 414 kcal
kcal/g prepared diet = 1.92 kcal/g diet

Nutrient	DM%[a]	As-Fed (g/100 g diet)	ME% (g/100 kcal)	% of total kcal
Protein	29	10.7	5.5	22
Fat	27	10.0	5.2	49
Carbohydrate	38	14.1	7.3	29
Fiber	0.5	0.2	0.1	—
Phosphorus	0.48	0.18	0.09	—
Sodium	0.40	0.15	0.08	—

[a]DM%, dry matter percent. If all the water was removed from this diet, this is the percentage of nutrient that would be present.

Diet: Salmon and Couscous

Species: Cat
Life Stage: Adult
Special Conditions: Renal disease. This diet is NOT complete and balanced and should only be used in cats with renal failure under the direct supervision of your veterinarian.

Ingredient	Quantity	Measure
Salmon, wild, fillet, baked	3	ounces
Couscous, cooked	¾	cup
Canola oil	4	tsp
Salt substitute (potassium chloride)	⅛	tsp
Salt, iodized (sodium chloride)	⅛	tsp
Bone meal powder	¼	tsp
Baking soda (calcium carbonate)	⅛	tsp
Multivitamin & mineral tablet, kids complete	½	each
Vitamin K, 100 mcg vitamin K per tablet	1	tablet
Taurine powder, 1000 mg per ¼ tsp	¼	tsp

Prepared weight (approximately) = 227 g
Total kcal as prepared = 454 kcal
kcal/g prepared diet = 2.00 kcal/g diet

Nutrient	DM%[a]	As-Fed (g/100 g diet)	ME% (g/100 kcal)	% of total kcal
Protein	29	11.5	5.8	22
Fat	28	11.4	5.7	54
Carbohydrate	31	12.3	6.1	24
Fiber	1.8	0.7	0.4	—
Phosphorus	0.44	0.18	0.09	—
Sodium	0.38	0.15	0.08	—

[a]DM%, dry matter percent. If all the water was removed from this diet, this is the percentage of nutrient that would be present.

Diet: Chicken and Rice

Species: Cat
Life Stage: Adult
Special Conditions: To prevent recurrence of oxalate urinary stones.
Use only under the supervision of your veterinarian. Urinary pH must
be monitored.

Ingredient	Quantity	Measure
Chicken, breast, without skin, cooked	6	ounces
Rice, white, long-grain, cooked	½	cup
Canola oil	1	tbsp
Salt substitute (potassium chloride)	⅛	tsp
Bone meal powder	½	tsp
Salt, iodized (sodium chloride)	⅛	tsp
Baking soda (calcium carbonate)	⅛	tsp
Multivitamin & mineral tablet, kids complete	½	each
Vitamin K, 100 mcg vitamin K per tablet	1	tablet
Taurine powder, 1000 mg per ¼ tsp	¼	tsp

Prepared weight (approximately) = 269 g
Total kcal as prepared = 509 kcal
kcal/g prepared diet = 1.89 kcal/g diet

Nutrient	DM%[a]	As-Fed (g/100 g diet)	ME% (g/100 kcal)	% of total kcal
Protein	53	20.4	10.8	43
Fat	19	7.5	4.0	39
Carbohydrate	22	8.4	4.5	18
Fiber	0.3	0.1	0.06	—
Phosphorus	0.7	0.26	0.14	—

[a]DM%, dry matter percent. If all the water was removed from this diet, this is the
percentage of nutrient that would be present.

Diet: Ground Beef and Rice

Species: Cat
Life Stage: Adult
Special Conditions: To prevent recurrence of oxalate urinary stones.
Use only under the supervision of your veterinarian. Urinary pH must
be monitored.

Ingredient	Quantity	Measure
Ground beef, 10% fat, cooked	8	ounces
Rice, white, long-grain, cooked	⅔	cup
Canola oil	½	tsp
Salt substitute (potassium chloride)	⅛	tsp
Bone meal powder	¾	tsp
Salt, iodized (sodium chloride)	⅛	tsp
Baking soda (calcium carbonate)	⅛	tsp
Multivitamin & mineral tablet, kids complete	½	each
Vitamin K, 100 mcg vitamin K per tablet	1	tablet
Taurine powder, 1000 mg per ¼ tsp	¼	tsp

Prepared weight (approximately) = 342 g
Total kcal as prepared = 682 kcal
kcal/g prepared diet = 1.99 kcal/g diet

Nutrient	DM%[a]	As-Fed (g/100 g diet)	ME% (g/100 kcal)	% of total kcal
Protein	49	19.7	9.9	40
Fat	22	8.8	4.4	42
Carbohydrate	22	8.9	4.4	18
Fiber	0.3	0.12	0.06	—
Phosphorus	0.7	0.30	0.15	—

[a]DM%, dry matter percent. If all the water was removed from this diet, this is the
percentage of nutrient that would be present.

Diet: Salmon and Rice

Species: Cat
Life Stage: Adult
Special Conditions: To prevent recurrence of oxalate urinary stones.
Use only under the supervision of your veterinarian. Urinary pH must
be monitored.

Ingredient	Quantity	Measure
Salmon, wild, fillet, baked	6	ounces
Rice, white, long-grain, cooked	⅔	cup
Canola oil	1	tbsp
Salt substitute (potassium chloride)	⅛	tsp
Bone meal powder	½	tsp
Salt, iodized (sodium chloride)	⅛	tsp
Baking soda (calcium carbonate)	⅛	tsp
Multivitamin & mineral tablet, kids complete	½	each
Vitamin K, 100 mcg vitamin K per tablet	1	tablet
Taurine powder, 1000 mg per ¼ tsp	¼	tsp

Prepared weight (approximately) = 296 g
Total kcal as prepared = 573 kcal
kcal/g prepared diet = 1.93 kcal/g diet

Nutrient	DM%[a]	As-Fed (g/100 g diet)	ME% (g/100 kcal)	% of total kcal
Protein	38	15.6	8.0	32
Fat	23	9.5	4.9	47
Carbohydrate	25	10.2	5.3	21
Fiber	0.3	0.1	0.07	—
Phosphorus	0.62	0.26	0.13	—

[a]DM%, dry matter percent. If all the water was removed from this diet, this is the percentage of nutrient that would be present.

Diet: Chicken and Rice

Species: Cat
Life Stage: Adult
Special Conditions: To prevent recurrence of struvite urinary stones.
Use only under the supervision of your veterinarian. Urinary pH must
be monitored.

Ingredient	Quantity	Measure
Chicken, breast, without skin, cooked	4	ounces
Rice, white, long-grain, cooked	½	cup
Canola oil	4	tsp
Salt substitute (potassium chloride)	⅛	tsp
Bone meal powder	¾	tsp
Salt, iodized (sodium chloride)	⅛	tsp
Multivitamin & mineral tablet, kids complete	½	each
Vitamin K, 100 mcg vitamin K per tablet	1	tablet
Taurine powder, 1000 mg per ¼ tsp	¼	tsp

Prepared weight (approximately) = 218 g
Total kcal as prepared = 457 kcal
kcal/g prepared diet = 2.10 kcal/g diet

Nutrient	DM%[a]	As-Fed (g/100 g diet)	ME% (g/100 kcal)	% of total kcal
Protein	42	17.1	8.2	32
Fat	26	10.5	5.0	48
Carbohydrate	25	10.5	5.0	20
Fiber	0.4	0.2	0.07	—
Phosphorus	0.78	0.3	0.15	—

[a]DM%, dry matter percent. If all the water was removed from this diet, this is the
percentage of nutrient that would be present.

APPENDIX 1

Dog Diets by Protein Source

Beef, Ground

Chicken

Tuna

Turkey

Venison

Whitefish

APPENDIX 2

Cat Diets by Protein Source

Beef, Ground

Chicken

Whitefish

INDEX

Printed and bound by CPI Group (UK) Ltd, Croydon, CR0 4YY

27/10/2024

14580240-0002